MAKING

THE BODY

Beautiful

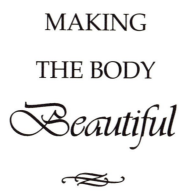

MAKING
THE BODY
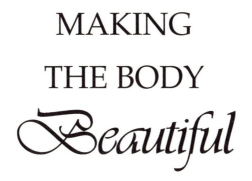
A CULTURAL HISTORY
OF AESTHETIC
SURGERY

Sander L. Gilman

PRINCETON UNIVERSITY PRESS

PRINCETON, NEW JERSEY

This book has been composed in Palatino

Library of Congress Cataloging-in-Publication Data

Gilman, Sander L.

Making the body beautiful : a cultural history of aesthetic

surgery / Sander L. Gilman.

p.   cm.

Includes bibliographical references and index.

ISBN 0-691-02672-6 (CL : alk. paper)

1. Surgery, Plastic—Social aspects—History.   2. Body

image—Social aspects—History.   I. Title.

RD118.G55   1999

617.9′5—dc21   98-48423   CIP

The paper used in this publication meets the minimum requirements

of ANSI / NISO Z39.48-1992 (R1997) (*Permanence of Paper*)

http://pup.princeton.edu

Printed in the United States of America

1   3   5   7   9   10   8   6   4   2

THIS BOOK IS DEDICATED TO

Philip Gossett

DEAN OF DEANS AND MUSICOLOGIST

EXTRAORDINAIRE

CONTENTS

ILLUSTRATIONS

Johannes Scultetus's image of the medical interventions involved in operating on the nose and mouth. From *Kheiroplotheke Seu D. Ioannis Sculteti . . . Armamentarium Chirurgicum: XLIII. Tabulis* (Venice: Typis Combi, & La Nou, 1665). (Bethesda, Md.: National Library of Medicine) 9

Dr. Keith's restoration of a lost nose. From the *London and Edinburgh Monthly Journal of Medical Science* 4 (1844): 112. (Bethesda, Md.: National Library of Medicine) 11

Humphrey Bogart in *Dark Passage* (1947). (New York: Museum of Modern Art) 28

Vilray Papin Blair's rebuilding of an underdeveloped lower jaw (1909). From Blair's "Underdeveloped Lower Jaw, with Limited Excursion," *Journal of the American Medical Association* 53 (1909): 178–83. (Bethesda, Md.: National Library of Medicine) 38

Noseless infant born with congenital syphilis. From J. Jadassohn, ed., *Handbuch der Haut- und Geschlechtskrankheiten,* 23 vols. (Berlin: Julius Springer, 1927), 19:88. (Chicago: private collection) 52

Lon Chaney as the Phantom of the Opera (1925). (New York: Museum of Modern Art) 53

Profile of the "insane" patient with congenital syphilis. From Emil Kraepelin, *Psychiatrie,* 8th ed., 4 vols. (Leipzig: J. A. Barth, 1909–1915), 2:336. (Bethesda, Md.: National Library of Medicine) 56

Ambroise Paré's artificial nose. From *Les oeuvres d'Ambroise Pare . . . en plusieurs endroicts, & augm. d'un fort ample Traicte*

$\mathcal{D}$URING the academic year 1990–91, I was the visiting historical scholar at the National Library of Medicine in Bethesda, Maryland. It was a rare occasion to work in a setting where serious scholars, both visitors and staff, were focused on specific questions in the history of medicine. It was an extraordinary experience to be in one of the world's great libraries and to be working with the resources of that collection as intensively as I have ever worked anyplace else. At the end of my stay, I turned to one of the senior librarians over lunch and commented that I had been unable to find what I was looking for that morning. I was searching for a good overview of the field of aesthetic surgery and what I found was often skeletal or quite narrowly conceived. His answer was laconic: "Well, write one then."

This is the result. It is not quite a comprehensive internal history of "aesthetic surgery," because such an account would drown in superfluous details what I consider to be the inner story of the field. One can write a history of any specialty of medicine and chart its history, procedure by procedure or nosological description by nosological description. The end result is, not surprisingly, always the same—with enough details, some can be selected to show how things improve over time. Errors are minutely corrected, and the cumulative effect is a movement forward. Medicine becomes a litmus test for the history of progress. But the cultural history of aesthetic surgery presented here does not rest on a theory of progress. It tries to puzzle out the meanings associated with bodies, doctors, and patients, using an argument that is thematic as well as chronological. I see the history of modern aesthetic surgery from the nineteenth century to the present moving from surgery on the face to correct what were seen as signs of "racial" difference to a much broader alteration of other forms of bodily difference. After trying to answer some of the basic questions—what are the procedures? which are aesthetic and why are they considered so? how did the field get its name? who are the patients? how does aesthetic surgery fit into the pattern of what has come to be called the "modern"?—the book focuses on the nose. This emphasis on the nose may at first seem excessive, but it is a consideration of this organ that best provides not only the basic history of aesthetic procedures across time and space but also the ground for understanding the basic motivation for aesthetic surgery—the desire to "pass."

Why begin with the nose?[1] Aesthetic surgery deals with an imagined body and an imagined psyche, yet it is the visible body that, at least initially, captures the attention of the surgeon. Aesthetic surgery deals with the face first because (along with the hands) it is the part of the body that is "uncovered" in the West.[2] We see the face, and the act of seeing the face is immediately loaded with multiple layers of meaning. The face is read "scientifically," Charles Darwin noted, as marking the boundary between civilization and barbarism: "As the face with us is chiefly admired for its beauty, so with savages it is the chief seat of mutilation."[3] Darwin gave the face meaning within his system of representations. Such meanings shape the visualized body, and it is this spectral body that is central to the pursuit of aesthetic surgery. In the 1890s, as modern aesthetic surgery began, it was commonplace to hear the shape of the nose associated with qualities of character: "a well-formed nose is a distinctively human feature." Or commentators noted that "it is certain that the shape of the nose is generally regarded not alone from an aesthetic point of view, but that to many minds it conveys an idea of weakness or strength of character, and also of social status. Certain types of nose are 'better bred' than others, and, other things being equal, a man with a 'good nose' is more likely to gain immediate respect than one with a 'vulgar' nose."[4] This focus on the "beautiful" face is understood as a quality of the modern, civilized world.

Oswald Spengler (1880–1936), in *The Decline of the West* (1918), called the fascination with the meaning of the face a sign of the triumph of the "science" of physiognomy and the movement toward a "single uniform overarching physiognomy of all human beings."[5] Spengler's view comes well into the "age of physiognomy." Richard Sennett, commenting on the claims of late nineteenth-century culture, notes that "sight itself has the power to create a moral indictment; all society's ills are *visible*."[6] And they are especially visible on the face. The face and the sciences that contribute to its reading are given specific priority as signs of the modern.

The breast, buttocks, and belly quickly became additional sites for the modern aesthetic surgeon. In the West, we continue to fantasize about the body under the clothes and thus see it powerfully in our imagination. (It is of little surprise that the fashion of modern aesthetic surgery parallels the fashion of clothing and cosmetics.) Both acts of seeing are colored by our imaginary construction of the body image we are "seeing," especially if that person is ourselves. First the face and then the body—this is the trajectory of aesthetic surgery as it begins to "remedy" the ills of the modern world as inscribed on the human form.

When we examine the history of noses and nose jobs, we immediately understand that the existing line between reconstructive and aesthetic surgery is quite tenuous. Blair O. Roger, one of the most prolific surgeon-historians of aesthetic surgery, commented that "the history of corrective rhinoplasty cannot be divorced from the history of reconstructive rhinoplasty."[7] The question here is to determine what meaning is given to the move from "reconstruction" to "correction" in the course of the late nineteenth century. The answer lies in understanding the unalterable link between psyche and body, between character and the nose, which is central to the rise of the aesthetic surgeon and the profession of aesthetic surgery. But this model of the relationship between mind and body must be understood in the light of what the physician and the patient imagine can and should be done to the body. How a culture produces such an understanding of the psyche and the body is central to any history of aesthetic surgery.

The history of the nose must be written as part of the history of the face. And we have a long tradition in the West of giving meaning to the face and its parts.[8] One can imagine (as Charles Darwin has done) that the nose defines the human face. We can "see" it as central to the face. The face, in terms of a psychology of perception, is not a face without a nose. One can read the culture of the nose and its centrality to the study of physiognomy. One can stress that the face is the one part of the modern body (along with the hands) that is usually uncovered and therefore available for scrutiny and analysis. A society in which all of its members wore masks might stress an imagined nose, much as Western society stresses an imagined breast or buttock. The West "sees" the nose and thus imagines that it is real and immediate. The more immediate and concrete it is, the more it becomes a place for fantasy. Noses are thus the ideal space to begin a history of the imagined body and the surgical interventions that alter it.

This book shall focus on two "noses," first the too-short nose and then the too-long, each of which can be read in a number of ways. These noses are examined in terms of their historical priority as the object of the surgeon's intervention. The too-long nose covers a period slightly later, but overlapping that of the too-short nose. It is not that there was a pure periodization of noses, with long noses succeeding short noses in the public imagination, although such a notion is amusing. Rather the concern with the too-tiny nose demands greater public and medical attention prior to the "discovery" of the too-long nose as a cultural and surgical problem. The syphilis epidemic of the sixteenth century overlapped with the debates about race and gave them specific nuances. The anxieties that marked the missing nose as a sign of sexual stigma came to be translated into the anxieties about the "too-small" nose with its racial implications. All concerns with the anomalous nose existed simultaneously; it was only a question of emphasis and priority, and the too-short nose won—by a nose.

By beginning with the history of the pathological nose, I can show how the expectations of aesthetic surgery rest on the history of race and racial science. Central to the overlap is the concept of "passing," which extends from "passing" in a racial sense into "passing" into other categories such as "sexuality" and "youth."

Such a notion of "passing" is not becoming "invisible" but becoming differently visible—being seen as a member of a group with which one wants or needs to identify. Racial science had already borrowed this idea of "passing" from the putative act of repairing the damaged visage of the syphilitic. The fear felt by society in no longer being able to identify those members who are dangerous and the desire of those seen as dangerous no longer to be identified as different both are intrinsic to the ideology of aesthetic surgery. The idea of choosing to "pass," with its implication of the autonomy of the individual, is also central to all notions of "passing." And this too becomes part of the basic ideological structure of aesthetic surgery.

Aesthetic surgery has a major, expanding role in modern medicine, and how it claimed that place is an important part of the history of modern culture. The goal of this book is neither a "positive" nor a "negative" history of aesthetic surgery. It is also not a comprehensive overview, for such an overview by definition would claim to chart a single story. This book does not name all of the names; it does not list all of the actors or all of their stages; it does not even attempt to be exhaustive in describing the history of all of those surgical procedures called "aesthetic." What it does try to do is to tell an interlocking set of stories that readers interested in other aspects of modern culture will find useful, if not familiar; think of it as a cyber-jigsaw puzzle into which infinite numbers of new pieces are constantly being generated that can be fitted together in myriad ways, each piece changing every story ever so slightly. This is not a "postmodern" model of writing history. As the great British social historian George M. Trevelyan noted almost a century ago, "in the most important part of this business, history is not scientific deduction but an imaginative guess."[9] The imaginative guess of this volume is rooted in readings of surgical textbooks and papers (with their images) as well as of literature, art, and films. These sources are spaces in which certain shared cultural assumptions about bodies and minds are played out. These sources, too, are not exhaustive. They present fragments of a story about aesthetic surgery. As a reader you can use these fragments to make sense of other aspects of aesthetic surgery or of the modern that I do not or cannot write about.

This book draws on some of my earlier work, specifically discussions of aesthetic surgery in *The Jew's Body* (1991) and *Health and Illness* (1995). It adds much to what was written there and expands the number of pieces in the cyber-jigsaw puzzle just a bit more.

What you will read has had the benefit of discussions with friends and colleagues (sometimes the same people) at the Cornell Medical College, the University of Chicago, the Wellcome Institute for the History of Medicine (London), the University of Michigan, the Courtauld Institute (London), the School of Oriental Studies (London), the Center for Advanced Study in the Behavioral Sciences, and the National Library of Medicine. Sections of this book have been given as talks at numerous universities in North America and Europe. My research assistants, Rhoda Rosen, Veronika Furchtner, Katja Garloff, and Anke Pinkert, were of great help in putting this project on track. I am grateful to my editor, Brigitta van Rheinberg, for her detailed comments on the manuscript. Hilary Hinzmann read and commented on every word in this manuscript and Madeleine Adams copyedited it. I am indebted to them for many stylistic and critical suggestions. This volume was completed while I was a Fellow at the Center for Advanced Study in the Behavioral Sciences at Stanford, California. I am grateful for financial support provided by the Andrew W. Mellon Foundation. The images have been gathered from a number of sources, all identified in the list of illustrations.

Stanford, California
June 1, 1997

MAKING

THE BODY

Beautiful

❧

CHAPTER ONE

Judging by Appearances

WHAT IS AESTHETIC SURGERY?

ON A WORLD in which we are judged by how we appear, the belief that we can change our appearance is liberating. We are what we seem to be and we seem to be what we are! All of us harbor internal norms of appearance by which we decide whom to trust, like, love, or fear. We act as if these internal norms are both fixed and accurate. But we constantly redraw these visual maps as we negotiate the world with all of its complexities. And as we see the world, the world is also seeing us, judging us by our appearance. To become someone else or to become a better version of ourselves in the eyes of the world is something we all want. Whether we do it with ornaments such as jewelry or through the wide range of physical alterations from hair dressing to tattoos to body piercing, we respond to the demand of seeing and being seen. Such visual judgments are ubiquitous and perhaps even necessary. But they also trap us. In the past hundred years we have increasingly turned to those whom we believe can permanently alter the way we look to others—to the aesthetic surgeons.

As we come to the close of the twentieth century, modern aesthetic surgery is celebrating its centenary. Most of the modern procedures employed in aesthetic surgery date to the 1880s and 1890s. Since then, the rise in the number of aesthetic surgery patients and procedures has been spectacular.[1] The past two decades alone show startling growth. In the United States in 1981, 296,000 such procedures were undertaken; in 1984 there were

477,700 "aesthetic" operations; in 1996 the American Academy of Facial Plastic and Reconstructive Surgery's (AAFPRS) survey stated that 825,000 plastic and reconstructive procedures had been performed on the face alone in 1995, an increase of 9 percent since 1993.[2] And the line between "reconstructive" and "aesthetic" procedures, as we shall discuss, is blurry. Moreover, as testimony to the popularity and growth of aesthetic surgery, in 1994 65 percent of these procedures were done on people with family incomes less than fifty thousand dollars a year, even though neither state nor private health insurance covers aesthetic surgery.[3] To provide some sense of the relative scope of these statistics: during 1993, one out of thirty-five surgical procedures was "aesthetic," and of those, one in twelve was a nose adjustment; one in thirty, a face-lift; one in 1,992, a buttock implant. Surgery of the eyelid and hair transplants both enjoyed big increases from 1993 to 1995. Eyelid surgery (blepharoplasty) increased 37 percent and hair transplants increased 6l percent. (It remains to be seen whether the new over-the-counter pharmaceutical treatments for hair loss will put a dent in the hair transplant business.) The most frequently performed aesthetic surgery for women in 1995 was eyelid surgery (blepharoplasty); for men, nose jobs (rhinoplasty).[4]

Such surgery is elective by definition. Elective procedures are unnecessary, or at least not immediately necessary. National health schemes or private insurers in basic coverage rarely cover them. And aesthetic surgery patients are seen as not really sick. Indeed, according to the definition of the "patient's role" by the influential American sociologist Talcott Parsons (1902–79), aesthetic surgical patients are not really patients at all.[5] (This is another reason why insurers do not want to cover them.) Among the central qualities Parsons ascribed to the role of the patient was a "gain from illness." What do we get from admitting we are sick? The attention of a loved one or employer, a day off from work, flowers delivered to the sick room? There is little "gain from illness" for aesthetic surgery patients. Indeed, many of them keep their treatment a secret and thus forfeit all of the sympathy one gains from being ill. In addition there is none of the sense of mortality that defines Parsons's normal patient. For aesthetic surgery patients, the prognosis in terms of morbidity and mortality is almost ideal: people rarely are incapacitated or die from such procedures. There is little anticipated pain, and it is the patient, not the physician, who is supposed to judge the success of the procedure. Although consumer activists may urge us all to think of ourselves in relation to our doctors as clients rather than as patients, aesthetic surgery is the one area of medicine that makes widespread use of the term *client* rather than *patient*. I shall refer to these "clients" as "patients" throughout the book, although I am well aware that this is problematic. In spite of health coverage limitations, the expansion of the number of procedures understood as aesthetic surgery at the close of the twentieth century is immense. Aesthetic surgery has clearly become a potent force in contemporary attitudes to the body.[6]

The growth of aesthetic surgery may also be gauged through the increased professionalization of aesthetic surgeons. In North America in 1997, three different "professional" groups invested colleagues with special credentials for aesthetic surgery: the plastic, aesthetic, and reconstructive surgeons, ear-nose-throat (otorhinolaryngologic) surgeons, and eye (ophthalmologic) surgeons.[7] This credentialing is called "board certification"; the first of these boards for aesthetic surgery was the American Board of Plastic Surgery, which was organized in 1937 and admitted to the American Board of Surgery the next year. A board-certified surgeon is eligible to join one of the professional organizations of aesthetic surgeons. A number of professional groups of "board-certified" surgeons exist today. The oldest such association for aesthetic surgery in the United States, the American Association of Oral Surgeons, was founded in 1921. It became the American Association of Plastic Surgeons in 1942, and today is known as the American Society of Plastic and Reconstructive Surgeons, comprising 97 percent of all plastic surgeons certified by the American Board of Plastic Surgery. In addition there are the American Academy of Facial Plastic and Reconstructive Surgery, an organization predominantly made up of otolaryngologists; the American Academy of Cosmetic Surgery, an organization of a wide variety of medical specialists who are boarded either by the

American Board of Medical Specialties (ABMS) or by the American Osteopathic Association; the American Society for Aesthetic Plastic Surgery, the self-acknowledged organization of aesthetic surgeons, which was founded only in 1967; the American Society for Dermatologic Surgery, an organization of ABMS-boarded dermatologists; the American Society of Ophthalmic Plastic and Reconstructive Surgeons; and the American Association of Oral and Maxillofacial Surgeons. But, of course, any physician, whether acknowledged as a specialist by his peers or not, can undertake aesthetic surgery. More and more non-"board-certified" physicians undertake aesthetic procedures every day, even dentists doing hair transplants.[8]

Aesthetic surgeons of every description do a truly astounding number of procedures. In 1996 the total number of all aesthetic surgical procedures such as "nose jobs, tummy tucks, and other improvements" exceeded 1.9 million, up from 1.3 million in 1994.[9] This is about one procedure for every 150 people in the United States every year; those who have had such a procedure are still a minority, but one that grows extensively each year. Part of what is so astonishing about this growth is the range of surgical procedures now offered under the rubric of aesthetic surgery. A list of common aesthetic procedures today would include the following operations on the face:

- Cheek implants, which use malar implants for the augmentation of the face
- Chin augmentation (mentoplasty), which uses implants
- Collagen and fat injections, which enhance the lips or plump up sunken facial features
- Ear pinback (otoplasty), which brings the ears closer to the head
- Eyelid tightening (blepharoplasty), which tightens the eyelids by cutting away excess skin and fat around the eyes, eliminating drooping upper eyelids and puffy bags below
- Face-lift (rhytidectomy), which tightens the jowls and neck
- Forehead lift, which tightens the forehead and raises the brow to minimize creases in the forehead and hooding over the eyes
- Hair transplantation, which treats male pattern baldness with a variety of techniques, among them scalp reduction, tissue ex-

pansion, strip grafts, scalp flaps, or clusters of punch grafts (plugs, miniplugs, and microplugs)

- Nose job (rhinoplasty),which changes the appearance of the nose
- Scar revision and the removal of common birthmarks (such as capillary nevus and port wine nevus), tattoos, and scar tissue (such as keloids, thick scar tissue that forms on an otherwise normally healing wound)—all now undertaken by means of surgery or laser treatment
- Skin resurfacing (laser, chemical face peel, and dermabrasion— sanding of the skin), which smoothes the skin, removing fine wrinkles, minor skin blemishes, and acne scars

and operations on the body:

- Arm lift (brachioplasty), which tightens the skin of the upper arm
- Breast augmentation, which can either increase the size of existing breasts or replace breasts removed through mastectomies
- Breast implant removal
- Breast reduction (mammaplasty), which reduces the size of the breast
- Breast tightening (mastopexy), which tightens the skin of the breast
- Buttock-lift and thigh-lift, which tighten the buttocks and thighs
- Calf and other implants, which shape the body
- Foreskin reconstitution (epispasm or posthioplasty)
- Liposuction (as well as lipectomy), which removes fat
- Male breast reduction (gynecomastia)
- Penile enlargement and implants
- Transgender surgery, which alters the form of the primary and secondary sexual characteristics
- Tummy tuck (abdominoplasty), abdominal apronectomy, or dermolipectomy, which reduce body size due to obesity, tighten skin, and remove fat (adipose tissue)

This is certainly not an exhaustive list, but it does give the reader some sense of the wide range of such procedures available today.

But this is not simply an American phenomenon. People all over the world are having aesthetic surgery in greater and greater numbers. The globalization of aesthetic surgery has spawned numerous centers that link surgery and tourism. North Americans have long gone to Mexico, the Dominican Republic, and Brazil; now the United Kingdom has started to offer "aesthetic surgery" tours for Americans as well. People in the United Kingdom still flock to Marbella in Spain for discreet face-lifts, but Poland and Russia are now competing for this market. For medical tourists in the Middle East, Israel has become the country of choice for many procedures, even for citizens of countries that do not have political ties to Israel; Germans visit South Africa for breast reductions and penis enlargements as well to see the Kruger National park; South Korea and Singapore are important for the Asian market; and Beirut, Lebanon, is the place to go for quick, no-questions-asked transgender surgery.[10] Medical tourism has become big business, and aesthetic surgery, because of its elective nature, is a large part of the action. For every procedure recorded in one country, similar procedures are being undertaken on that country's citizens elsewhere. The International Confederation for Plastic Surgery and Aesthetic Surgery, which had its first meeting in Uppsala in 1955, comprises seventy-eight national societies, ranging from the Argentinean Society of Plastic Surgery to the Yugoslavian Society of Plastic and Reconstructive Surgery. Aesthetic surgery has become a worldwide phenomenon in the past few decades.

Why Is It *Aesthetic* Surgery?

From these statistics, the burgeoning popularity of "aesthetic" surgery is evident, but why is it called "aesthetic surgery"? The name *aesthetic surgery* seems to be a label for those procedures which society at any given time sees as unnecessary, as nonmedical, as a sign of vanity. "Aesthetic" surgery is the opposite of "reconstructive" surgery, which is understood as restoring function. In the Middle Ages there was no discussion of either type of surgery.[11] And yet noses and other body parts were certainly lost to war, accident, and disease in the Middle Ages.[12] Only with the

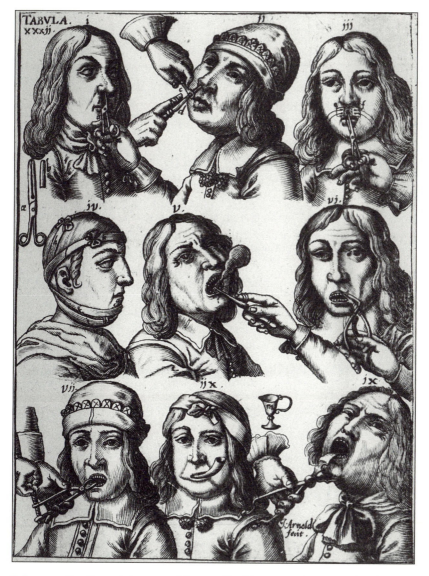

Johannes Scultetus's image of the medical interventions involved in operating on the nose and mouth, 1665. This is both reconstructive as well as aesthetic surgery in the discourse of the time.

Renaissance did surgeons begin to speak of aesthetic or beauty surgery.[13] The Renaissance distinction between the "reconstructive" and the "aesthetic" reappears in the course of the nineteenth century.

The rise of aesthetic surgery at the end of the sixteenth century is rooted in the appearance of epidemic syphilis. Syphilis was a highly stigmatizing disease from its initial appearance at the close of the fifteenth century. The role of the new *chirurgia decoratoria* was to rebuild the noses of syphilitics so that they could become less visible in their society. An early historian of aesthetic surgery, Otto Hildebrand (1858–1927), himself a reconstructive surgeon, noted the relationship between the new aesthetics of the Renaissance, the outbreak of syphilis, which caused defects of an "unaesthetic" nature, and the rise of aesthetic surgery.[14] But the innovations in aesthetic surgery that were developed in the sixteenth century vanished in Europe until the late eighteenth century, when a new age of syphilophobia began in Europe. After that point, surgeons began to seek a new name. Philippe Frédéric Blandin (1798–1849) suggested the term *autoplasty* for procedures in which skin is taken from the same individual for grafting purposes.[15] Such grafting procedures to alter the form of the body were clearly understood as reconstructive in nature.

It was *plastic surgery*, not *autoplasty*, that became the dominant label for all featural and reconstructive surgery by the early nineteenth century. Pierre Joseph Desault (1744–95) proposed *plastic surgery* (from the Greek *plastikos*, meaning "fit for molding") in 1798 as the label for those procedures that repaired deformities and corrected functional deficits.[16] Such surgery was to restore the body to its ideal prior state; it was understood as reconstructive. The term *plastic* became commonplace after Carl Ferdinand von Graefe (1787–1840) entitled his monograph on reconstruction of the nose *Rhinoplastik* (1818).[17] Plastic surgery was initially understood as surgery on the nose. Following Graefe, there was a surge in the number of " . . . plasties," such as blepharoplasty, surgery on the eyelid. To avoid a plethora of such terms, Eduard Zeis (1807–68), in his 1838 survey of the state of the field, disavowed the continuous labeling of specific procedures after the

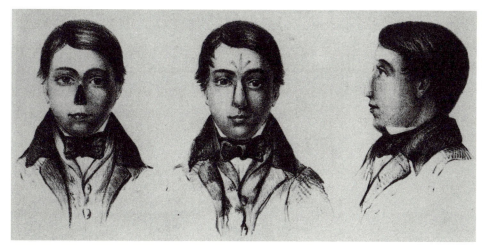

Dr. Keith's restoration of Donald MacKenzie's nose, lost from a case of lupus, 1841.

model of "rhinoplasty."[18] He wanted a single category for all reconstructive procedures on the face and body, and adopted Desault's term *plastic surgery* to encompass them.

Nevertheless the explosion of " ... plasty" terms following Graefe did not and does not let up. I shall refer to the various categories and labels employed by the surgeons I will be discussing without giving any specific weight to them. Many of these terms are attempts to create priorities for specific techniques through the creation of new "plasties." At least one contemporary American aesthetic surgeon has commented that "the evocation of Greek roots is indicative of insecurity, frequently unconscious, among many cosmetic surgeons. In my presence, the head of a prestigious plastic surgery service chastised a resident who listed the procedure as a face-lift instead of a rhytidectomy, which the chief said 'would look better to our colleagues.' "[19] As with the proliferation of technical terms in clinical psychiatry, the status of the medical subspecialty determines the nature of the field's discourse. The lower the perceived status of a field within the general culture as well as within the culture of academic medicine, the more complex and "scientific" the discourse of the field becomes.

The Renaissance label *beauty surgery* was resurrected as early as the 1840s by the innovative German facial surgeon Johann Friedrich Dieffenbach (1792–1847). He used it with evidently pejorative overtones in order to contrast it with "real" reconstructive surgery.[20] Dieffenbach, the "father of plastic surgery" (as most histories of reconstructive surgery consider him), again draws the line between reading a procedure as having a "real medical" as opposed to merely an "aesthetic" function.[21] The history of aesthetic surgery evolves from a conscious or unconscious juxtaposition with reconstructive surgery. This juxtaposition is often (as with Dieffenbach) seemingly arbitrary, but always meaningful.

Certainly the most widely used popular designation for aesthetic surgery today is *cosmetic surgery*. (In the database of general newspapers and magazines for the past two years on Lexis-Nexis, *reconstructive, plastic,* and *cosmetic surgery* each have more than the maximum of one thousand citations; *aesthetic surgery* occurs only 126 times.) The term *cosmetic* in medicine has its origin in the subspecialty cosmetic dermatology.[22] This field developed at the close of the nineteenth century and dealt with the improvement of "abnormal" appearance resulting from pathologies or trauma, including the use of corrosive cosmetics (such as lead compound face powder). Its antecedents can be found in the conflation of medicine and cosmetics in classical Egyptian and Greco-Roman medical texts, which will be discussed throughout this volume. The development of medical cosmetics in the late nineteenth century had its own specific form. Growing out of the popular racial ideology of lay writers such as Hermann Klencke (1813–81) during the 1860s, it was clearly intended to improve or preserve the attractiveness of the individual and thus improve the breeding of the race.[23] This racial tradition maintained itself through the beginning of the twentieth century within the ideology of bodybuilding. This is closely related to cosmetology through the bodybuilder's emphasis on "sensible skin care."[24] The racial view was an intrinsic part of the discourse used by medical dermatologists at the end of the century. This field

quickly developed into a major part of what physicians were supposed to do—and beauticians were not![25]

Aesthetic or *cosmetic* or *beauty surgery* began to appear sporadi-
cally in the course of the nineteenth century as labels for an alternative model of therapy, first within the tradition of reconstructive surgery, and then as its antithesis. Those who used these
labels were aware that "cosmetic" or "beauty" or "aesthetic"
surgery bore the pejorative overtones used by Dieffenbach. During and following World War I, there was a movement to expand
the patient base by using for "aesthetic" purposes those techniques evolved in the treatment of soldiers. Even though early
twentieth-century "reconstructive" procedures, such as the rebuilding of the "harelip," had been understood as "aesthetic" in
the mid nineteenth century, the division between "plastic" and
"aesthetic" surgery was made to seem absolute.[26]

The self-conscious rise, during the closing decades of the nineteenth and the opening decade of the twentieth century, of surgeons who saw themselves as "beauty" surgeons was challenged
by the postwar reconstructive surgeons, who saw aesthetic
surgery as incidental to their practice. The best-known Allied reconstructive surgeon, the New Zealander Harold Delf Gillies
(1882–1960), advocated seeing "aesthetic surgery" as a natural
subordinate extension of "reconstructive surgery." In 1934 he
called the field: "aesthetic, reconstructive surgery." He also condemned the "poorly qualified and very well advertised surgeons
[who] have adopted the term, plastic surgery, without any true
training in surgery and without any other surgical ability than to
remove a few folds of skin or a small hump of the nose. . . . It is
so easy to agree to do some cosmetic operations which may in fact
not be justified, and it is so troublesome, sometimes, to decide
whether in a particular patient the proposed operation will give
that pleasure and satisfaction which it would in another."[27] Many
of the surgeons involved in rebuilding the fractured faces of soldiers came out of the newly developing world of aesthetic
surgery, and they continued their practices following the war.

As a "positive" label, *beauty surgery* had begun in earnest in the opening decade of the twentieth century, but this term evidently was soon tainted, as Gillies's comments showed. The "beauty" surgeons were often simply denounced as quacks by the medical profession. In 1934 Jacques W. Maliniak (1889–1976) attacked the "brazen quackery that has attended the development of modern plastic surgery."[28] This "quackery" was, however, not much different in its approach and success from the procedures developed and used by physicians within the medical establishment. The label *quack* was used to limit the investiture of those permitted to undertake "serious" interventions. The relationship of quacks with beauty surgery has a long history, stretching back into the eighteenth century, to the rise of anxiety about disease and its disguise.

In the eighteenth century, the Edinburgh "quack" John Taylor (1703–72), according to his own account, removed scar tissue from the lower lid of a burn victim's eye. The pain was excruciating, and the patient repeatedly shouted, "You hurt me, you hurt me!" to which Taylor replied, "Remember, Lady, Beauty! Beauty!"[29] When he was finished, the woman's friends "were astonished and it looked as if the business had been done by some miracle." Taylor performed a number of *aesthetic* procedures, including removing part of the upper eyelid in a patient who suffered from a drooping eyelid (ptosis), using a procedure that would become commonplace a hundred years later in the age of Dieffenbach. Despite his evident skill, Taylor was a "quack" according to the Edinburgh Royal College of Physicians, which excoriated him in print. This was to no little degree because his stated goal was "beauty." For "beauty doctors," as William Hogarth showed in his *Marriage à la Mode,* offered the means of masking illnesses such as syphilis as well as restoring beauty. They provided the means by which diseased faces could "pass" as healthy. "Natural" beauty was a guarantee of the health of the individual as well as the health of the state.

The term *beauty* again became pejorative in American feminist rhetoric against aesthetic surgery in the 1980s.[30] *Beauty doctors* and *the beauty industry* were not terms of endearment. In order to maintain the idea of the "beautiful" without using the terms *beauty* or *cosmetic,* the profession turned to the classical label *aes-*

thetic. The term *aesthetic surgery,* although used in 1903 to describe paraffin therapy, which shall be discussed in detail later, came into more common use only after 1934.[31] This term, which differentiates the field from "reconstructive" surgery, is most commonly used today to describe elective procedures that alter the surface and shape of the body. The stress on the spelling *aesthetic* (rather than the less "literary" *esthetic)* has been noted by one commentator as helping to establish the "seriousness" of the field: "The 'a' that precedes 'esthetic' in most communications from official organizations of surgeons doing this type of operation also serves to upgrade the image by conferring on it a classical lineage."[32] The irony is that over the past few years beauty parlor workers in the United States, earlier called cosmeticians, have begun to call themselves "estheticians."[33] The classical lineage, with its conflation of health and beauty, is indeed part of the complex history of aesthetic surgery.[34]

The debate about "priorities," which haunts most realms of modern science and medicine, takes on a special meaning in the case of aesthetic surgery. Who undertook the first modern face-lift, nose job, tummy tuck, and so forth? This is not an "academic" question of who gets mentioned in the histories of the discipline. No medical subspecialty except psychiatry has spent as much time and effort documenting its own history. In creating an archaeology that places modern "aesthetic" procedures in historical line with (and parallel to) "reconstructive" procedures, aesthetic surgeons and their historians attempt to provide a "serious" medical context for aesthetic procedures. This is analogous to the creation of medical terminology. Within surgery, aesthetic surgery may well be unique in its concern for its own history. This concern parallels the modern creation of the field, certainly as far back as Dieffenbach and Zeis in the mid nineteenth century.[35] The priorities debate among the historians of aesthetic surgery often turns on moments of transition from a self-consciously "medical" model, which does not acknowledge "beauty" as one of its goals, to a competing model of "aesthetic" surgery, in which the creation of a "beautiful" face and body is asserted as a legitimate medical goal. Such a movement takes place in the Renaissance and again in the nineteenth century. In the latter period surgeons not only tried to correct the ugliness that results from diseases such as syphilis, but they also tried to correct the "ugliness" of nonwhite races. Medicine's job became correcting the appearance of illness as well as its pathology. Racial science used appearance as a means of determining who was fit and who was ill, who could reproduce and "improve" the race and who should be excluded and condemned. In a world based on Enlightenment ideals of "disciplining the body and of regulating populations,"[36] to cite Michel Foucault, aesthetic surgeons began to offer ways of altering the body to make it appear "healthy" by making it appear racially acceptable. This took place in the 1880s and 1890s, in operations on the ear, the nose, and the breast. Only after this possibility of correcting the "ugliness" of disease and race had been established did other forms of "beauty" surgery begin to be a conceptual possibility. Once you can change what a society understands as unchangeable, such as racial markers, then it is possible to imagine altering other aspects of the body that seem permanent, such as signs of aging. The historical development of specific procedures mirrors the unique double face of aesthetic surgery as parallel to and different from reconstructive surgery.

REMAKING THE SELF

Central to the growth of aesthetic surgery at the close of the nineteenth century was the ability of physicians to eliminate the pain of the operations and reduce the risk of infections. These changes emboldened patients to undertake such procedures more frequently. They could now cease to be mere patients and create the new and different role of medical client. Anesthesia became generally accepted and central to the practice of surgery after the discovery of ether anesthesia by William Thomas Green Morton (1819–68) in 1846. By the 1880s, the further development of local anesthesia, in the forms of cocaine for surgery of the eye, spinal (subarachnoid) anesthesia, and epidural anesthesia, meant that the greater risk of dying under general anesthesia could be avoided. Local anesthesia has played a central part in the development of aesthetic surgery as a widely practiced specialty. It is one of the primary factors in the successful outcome of the patient, who can follow the procedure and, unlike the patient under general anesthesia, does not morbidly fantasize about the opening of the body while unconscious.[37] Under local anesthesia, aesthetic surgery can be experienced as a procedure a patient actively chooses, not a cure to which he or she passively submits under general anesthesia, giving up all control of the self. The patient's perception of autonomy is central to the popularity of aesthetic surgery.

The movement toward antisepsis paralleled the development of anesthesia. In 1867 Joseph Lister (1827–1912) provided a model for antisepsis that became generally accepted by the end of the century.[38] The potential avoidance of infection meant that patients' anxiety about cutting the skin was lessened. The acceptance of antisepsis was relatively slow, but was strongly encouraged by aesthetic surgeons. On November 26, 1877, Robert F. Weir (1838–94), one of the major figures in the creation of American aesthetic surgery, said in a talk before the New York Medical Association that the acceptance of antisepsis in Britain and Germany had outpaced that in the United States. He urged that the smallest detail of the cleansing of patient, surgeon, instruments, and surgical theater be carried out so that the patient not be placed at needless risk.[39] Once this was done, the risks attendant on aesthetic surgery decreased sharply because of the reduction in the high incidence of infection.

With pain and infection removed or reduced, aesthetic surgery came into its own. Yet anesthesia and antisepsis were necessary but not sufficient to mark the beginning of the modern history of aesthetic surgery. It was the Enlightenment ideology that each individual could remake him- or herself in the pursuit of happiness that provided the basis for the modern culture of aesthetic surgery. Indeed, it is remarkable how often aesthetic surgeons cite "happiness" as the goal of the surgery.[40] "Happiness" for aesthetic surgeons is a utilitarian notion of happiness, like that espoused by John Stuart Mill (1806–73), who placed the idea of happiness within the definition of individual autonomy.[41] You can make yourself happy through being able to act in the world. This was mirrored in the rise of modern notions of the citizen as well as the revolutionary potential of the individual. Autonomy stands as the central principle in the shaping of aesthetic surgery. "Sapere aude!" wrote Immanuel Kant (1724–1804), " 'Dare to use your own reason'—is the motto of the Enlightenment."[42] The ability to remake one's self is the heart of the matter.[43]

The Enlightenment self-remaking took place in public, and was dependent on being "seen" by others as transformed. This extended to the reshaping of the body, even within the world of fashion: "At home, one's clothes suited one's body and its needs; on the street, one stepped into clothes whose purpose was to make it possible for other people to act as if they knew who you were. One became a figure in a contrived landscape; the purpose of the clothes was not to be sure of whom you were dealing with, but to be able to behave as if you were sure."[44] The rise of aesthetic surgery required the physician and the patient to accept an ideology of the medical alteration of the body and the state. And yet, as we shall see, there is an inherent tension between the Enlightenment promise—You can become one of us and we shall be happy together—and the subtext—The more you reshape yourself, the more I know my own value, my own authenticity, and your inauthenticity. You become a mere copy, passing yourself off as the "real thing."

Happiness, the central goal of aesthetic surgery, is defined in terms of the autonomy of the individual to transform him- or herself. Thomas Jefferson famously included the pursuit of happiness in his Enlightenment list of the ideal goals of the autonomous citizen. Happiness in this context is a "peculiarly modern, Western idea," as Richard Sennett comments.[45] By the late nineteenth century the belief that the surgeon can cure unhappiness is entrenched in aesthetic surgery. A generation later, in 1929, the Portland, Oregon, "beauty" surgeon Adalbert G. Bettman (1883–?) took it as given that aesthetic surgery "has been perfected to such a degree that it is now available for the improvement of patients' mental well-being, their pursuit of happiness."[46] The Enlightenment debate about the individual's autonomy to remake him- or herself is linked to the power of the institutions of medicine and to the new role of the aesthetic surgeon, not just to heal illness but to fulfill the patient's desires.

All of these changes in aesthetic surgery took place following the most wrenching political revolutions (from the American and French revolutions to those of 1848 and the American Civil War). The revolutions continued, however, in the fields of "science" from Louis Pasteur (1822–95) to Robert Koch (1843–1910) to Thomas A. Edison (1847–1931). The transformation of the Enlightenment notion of self-improvement moved from the battlefield of liberalism to the laboratories and surgical theaters of the later nineteenth century. This is the further context of aesthetic surgery. This age prefigures the revolutionary movements of the late nineteenth and early twentieth centuries. All of the destabilization that had been experienced and repressed following mid-century came to be experienced again in a sea change in imagining who we are and what our bodies are. It is not that the reconstructed body was "invented" at the end of the nineteenth century, but rather that questions about the ability of the individual to be transformed, which had been articulated as social or political in the context of the state, came to be defined as biological and medical. The political "unhappiness" of class and poverty, which led to the storming of the Bastille, came to be experienced as the "unhappiness" found within the body. In each case, the body was the location of the "unhappiness." In the former, it was revolutionary change that would cure the body; in the latter, it was the cure of the individual by which the unhappiness would be resolved.

In the great political movements of the late nineteenth and early twentieth centuries, these dynamic patterns again merged. George Mosse has shown that the revolutionary movements of the late nineteenth century, Zionism, Communism, and Fascism, also reworked the notion of the body as one of their core beliefs.[47] Each wanted to create, for its own purposes, new bodies, which represent the potential of the new system. This political transmutation of the body is also central to the culture of aesthetic surgery. You can become someone new and better by altering the body. In liberal societies it is often imagined as the transformation of the individual, such as the immigrant, into a healthy member of the new polis. The individual can be transformed and made happy. Aesthetic surgery accepts this premise, and adds that such happiness also can be the result of medical practice.

The happiness of the physician parallels that of the patient. The surgeon's happiness comes to be a sign of his ability to transform himself. The rise of aesthetic surgery marked the professionalization and organization of modern medicine.[48] The increase in the social status of the physician/surgeon in the Enlightenment meant an increase in the financial rewards associated with becoming a medical professional. If you were a "real" doctor, you had status and money. Not being a real doctor meant you were a "quack" and were economically marginalized. One could simply not risk being called a "quack," a term often used for the early aesthetic surgeons as well as the syphilis doctors, because it marked one as beyond the boundaries of social and professional status. By the middle of the nineteenth century, the reconstructive or aesthetic surgeons and the syphilologists were all elbowing their way into the medical establishment. They did not want to be seen as doing the work of the beautician or "quack," but that of the medical practitioner. But their ability to enable people to "pass" as different made their position marginal. *Passing* was the nineteenth century's pejorative term for the act of disguising one's "real" (racial) self. It was also the ultimate articulation of the Enlightenment notion of transformation. The transgressive act of "passing" showed how tenuous the boundaries in the social order really were. The newly enfranchised physicians derived their status and income from escorting patients across these boundaries.

When the successful American surgeon Maxwell Maltz (1899–1975) remembered deciding to become a "plastic surgeon," he set his memory in a dialogue with his Jewish mother in New York City in the 1920s. "What was a plastic surgeon anyway? . . . From what I told her it seemed nothing more or less than a beauty doctor, a movie-picture kind of doctor, not a real doctor like the man who pulled out tonsils and cured scarlet fever. So you don't like your nose so you cut it off?"[49] That Maltz in 1953 imagines such a conversation (accompanied by "steaming golden soup") set before World War I is an indicator of how racial models of "passing" accompanied the stigma of the "aesthetic quack." Quackery lay not in being a "beauty" doctor, but in making it possible for others to disguise themselves through surgery. Such a role put the aesthetic surgeon, no matter how skilled or how well trained, beyond the pale of the new field of reconstructive surgery.

But in the Enlightenment ideology of nineteenth-century medical science, the hygiene of the body became the hygiene of the spirit and that of the state. A concern with "hygiene" in the broadest sense and aesthetic surgery's role in the physical alteration of the "ugliness" of the body led the aesthetic surgeon to become the guarantor of the hygiene of the state, the body, and the psyche. He (with one exception, all of the early aesthetic surgeons were men) provided a type of surgical eugenics, a means of improving the individual and, through the individual, the state. Daniel Kevles defined a tension between the "old eugenics" of selective breeding and a "new genetics" of genetic manipulation.[50] Aesthetic surgery is, as we shall see, more closely allied to the latter than to the former. Eliminate or transform—this was and is the dilemma of nineteenth- and twentieth-century biological science and its cousin, medical practice. Aesthetic surgery could transform the body into a new and happier one, one that fulfilled the expectations of a new society and changed as these expectations changed.

"Passing"

The pursuit of happiness through aesthetic surgery presupposes decisive categories of inclusion and exclusion. Happiness in this instance exists in crossing the boundary separating one category from another. It is rooted in the necessary creation of arbitrary demarcations between the perceived reality of the self and the ideal category into which one desires to move. It is the frustration or fulfillment of this desire that constitutes "unhappiness" or "happiness." The patient and the surgeon know that there is a group that the patient wants to join, and that the surgeon can help him or her to do so. The surgeon can enable the patient to "pass" as a member of the desired group. The categories defining such groups seem to be "real." They seem not to be invented, and thus appear to be quite separate from the imaginations of both patient and surgeon. Yet they are as much a product of the desire of both as any reality beyond them. The nineteenth-century "Jew" who desired to be a "German" assumed that "German" was a real category defined in nature rather than a social construct. "Passing" is thus moving into and becoming invisible within a desired "natural" group. The model of "passing" is the most fruitful to use in examining the history and efficacy of aesthetic surgery. Taken from the history of the construction of race, not gender, it provides the most comprehensive model for the understanding of aesthetic surgery.

The patient believes that there is a desirable category of being from which he or she is excluded because of reasons that are defined as physical. The results of this exclusion are symptoms of psychological "unhappiness." Other signs present in the external world may well mark the exclusion, but they are seen as corollaries of physical difference. The individual desires to join a new community defined economically, socially, erotically (or in all three ways), but this group is primarily defined physically. The surgeon believes that with ever more innovative medical interventions, the patient can be enabled to "pass." The surgical techniques must constantly evolve so as to perfect the illusion that the boundary between the patient and the group never existed. The individual must seem to have always been a member of the cohort. Each set of procedures enables individuals to "pass." The problem with this is that beauty is culturally constituted, and so that which made you (in)visible in one generation or in one place marks you as visible in another.

Each physical category must be so constructed that it has a

clearly defined, unambiguous antithesis (hairy/bald, fat/thin, large-breasted/small-breasted, large nose/small nose, male/female). These categories are all socially defined so as to make belonging to the positive category more advantageous than belonging to the negative category. The advantage of each constructed category changes as the society that recognizes it changes. "Fat" has a positive value in certain societies at certain times, for example, as a sign of prosperity. In other societies at other times "fat" has a negative value as a sign of ill health. Indeed, definitions of "fat" and "thin" change from time to time and place to place. What remains constant is the idea that the external body (with whatever qualities are ascribed to it) reflects the values of the soul. To "pass," one must be able to move from a negative category (bald) to a positive category (hairy), which means moving from a negative character to a positive one. Although such categories are subject to continual change, surgeons and patients act as if they are permanent. Indeed, in the construction of ever finer differentials (such as we shall see in the creation of "ethnic appropriate aesthetic surgery" in the 1980s) the antitheses are simply made more specific.

Since the early nineteenth century these categories of inclusion/includability and exclusion/excludability have been defined in terms of "pariah" groups constructed in categories such as race, gender, and class.[51] At any given moment we each know to which group we belong and to which we do not. The gendering of aesthetic surgery is only one aspect of these social constructions of ideal (read: beautiful) groups. Its importance lies more with the nature of the category than its gender specificity. The dichotomy between the "large-nosed" and the "small-nosed" presents an analogous antithesis to the constructions of gender as in male/female, butch/fem, gay/straight, and so on. Within the history of aesthetic surgery the categories are initially those of "pathology" (healthy/diseased) and "race" (Jew/Aryan, Irish/English, black/white). Operations on ears and noses are pejoratively labeled aesthetic in the late nineteenth century because they enable individuals to "pass" as "normal," that is, as neither Irish nor Jewish. The initial operations to mask pathological and/or racial signs are only then followed by the development of other "aesthetic" operations to remove signs of aging or to transform the structure of the genitals. These enable individuals to pass into other cohorts, to become young or female. Many of these categories, such as breast reduction, become "aesthetic" when they are tied to the alleviation of perceived racial "stigmas." The alleviation of these sources of perceived unhappiness is undertaken so that the individual can "pass" and become "happy." Categories of unhappiness such as looking too old are tied to class or at least economic definitions of happiness. These all (in complex ways) are defined by and define the bipolar notions of "beauty" and "ugliness," "happiness" and "unhappiness."[52]

American racial literature of the turn of the last century asserted that "a face can be said to be indisputably beautiful only when it unites features befitting the bearer's age, sex, and race, with the signs of blooming health, and if it be disfigured neither by deformity nor by the traces of some or other impairment nor by the reflection of spiritual disharmony."[53] Such idealized notions of "beauty" demanded eugenic controls to avoid the pollution of the body politic by the ugly and deformed. Thus, in addition to the legal bars against "racial" categories, such as those that kept the Irish, Jews, and African Americans, as well as the "contagious" (as Judith Walzer has shown in her study of Typhoid Mary),[54] from appearing in specific social environments, there have been laws against the "ugly." These "ugly laws" were generally part of vagrancy laws, which imposed fines on "unsightly" people who were seen in public places. In my home city of Chicago, the infamous Chicago municipal code 36-34 (1966) (repealed in 1974) imposed fines on persons who appeared in public who were "diseased, maimed, mutilated, or in any way deformed so as to be an unsightly or disgusting object."[55] Such laws are the equivalent of the "Jim Crow" laws in the South or the Nazi posting of signs ordering Jews not to enter parks. They heighten the sense of one's visibility. No wonder individuals desired to become "(in)visible" by looking like the group in power.

The discourse of "passing," which comes out of the racialization of nineteenth-century culture, is the very wellspring of aesthetic surgery. The boundary between reconstructive and aesthetic surgery was distinguished on the basis of the introduction of procedures that were seen as enabling individuals to "pass." "Aesthetic" procedures were and are those that enable individuals to pass into a category that they perceive as different from themselves. Given a general scientific acceptance in the nineteenth century of a permanent human constitution, which intimately connected the internal and external qualities of a human being, aesthetic surgery could not be seen as "real" medicine. A medical procedure that attempts to "correct" the "uncorrectable" simply masks the reality of the individual. The attempt to alter the unalterable, to change the psyche of the individual by changing his or her physiognomy meant creating a simulacrum of a human being rather than a "new person." But, of course, those wanting to "pass" had to believe that changing the exterior also changed the inner reality or at least that society would accept the external appearance as a true indication of the internal reality. Following the Enlightenment notion of human autonomy, "passing" not only was possible but also became an imperative for some members of certain race, class, and gender groups in the nineteenth century.

These groups placed what Lawrence Haworth has called "critical competence" at the center of their definition of the human being.[56] Each individual must be autonomous, which Thomas Scanlon defines as seeing "himself as sovereign in deciding what to believe and in weighing competing reasons for action."[57] You are the sum total of what you believe yourself able to become. This is the ideological underpinning of "passing." It is what Isaiah Berlin has called "positive liberty": "I wish to be somebody, not nobody . . . self-directed and not acted upon by external nature or by other men as if I were a thing, or an animal . . . incapable of playing a human role, that is, of conceiving goals and policies of my own and realizing them."[58] The parallel between refusing the constraints of "external nature" (the ill or deformed body) and the desire to play a "human role" lies at the very heart of aesthetic surgery as a means of expressing autonomy and thus "passing." But if claiming the right to change one's body is a claim of autonomy, relying on a surgeon to execute the change is a surrender of autonomy. This tension marks the history of aesthetic surgery from its inception and continues to define it today.

Following the influential sociologist Max Weber's (1864–1920) argument about the construction of validity through group consensus, one can see "passing" as a type of silent validation.[59] Belonging to a new group must evoke certain responses by third parties (such as erotic or economic acceptance), and the most important of these are silent. The person with a "too-small" nose who has had aesthetic surgery is accepted *without comment* into the world of the large-nosed people, and the small-breasted person after a surgical procedure *silently* enters into the cohort of the large-breasted. *Silence is acquiescence.* If there is any sign that one is unable to "pass," then the procedure must be considered a failure. If the cohort is able to detect the alteration, it will make some further distinction between "authentic" and "inauthentic" bodies, and "passing" becomes impossible. Each age recognizes the reconstruction of the body in its own time. Such rejection, however, is usually not because of the surgeon's limits but because of the psychological makeup of the patient or of the cohort. Belief is everything, and once one begins to recognize in others or in oneself the marks of transformation, no silent acceptance is possible.

CRIMINAL BODIES

The ambiguity associated with ideas of "passing" through aesthetic surgery can be found in social attitudes toward criminality. Criminality posed an interesting question for aesthetic surgeons. In a world in which psychopathology and sociopathy are reflections of character, can the psyche truly be altered through interventions that change the body, or does the soul remain unchanged? If "good" character is reflected in the beautiful body and the happy psyche, is "bad" character mirrored in the deformed body and the unhappy soul? An ancient but still vital trope associates ugliness with bad character. Franciscus Vellesius, physician to Phillip II in sixteenth-century Spain, could write, "Si duo homines inciderunt in criminis suspicionem, is primus torqueatur, qui sit aspectu deformia."[60] (The very face of the criminal reveals his soul.) One great social fear in early twentieth-century Europe and the United States was that the criminal, especially the Jew or black as criminal, would alter his appearance through the agency of the aesthetic surgeon and vanish into the crowd. Thus the suggestion, first made in Germany in the eighteenth century, that criminals be tattooed. Cesare Lombroso in the mid nineteenth century, like Johann Caspar Lavater in the previous century, provided detailed images of criminal types as a means of identifying them even before they could commit a crime.[61] His prime concern was with "criminal men"; it was only at the very end of his career that he turned to documenting the physiognomy of "criminal women." Indeed, the discourse on aesthetic surgery and criminality is gendered male. Criminality does not vanish with the introduction of aesthetic surgery, only "our" ability as observers using the nineteenth-century Bertillon method, which recorded external signs and physical measurements such as height, weight, eye color, and so on to codify criminality.

When popular fantasy imagines the falsely accused criminal "passing," it is through aesthetic surgery. In Delmer Daves's *Dark Passage* (1947) with Humphrey Bogart (as Vincent Parry) and Lauren Bacall (as Irene Jansen), Bogart plays a man wrongly convicted of murdering his wife, who escapes from prison in order to prove his innocence.[62] Bogart finds that his features are too well known, and he is forced to seek some illicit backroom aesthetic surgery (performed by Houseley Stevenson as Dr. Walter Coley). The entire presurgical part of the film is shot from a Bogart's-eye view, with the audience seeing the fugitive for the first time as he starts to recuperate from the operation in the apartment of a sympathetic young artist (played by Bacall) with whom he falls in love. Our identification with Bogart is complete. We literally see the world through his eyes and when his face is revealed—it is the face of Humphrey Bogart! This is a film of innocence violated and of aesthetic surgery rectifying injustice. Bogart's "passing" as innocent enables him to prove himself in-

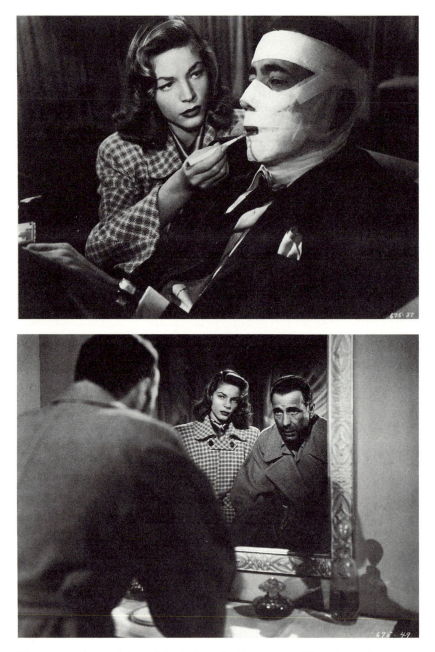

The escaped convict as object of aesthetic surgery. The viewer becomes the patient. Humphrey Bogart (and Lauren Bacall) in *Dark Passage*, 1947.

nocent, but only to Bacall and to the viewer. Society continues to see him as criminal.

Other models of "passing" exist within this narrative. For if Bogart is innocent and aesthetic surgery enables him to prove it, then "real" criminals, too, can turn to aesthetic surgery to "pass" as innocent by masking their countenance, as did John Dillinger a decade before the film.[63] This view continues across the century. In 1997, Richie Ramos, a major drug trafficker, had his nose "reshaped, [had] fat vacuumed from his waist and cheeks, and [had] gunshot scars removed from his face and . . . a bulging bullet fragment from his head."[64] Jose Castillo, the surgeon who Ramos claimed undertook these procedures, was charged with harboring a fugitive and obstructing justice in February 1997.

The corollary theory also exists—that criminality itself could be a reflex of feeling "different" because of the perception of the criminal as "ugly" and therefore as "bad."[65] In 1921 the *San Francisco Examiner* commented that 11 percent of the two thousand men who entered San Quentin after 1917 had "crooked noses."[66] Convicts in the United States, according to the *New York Times* in 1927, began to demand the right to have aesthetic surgery. In one case, a cauliflower ear, a dented nose, and wrinkles were removed from a fifty-year-old convicted felon. The commentator noted that one felt a "thrill of reform through face-lifting."[67] As late as 1949, one French commentator was surprised that Americans believed in "operating on inferiority" as a means of reforming criminals.[68] Psychological theory, especially the concept of the "inferiority complex" developed by Alfred Adler, was used to provide a further rationale for the relationship between an ugly physiognomy and an unhappy psyche.

Both of these views have cultural currency at the close of the twentieth century in the "real" world of crime and courts—as well as in popular fiction such as Carl Hiassen's satire of the hard-boiled detective and the aesthetic surgery industry in Florida, *Skin Tight* (1989), in which the villain, Rudy Graveline, actually kills a patient while incompetently performing a routine rhinoplasty, and then employs a man who had been badly deformed by another aesthetic surgeon to murder the detective pursuing the case. The satire lies in the depiction of the world of Miami's aesthetic surgery culture as well as the extraordinary visibility of the deformity of the murderer, which was caused by aesthetic surgery. He has become so monstrous that he is unable to "pass" under any circumstance. Hiassen's fiction eerily became reality when in 1994 the Miami aesthetic surgeon Dr. Ricardo Samitier Jr., known locally as "Dr. Lips," was convicted of manslaughter and sentenced to five years in prison for the death of his patient, the lounge singer Claudio Martell, who bled to death in 1992 while undergoing penis-enlargement surgery to surprise his wife.[69]

In a world in which the beautiful is the exception, the question remains whether it is desirable to be beautiful. Certainly, setting oneself apart from the norm means that one is understood as exceptional, and yet this end of the "bell curve" of the beautiful is certainly more desirable than the other end, at which the ugly (and its associated concepts) dwell. In the fantasy of the Enlightenment, the reconstruction of the face became a way of reconstructing the aesthetic and moral sensibility of the new citizen, of making modern man beautiful and moral and healthy. Yet for all of the desire to set up antitheses of moral and immoral, beauty and ugliness, good and bad character, all of the systems of physiognomy understood the problem of disguise, of "passing." Indeed the questions of the representation of race and the aesthetics of beauty are closely intertwined.[70] There are "beautiful" races and "ugly" races in the racial theory of the nineteenth century.

Superficial changes in the body could lead the innocent observer to misconstrue the true nature of the inner (or even the outer) appearance of the individual. As the seventeenth-century divine Thomas Walkington (?–1621) notes in his *Optick Glasse of Humours*, "All is not Gold, that glistereth; every Persian Nose argues not a valiant Cyrus. We often see *plumbeam machaerum in aurea vagina*, a leaden Rapier in a golden Sheath. The fair-branch'd Cypress-tree fruitless, and barren; a putrefied nutmeg gilded over . . . Many a gaudy outside, & a baudy deformed inside."[71] Does the alteration of the surface cause the soul to change, or does the soul maintain its inviolate nature no matter what happens to the surface? Can we truly make someone happy by altering his/her appearance or do we merely shift this unhappiness to other aspects of the person? Does one "pass" when one has aesthetic surgery, or does one become a new person? Such questions shape the desire of patients to undertake aesthetic surgery and of surgeons to develop procedures that try with ever more sophistication to create "new" and thus "happier" people.

Gender Questions

Many of the recent studies of aesthetic surgery have been critiques of the social construction of "female beauty." Often the ideological position of such studies stresses the invidious effect of the patriarchal institutions of medicine on women who have been made insecure about their bodies and who seek to "cure" their "unhappiness" through surgery. Society makes women "unhappy" about their bodies and then supplies the "cure" through the hand of the surgeon. Such a simple victim/perpetrator model does not come close to the complexity reflected in the history of aesthetic surgery in regard to gender. From its earliest moments, the claim of aesthetic surgery to creating mental "happiness" does not privilege any specific category, including gender.

As many contemporary theorists following Judith Butler have been at pains to point out, gender is a socially constructed set of categories that are as much determined by as determinant of other social classifications. A history of aesthetic surgery solely from the perspective of gender would distort the role and definition of the patient as well as the surgeon. Let us imagine that gender is but one of the categories that must be understood as shaping one's sense of one's body and one's psyche. In some historical and social contexts it may be the primary defining quality of the body, in others an ancillary and dependent one. In the final stage of this study "gender" plays an overt role, and yet, as we shall see, it is a concept of gender highly modified by the importance of racial science. Gender is a consistent presence in the history of aesthetic surgery, yet with constant shifts of meaning and nuances.

Most of the patients on whom late nineteenth-century surgeons exhibited their procedures were men. Aesthetic surgery came, by the 1990s to be gendered female: "Americans think it's more appropriate for a woman to surgically alter her appearance than for a man to do the same. Once again, young adults (under 30) are most conservative, with just 16 percent saying that cosmetic surgery is equally acceptable for men or women, while 28 percent of people 30 or older okay both."[72] Recent studies of "masculinity" reinforce this view. R. W. Connell, writing from a British perspective, notes that "true masculinity" is somehow antithetical to aesthetic surgery.[73] Such popular views had a powerful medical resonance. There was "something" wrong with men who wanted aesthetic surgery.

In 1972 one of the criteria for a poor outcome ("unhappiness") following aesthetic surgery was the observation that "the patient is a male and is likely to attribute a life history of multiple inadequacies to a single physical defect."[74] Two decades later such a statement would not be made. Men who seek aesthetic surgery are no longer assumed to be chronically more unhappy than women. Women are no longer seen as more easily able to separate out their general sense of self from their "unhappiness" over the form of a specific body part. There was a disproportionate increase (11 percent) in the number of men in the United States who had aesthetic surgery between 1990 and 1994. The 1995 figures report that men account for 33 percent of those undergoing facial plastic procedures, an increase of 9 percent since 1993.[75] The gender gap seems to be closing as we reconceptualize the idea of aesthetic surgery and the potential for individual transformation in the modern world.

This is not limited to the United States. There has been a marked increase in the number of men in the United Kingdom who have had or want to have aesthetic surgery.[76] In Brazil the number of men having aesthetic surgery has increased by 80 percent, from eight thousand in 1994 to fifteen thousand in 1995.[77] In Argentina the number of men having procedures soared when President Carlos Menem publicly acknowledged his numerous hair implants, two face-lifts, an eyelid reduction, and teeth replacement. "The president has shown absolutely no embarrassment regarding his own metamorphosis," Jorge Weinstein of the Organization of Argentine Plastic Surgeons says. "In fact, every time he has had a collagen injection everyone knows about it. He is not ashamed to show his vanity because it's simply part of the flamboyant and charismatic personality that makes him popular."[78] Men everywhere are no longer seen as psychopathic when they desire aesthetic surgery. Aesthetic surgery seems to be approaching a time when it will not be gendered at all. The stigmatizing quality of the procedures seems to be diminishing.

In the 1990s it is women having aesthetic surgery who are seen as more unhappy then men. Kimberly Ellena Bergman provided a generally accepted feminist reading of aesthetic surgery in the 1990s. She argued that "women's extreme concern with physical appearance is expressed in increased incidence of beauty-seeking behaviors such as eating disorders and addictive plastic surgery." In her dissertation she examined how "women's beliefs about physical attractiveness affect their lives." She concluded that women appear to be more dissatisfied with their physical appearance than previous research has reported. According to her, beauty-seeking behavior also seems motivated by women's fear of the rejection and contempt accorded unattractive women by themselves as well as others. Their choice to undertake aesthetic surgery was the result of "women's low self-esteem and its many consequences, obsessive concern with physical appearance, women's devaluing of their other qualities and traits, and lower aspiration levels for other accomplishments which would give them direct access to the rewards they seek with their beauty."[79] Views such as Bergman's see aesthetic surgery as the response to a patriarchal society's image of the woman and relates aesthetic surgery as a type of disease to other "pathologies" (such as eating disorders) that are gendered feminine at the end of the twentieth century. But the real number of women having procedures has increased radically over the past decades. The anxiety about being seen as "sick" seems to be contained within the world of feminist theory.

From the Enlightenment on, gender has played a major role in defining other categories of difference. Although all "men are created equal," women are held to have specific qualities, for example, an alleged heightened vanity, which give them special status. Women come to represent the unhealthy in the vocabulary of difference. It is not only women who are constructed as being vain.[80] Vanity is indeed one of the qualities ascribed to women, but it is also a quality ascribed to the (male) social parvenu in nineteenth-century European society. This too plays a role in the gendering of aesthetic surgery and its reading in modern culture. It is linked to the culture of authenticity through the claim that those who desire aesthetic surgery are self-deluded and, therefore, inauthentic. In the 1950s the accusation was made that "the surgeons who perform such operations, it is urged, merely pander to vanity, which is an offshoot of the Deadly Sin of pride."[81] For as Lionel Trilling noted, we need authenticity most in a world devoid of powerful beliefs, especially in ourselves.[82] And the construction of this belief in the authentic may be fixed historically to the Enlightenment. For Trilling the present world is one in which a direct experience of another person's emotional affect is understood as possible. For him this marks a shift from the world of sincerity, the self-conscious public exposure of private feelings and this shift takes place following the Enlightenment. The claim for authenticity, which haunts aesthetic surgery, is linked to its opposite, hypocrisy. We imagine that someone is "authentic," and if the person is revealed in our eyes not to be so, we condemn that person as shaming authenticity, as being a hypocrite.

Hypocrisy, the kissing cousin of vanity in a gendered philosophical discourse, is as often represented as male as female. For the late nineteenth century, the name Uriah Heep evoked the hypocrite incarnate. Hypocrisy, as Friedrich Nietzsche (1844–1900) noted in his *Twilight of the Idols* (1889), written during the age of the construction of modern aesthetic surgery, "has its place in the ages of strong belief: in which even when one is compelled to exhibit a different belief, one does not abandon the belief one already has. Today one does abandon it; now, which is even more common, one acquires a second belief—one remains honest in any event. . . . That is the origin of self-tolerance."[83] Can one acquire a new nose as easily as a second belief? Can one abandon the old nose, with all of its associations? Or, as Nietzsche suggests, is one merely a hypocrite—a person with two noses, one worn in public, one hidden within the psyche? Such a hypocrite is not "naturally" gendered. It is certain that misogynist thinkers of the late nineteenth century, such as Otto Weininger (1880–1903), would figure such hypocrisy "female." But Molière (1622–73) would not have done so.

For all of the problems of the gendered representation of aesthetic surgery, the social reality is that substantially more women than men undertake aesthetic surgery at this moment in the twentieth century. According to the American Society of Plastic and Reconstructive Surgery, in 1996 substantially more women than men had aesthetic procedures performed by the society's members (see table).

Overall in 1996 the society's members performed 73,921 procedures (11 percent) on men and 622,982 (89 percent) on women.

Gender Breakdown of Patients Undergoing Aesthetic
Surgery Procedures (1996)

	Percentage of Patients by Gender	
Type of Procedure	Women	Men
Breast augmentation	100	0
Breast reduction in men	0	100
Buttock lift	96	4
Cheek implant	86	14
Eyelid surgery	85	15
Face-lift	91	9
Forehead lift	92	8
Hair transplant (male-pattern baldness)	0	100
Liposuction	89	11
Nose reshaping	76	24
Thigh lift	99	1
Tummy tuck	95	5

Source: Data from American Society of Plastic and Reconstructive Surgeons' National Clearinghouse of Plastic Surgery Statistics, "1996 Gender Distribution: Cosmetic Procedures" (www.plasticsurgery.org/mediactr/gendis96.htm).

Since aesthetic procedures (elective surgery) are understood as
the sign of vanity during the period we are examining, they seem
to be automatically associated with the feminine. Males who undertake aesthetic surgery are thus feminized or, as we shall see,
feminized males in European society undertake aesthetic procedures to "pass" as "real" men.

In modern Western culture the acquisition of beauty seems to
be gendered feminine whether women undertake it or not. But
do "real" men have aesthetic surgery? Other elective procedures,
not labeled aesthetic, may come to have the same end result, the
"improvement" of the somatic body in order to cure the unhappy
psyche. But they are not labeled "aesthetic surgery." As the Hungarian surgeon Alfred Berndorfer has observed: "if we accept the
patients' answers to our detailed questioning, aesthetic causes
alone rarely play a part. The patients often complain of some disease; for example, they say that they cannot respire through the
nose, but when they push up the tip of the nose the respiration is
free. This may be true, but after further interrogation it is revealed
that this surgery would result also in a total aesthetic correction.
No patient has ever come back after the operation with the complaint that the respiratory difficulties are still present. These patients feel 'sickness' because of their nose deformity, even when
there is no disease."[84] Is this not hypocrisy in the commonest
sense? The desire among such patients to "pass" as different is
coupled with the anxiety about being seen as desiring this feminizing end. A man's desire for the "relief" of somatic problems
such as a deviated septum is seen to mask his desire for an
aesthetic procedure. This desire is in complex ways marked as
"feminine."

"Before and After"

Patient narratives in medical texts provide accounts of happiness,
and "before and after" photographs of patients document the
image of well-being created by aesthetic surgery procedures.[85]
The use of "before and after" photographs, like accounts of "pass-

ing," is evidence of a new invisibility—of appearing to have fit fully into the new category. In the late 1840s, less than a decade after the invention of photography, the American reconstructive surgeon Gurdon Buck (1807–87) began taking "before and after" photographs of his patients. Published in 1876, his photographs of the shattered and then rebuilt faces of Civil War soldiers were the first images of reconstructive surgery to enjoy wide circulation.[86] Aesthetic surgeons quickly followed suit. By the late 1880s their representations of the reconstitution of noses and faces were subtly altered to emphasize the new happiness of the aesthetic surgeon's patients. Every refinement of photographic technique and equipment, from the use of better lighting to the addition of fancier hair styling and cosmetics, has since been seized on to prove that a new and improved aesthetic surgery has dramatically increased the "happiness" of the patient. Nineteen seventy-nine saw the publication of a "psychological" study that determined that subjects who viewed "before and after" photographs of aesthetic surgical patients found the after images to have better personalities, be better potential marriage partners, and be "happier."[87] That was, of course, the intent of the "before and after" photograph in persuading future and present patients of changes in their mental and social status.

Documenting the line between the "before" state and the state into which one has now "passed" is vital for the aesthetic surgeon. Frederick Strange Kolle observed in 1911 that "patients who beg us to make them more beautiful, or less unsightly in the eyes of the ever-critical observer, are the most difficult to please . . . that the nose or the eyes or the ears have not been changed as much as they desired—in fact, so little that their closest friends have failed to evoke ecstatic remarks about the improvements."[88] Real change as measured by the patient is the sole proof of the success of the operation. And the way to give the patient this proof is through the photograph. Kolle advocated "properly and fully recording the case in a thorough and systematic manner." He suggested photographs or stencils or, best of all, casts of the body part—taken before and after. In all cases, he stressed that one must "look to contrast, and in pathological cases have the dis-

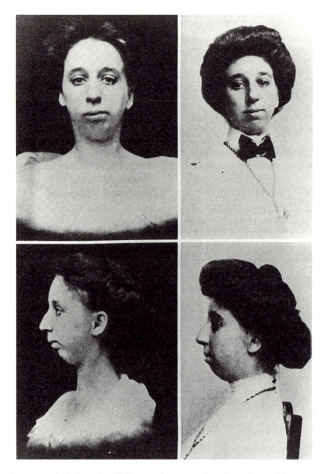

Vilray Papin Blair's rebuilding of an underdeveloped lower jaw, 1909. This is clearly an "aesthetic" as well as a "reconstructive" procedure. Blair comments on the "after" image (*below right*): "after the operation, the happier expression about the eyes is one of the results."

eased area printed so that it will stand out forcibly." He notes, by the way, that patients with hereditary defects and defects that were the result of age were loath to have such images taken "for fear their pictures will be used in some outlandish way." The act of "passing" is described here in detail: the procedure, the silent affirmation, the need for the physician to "show" the change from pathological to normal, and the fear of being revealed as "passing."

In one surgeon's practice, that of Max Thorek (1880–1960) in Chicago, the roles of photographer and surgeon come to complement one another. Thorek was a professional photographer and an innovative aesthetic surgeon.[89] His photography rested on strict principles of symmetry. Conservative in their form, his photographs provided a controlled and limited range of the "beautiful." This is especially true given the fact that his photographic work spanned the establishment of "modern" American art photography in the 1930s and '40s. For him the roles of surgeon and artist were one—evidence in the form of the photograph becomes evidence of the aesthetic improvement of the patient. One can evoke in this context Pierre Bourdieu's notion of photography as a "middle-brow" art.[90] His interest is in the middle class; and physicians as a caste are not usually thought of as bourgeoisie, even though they clearly are. Thorek's photography was artistic without being "arty." It was middle-class in its claims about the "beautiful" as the source of improvement, and thus it provided a clear continuation of his views concerning aesthetic surgery. The reliance of the physician caste on the norms and decorum of aesthetics is a measure of its need to be understood as middle-class. Photography in aesthetic surgery thus has a further purpose for the physician, an aesthetic one. It is greater than evidence of change; it is further evidence of the status of the "operator," the aesthetic surgeon as artist/sculptor.

The anxiety about evidence of this type was echoed in the 1977 guidelines for "ethics in aesthetic surgery" proposed by Salvador Castañares, who admonished his colleagues to use "only photographs representative of work performed by qualified plastic surgeons, preferably not those of the physician's own patients."[91] In her introduction to aesthetic surgery for potential patients, Elizabeth Morgan spends an entire chapter on the dangers of "before and after" photographs, illustrating how the illusion of change of character can be added to the photographs, so that "improvement" becomes a quality of the representation. It is no surprise that the "before and after" images reflect the prowess of the surgeon not only in altering the body but also in representing the altered state of mind of the patient. Morgan notes that a set of photographs of an "adorable girl" presents her first with a "close-up [which] distorts her face, and she has an anxious smile. The 'after' leaves the deceptive impression that surgery not only corrected her ears but made her prettier and more poised."[92] The boundary between the "unhappy" and the "happy" is documented as "fact" in the "before and after" photograph.

Morgan discussed only still photography. Aesthetic dentists are now encouraged to use "a live video camera" so that "patients could view themselves as others see them . . . "[93] (These should be juxtaposed with "photographs of 'ideal' smiles . . . to allow patients a basis of comparison.") Computer simulation has heightened the "before and after" problem because of the complex means of image manipulation it has made possible.[94] The ability to create proposed alternative images of the way the patient will appear using computer simulation is another means of heightening patient expectations. No image, static or moving, of the proposed altered appearance of a patient can be viewed except through the fantasy and expectations of the patient; no physician can do more than use the technology, no matter how sophisticated, to provide his/her aesthetic judgment with the window dressing of "fact."[95]

The story of the development of these techniques of documentation, as well as the institutionalization of images in medical specialties, comes to be part of the tale of "passing." Indeed the "before and after" photographs are "empirical proof" of the ability to "pass," to document that the patients have now entered into a new category of visibility. They are necessary because they elide the categories of the "beautiful" and the "happy" and offer a "scientific" representation of the constructed boundary that the patient has crossed.

Crossing boundaries raises one additional major question concerning the practice of photography in the history of aesthetic surgery. This concerns the representation of the unclothed body in medical photography.[96] This is a substantial problem because the function of photography within medicine and its nineteenth-century ancillary disciplines, such as physical anthropology, is clearly not without a voyeuristic quality. The "before and after" photographs of the breasts or buttocks are supposed to show the enhancement of the "erotic" and thus prove the increased happiness of the patient to both the patient and future patients.

There is a constant bleed between the world of the medical photograph and the general world of visual culture. Images did and do function in the worlds of high art and advertising as well as of aesthetic surgery. We shall discuss the use of these images as art at the conclusion of this book. The use of "before and after" photography in advertising has drawn the attention of the courts. The Minnesota Court of Appeals in 1990 found that implied contracts do exist between physicians and patients in regard to such photographs.[97] The use of "before and after" photographs without patient consent is a breach of the express warranty of silence arising from the physician-patient relationship. In this case, the physician had distributed copies of a promotional and educational publication containing unidentified "before and after" photographs of a patient's face without her consent. The brochure had also included similar unidentified photographs of other patients' breasts and abdomens in close proximity to the plaintiff's photographs. The meanings ascribed to these photographs were multiple. They were understood to be the patient's new erotic face and body; they were used to show the improved state of the body (and by extension, the happiness of the patient); and they were intended to serve as advertising.

In this study, the function of these images is to replicate and document the more general visual culture in which and from which such images function. Given the definition of aesthetic surgery as a means of altering the visible body in order to affect the psyche, it is vital to provide some set of analogous images from the general as well as from the medical culture.

At all of these moments, at every turn, there appears the question of why the patient sees his or her body as faulty. Also, how do physicians represent the body as abnormal? The Canadian aesthetic surgeon Benjamin Gelfant claims that his patients "merely wish to be normal . . . [they] simply want to 'fit in.' "[98] What is it that makes an individual so very unhappy with the appearance of aspects of his or her body, and how can this unhap-

piness be documented? How does the aesthetic surgeon undertake to lessen this unhappiness and document doing so? "Before
and after" photographs come to document the unhappy and the
happy state, the individual too visible to "pass" and the newly
(in)visible individual. The new face is there, and it is different
from the old; the new psyche must also be there, as different from
the old psyche as the new face is from the old face. Is the resulting face "real" or is it merely a "mask"? All of these questions
are intrinsic aspects of the field of aesthetic surgery and haunt its
history.

Thus "passing" remains central to all of the endeavors of the
surgeon as well as to the patient. To be seen or not seen as different, as criminal, as ugly, as sexually infectious is all part of the
promise of aesthetic surgery. You will look like everyone else, or
at least your fantasy of how everyone else looks. The ability to become (in)visible, seen but not seen, is the desire of the patient.
And the seeming proof of this lies in the "before and after" photograph, for it documents the journey from the world of the outsider to that of the insider, the successful "passing"—at least until
fashion changes, until the qualities ascribed to that in-group shift
and one is revealed as merely a surgical imitation of the original.

CHAPTER TWO

Victory over Disease

AMY AND THE PRINCESS

*Y*OUR NOSE shows the world the state of your soul. A too-short nose marks you as an unhappy soul. But does it represent the cause or the effect of your unhappiness? In Louisa May Alcott's (1832–88) novel *Little Women* (1868), which looks backward to the 1840s, the youngest daughter, Amy, is desolate—because of her nose.[1]

> If anybody had asked Amy what the greatest trial of her life was, she would have answered at once, "My nose." When she was a baby, Jo had accidentally dropped her into the coal-hod, and Amy insisted that the fall had ruined her nose forever. It was not big, nor red, like poor "Petrea's"; it was only rather flat, and all the pinching in the world could not give it an aristocratic point. No one minded it but herself, and it was doing its best to grow, but Amy felt deeply the want of a Grecian nose, and drew whole sheets of handsome ones to console herself. (pp. 62–63)

Amy experiences her inadequate nose as a character flaw. In this she follows the wisdom of her time. According to Samuel R. Wells's (1820–75) *New Physiognomy, or, Signs of Character: As Manifested through Temperament*, "a skillful dissembler may disguise, in a degree, the expression of the mouth; the hat may be slouched over the eyes; the chin may be hidden in an impenetrable thicket of beard; but the nose will stand out 'and make its sign' in spite of all proportions. It utterly refuses to be ignored, and we are, as it were, compelled to give it our attention."[2] Amy's sense of her nose as too flat internalizes the responses of people around her: "But Amy had not forgotten Miss Snow's cutting remarks about 'some persons whose noses were not too flat to smell other people's limes, and stuck-up people, who were not too proud to ask for them'" (p. 100). Her extreme unhappiness eventually prompts her to take corrective action: "Amy had capped the climax by putting a clothes-pin on her nose, to uplift the offending feature. It was one of the kind artists used to hold the paper on their drawing-boards, therefore quite appropriate and effective for the purpose to which it was now put. This funny spectacle appeared to amuse the sun, for he burst out with such radiance that Jo woke up, and roused all her sisters by a hearty laugh at Amy's ornament" (p. 178). It is through "art" that the body is to be altered, or at least through the artist's clothespin. This is a double pun. Not only does Alcott see the "aesthetics" of such an act as comic, but she also understands that the use of such materials is a sign of Amy's vain desire aesthetically to remake the body. Amy's vanity about her nose is a symptom of her overall vanity and, by the close of the novel, with the return of the children's absent father, Amy's vanity seems to have been tamed.[3] She no longer focuses on herself but strives to help others. Alcott uses Amy's nose to illuminate her psyche. The youngest child's vanity is what she has to "unlearn" by the close of the novel. In order to become an adult she must learn to accept her flat nose as a constitutional condition.

Such a flaw of character was to be corrected, not by the aesthetic clothespin, but by moral regeneration. Becoming "happy" in Amy's world could not be accomplished by turning to the physician, even though some American physicians of the time desired such a turn. John Peter Mettauer of Virginia penned the following sentiment in the late 1830s: "I am willing to hazard all that ignorance and presumption can possibly incur by any efforts which I might make in attempting to correct a natural deformity if the happiness and comfort of a fellow being could thereby be promoted even in an inconsiderable degree; and could I become a humble instrument of restoring to beauty its wonted comeliness, without which in many cases such as we are now considering, life would be a sense of endless sorrow, I should be more than compensated for exposing myself to the ridicule and sarcasm of short sighted if not invidious fatalism."[4] Mettauer did not build up too-short noses. His innovative work concentrated on cleft palate and hypospadias, a developmental error of the penis in which the opening of the penis is not at its end, and thus was reconstructive within the understanding of the nineteenth century. His struggle was against the American surgeons who lived by John Dryden's (1631–1700) admonition that "God did not make his Works for man to mend."[5] Defects of the body, like defects of character, were the work of God and should not be altered by a mere physician. Likewise, Alcott's narrative demands that Amy learn to live with her nose and presents this as a test of the maturity of her character.

Moral change was not yet to be the undertaking of the physician, even though it was becoming the role of the "insane asylum" director in the turn to moral management of the "insane" at the beginning of the nineteenth century. As in Alcott's world, the model for correcting and healing the soul was the family, and the (nonmedical) director of the reformed asylum took the role of the father. Lay people, not doctors, ruled the reformed asylum as moral models of rectitude and caring. The desire to shape the soul through the reshaping of the body remained a fantasy. Concerns with the body were expressed in terms of moral rather than physical transformation—following the dictates of the physiognomists who saw "permanent" (rather than acquired) physical signs as immutable exterior forms of the eternal nature of the human soul. Moral management, however, assumed or hoped that the soul was indeed changeable so that it could be reformed. This view of the potential of individual autonomy was at the core of the belief in the transformability of the unhappy soul.

Amy matures to young adulthood in the sequel to *Little Women*. She "is with truth considered 'the flower of the family,' for at sixteen she has the air and bearing of a full-grown woman, not beautiful, but possessed of that indescribable charm called grace. One saw it in the lines of her figure, the make and motion of her hands, the flow of her dress, the droop of her hair, unconscious yet harmonious, and as attractive to many as beauty itself. Amy's nose still afflicted her, for it never would grow Grecian, so did her mouth, being too wide, and having a decided chin. These offending features gave character to her whole face, but she never could see it, and consoled herself with her wonderfully fair complexion, keen blue eyes, and curls more golden and abundant than ever" (p. 23). Amy remains inherently unhappy with her "characterless" nose. She still does not understand that the features she hates give her physiognomy a unique quality. She focuses on the features that she perceives as "pretty" (eyes, hair, and complexion) rather on than those that are signs of a strong character. She never truly abandons her insecurity.

Amy's anxiety about her nose parallels the anxiety that Aylmer, "the man of science" in Nathaniel Hawthorne's (1804–64) short story "The Birth-Mark" (1846), feels about the blemish in the shape of a hand on the otherwise perfect face of his new wife.[6] The mark itself is so trivial an error in its "deeper shade of crimson" that it is hardly noticeable to the narrator. But it is noticeable enough to others that it becomes a source of erotic fascination to her suitors, and of horror to her eventual husband.[7] His obsessive focus on her one visible fault causes him to desire to remove it.

Aylmer first dreams that he will remove the birthmark surgically, "But the deeper went the knife, the deeper sank the Hand, until at length its tiny grasp appeared to have caught hold of Georgiana's heart." Surgery in Hawthorne's world, as in Alcott's, is so unthinkable that it can be imagined only as a dream (or nightmare). Aylmer then attempts a series of failed experiments to remove the blemish. Eventually he develops a potion to "cure" her "birth-mark." The potion is the "Elixir Vitae," the elixir of life, which can "cure" the "birth-mark of mortality," but such medicine cannot cure the spirit; it can only kill it. "As the last crimson tint of the birth-mark—that sole token of human imperfection—fade[s] from her cheek," she dies. The tools of medical science are as helpless to perfect the external nature of a human being, an external nature that mirrors the imperfect being within, as Amy's clothespin. Surgery is beyond realization, even for the obsessive lover and man of science.

In the figure of Amy we have a model for a nineteenth-century presupposition about aesthetic surgery. Her nose functions as a nose, but it is unaesthetic and is therefore read as a sign of "bad" character. According to the physiognomist Samuel R. Wells, such signs are fixed and naturally reflect the inner character. Alcott wants her characters to be capable of change. Yet she makes Amy incapable of transcending her physical difference. Not birth, but life is the cause of this difference. For this reason, she attributes the shape of Amy's nose to an accident. According to the narrator, Amy was dropped on her nose as an infant. But, like accidents of birth, accidents of life have consequences with which one must come to terms. No artificial interventions, not even the aesthetic clothespin, can change them. The clothespin is a parody of the notion of self-help which, in the form of self-reliance, was the central tenet of Louisa May Alcott's own education by her father, Bronson Alcott. Amy does not turn to another institution outside of the family, such as medicine, to repair her nose and her self-esteem; she tries to fix them herself. But, given the social laws of this fictive world, self-reliance cannot redeem persistent vanity. Amy's vanity is a character flaw, which magnifies the shape of her nose and makes it the center of her unhappiness. It is not the fixed quality of the face that determines character, but character that reads the body!

Not surprisingly, among those at the beginning of the nineteenth century who did not believe in a code of self-reliance or autonomy, the evident place to seek a "cure" was in the world of medicine, which was already associated with the "healing" of such damaged visages. Nikolai Gogol (1809–52), in his black fantasy of 1836 concerning the loss of a nose, has another character advise his Major Kovalyov, who awoke one morning without his nose: "you'd better see a doctor about it. I've heard there's a certain kind of specialist who can fix you up with any kind of nose you like."[8] Amy did not seek out a physician, even though physicians such as Mettauer were available in her America. Indeed, in the terms of the novel, it is evident that Louisa May Alcott (like Gogol) saw a preoccupation with the nose that would lead to visiting a physician as a type of vanity. In her world of fiction, vanity is equivalent to a moral defect. What Amy is supposed to learn by the end of the novel is that her self-centeredness is a fault to be overcome by her concentration on the needs of others in the family; and yet it is clear that even in Alcott's sequel, she does not really learn this lesson. Her nose remains her greatest weakness but it is a sign of the weakness of character. Her weakness parallels her sister Jo's extraordinary self-reliance and strength of character to create something of a balance in the closed world of this nineteenth-century family.

Louisa May Alcott's tale of Amy's nose stems from the world of moral fiction written for young women as models of self-reliance and autonomy. Alcott's novels set in the 1840s present Amy's problems with her nose as a comic interlude, but one with profound implications. For a moment, let us turn to another tale of a nose, from the 1820s, not too long before the real life experiences of the Alcott family that were transmuted into *Little Women.* Writing in a Heidelberg medical journal, Dr. von Klein tells us the rare story of one of his patients who requested his help in acquiring a "more beautiful" nose.[9] She was a young princess less than twenty years old who had what is technically called a "saddle nose," a nose that sagged at the bridge. This is the parallel to Amy's nose, which did not have a Grecian form. The princess suggested to her physician that a bridge of gold be inserted to build up and straighten the nose. The bridge had to be inserted through the skin and could leave scars. So she also proposed that the procedure first be tried on some poor individual to see whether infection and "ugly" scarring would result. Dr. von Klein proceeded to the local pauper's hospital, found an individual to volunteer—based on the payment of a thaler and the promise that he could keep the gold bridge once it was removed. To the doctor's surprise the operation was a success—no infection and a very small scar. But his original patient, the princess, vacillated when confronted with the possibility of such a procedure without any general or even local anesthesia. At one point, she actually got up and ran away with the chair to which she had been strapped for the procedure.

Unlike Amy's clothespin, Dr. Klein's insertion of a gold bridge would have scarred the nose. Scars tell the world the patient's secret. They are the shadow presence of what the patient wished to hide. In the tales of both Amy and the princess, a young woman who sees herself as ugly devises her own treatment. But whereas Amy treated herself, the princess turned to an expert from the world of medicine. Although his patroness did not in the end permit herself to be operated upon, von Klein reveals why she felt herself to be ugly and wanted surgical treatment—such an operation, he noted, should be thought of for those who had lost their noses through the pernicious actions of scrofula, lupus, or syphilis. The moral fault, however, is not that of the princess, but rather a sign of the collapse of the morality of the aristocracy. Born with a sunken nose, she was the "victim" of her infected parents, whose legacy to her was hereditary syphilis.

THE SYPHILITIC NOSE

The syphilitic nose marked the body as corrupt and dangerous. And this sign of "bad character" was literally written on the face. The collapse of the cartilage and the infection of the bone of the nose made the missing nose one of the most prominent and feared signs of the new disease of syphilis in the sixteenth century. As early as 1502 Juan Almenar (fl. 1500) wrote of the "passio turpis saturnina" (ugly, dark face and feelings) of the syphilitic.[10] The modern history of syphilis was not yet a decade old at that point. From the very beginning of the epidemic, the face of the syphilitic was understood as marked. William Shakespeare (1564–1616) put this curse in the mouth of Timon of Athens:

> Consumptions sow
> In hollow bones of man; strike their sharp shins,
> And mar men's spurring. Crack the lawyer's voice,
> That he may never more false title plead,
> Nor sound his quillets shrilly: hoar the flamen,
> That scolds against the quality of flesh,
> And not believes himself: down with the nose,
> Down with it flat; take the bridge quite away

Of him that, his particular to foresee,
Smells from the general weal.

(Timon of Athens, IV:iii)

The sunken nose and feminized voice became in the public's consciousness the ultimate signs of the syphilitic. In the medical literature of the late nineteenth century, the British syphilologist Jonathan Hutchinson (1828–1913) first described the "hutchinsonian facies" of the person with congenital syphilis.[11] This included the depressed nasal bridge. Although Hutchinson was the first modern physician to document the "stigmata" of syphilis, the signs of syphilis, in both its initial virulent and congenital forms, had long been recognized in popular consciousness. The missing nose came in the nineteenth century to be seen as a sign of the transmission of syphilis to the newborn. You can see the sign of corruption in their very faces and hear it in the syphilitic's very voice, unto the seventh generation.

The cultural representation of the too-small nose as a sign of the syphilitic and, therefore, the immoral, is seemingly ubiquitous. In Gaston Leroux's (1868–1927) novel *The Phantom of the Opera* (1911), the Phantom's masked face had "eyes . . . so deep that you can hardly see the fixed pupils. You just see two big black holes, as in a dead man's skull. His skin, which is stretched across his bones like a drumhead, is not white, but a nasty yellow. His nose is so little worth talking about that you can't see it side-face; and the absence of that nose is a horrible thing to look at."[12] This nose is so tiny that it seems to be missing. The Phantom's nose seems to be the locus of the horror felt by the viewers as well as by the ghost himself. He often sports a "long, thin, and transparent" nose, which is evidently "a false nose" (p. 30). "When he went out in the streets or ventured to show himself in public, he wore a pasteboard nose, with a mustache attached to it, instead of his own horrible hole of a nose. This did not quite take away his corpse-like air, but it made him almost, I say almost, endurable to look at" (p. 207). His missing nose led him to hate those with "real noses," and gave his face the aura of a death's head (p. 227). Indeed, the ghost "smelt of death" (p. 126). He felt himself as "built up of death from head to foot" with "his terrible dead flesh" (p. 129). We see his face very early on in the novel, and its physiognomy reveals what is at the center of Erik's horror—branded on his physiognomy are the scars of congenital syphilis. Rupert Julien's (1889–1943) American film (1925), starring Lon Chaney (1883–1930) as the Phantom, evokes Leroux's etiology in the "pity and horror" felt by the audience in seeing the Phantom's visage. Chaney adapted the standard physiognomy of hereditary syphilis for his makeup. Lon Chaney's careful makeup representing Erik's missing nose is a sign of the diseased soul. In the novel, it is a sign of congenital syphilis, for Erik is born looking the way he does.

Syphilis marked the face of the naive and the innocent as well as the lecher and hypocrite. Voltaire's (1694–1778) Candide finds his teacher, the incurably optimistic philosopher Dr. Pangloss, "all covered with scabs, his eyes sunk in his head, the end of his nose eaten off, his mouth drawn on one side, his teeth as black as a cloak, snuffling and coughing most violently, and every time he attempted to spit out dropped a tooth." His is the last face in a long litany of diseased physiognomies in the literature of the Enlightenment. The cause of his dilemma was "Pacquette, that pretty wench, who waited on our noble Baroness."[13] Whatever the cause, the too-tiny or missing nose of the syphilitic marks the evil and weakness of the flesh. It is a public sign of moral failing.

At the middle of the nineteenth century, as Louisa May Alcott wrote her novels, the meaning associated with the disfigured and sunken nose was specifically that of the syphilitic. The Berlin surgeon Johann Friedrich Dieffenbach (1792–1847), the central figure in nineteenth-century facial surgery, wrote in 1834 that "a man without a nose [arouses] horror and loathing, and people are apt to regard the deformity as a just punishment for his sins. This division of diseases, or even more their consequences, into blameworthy and blameless is strange. . . . As if all people with noses were always guiltless! No one ever asks whether the nose was lost because a beam fell on it, or whether it was destroyed by scrofula or syphilis."[14]

The surgeon's moral imperative was to correct and hide the

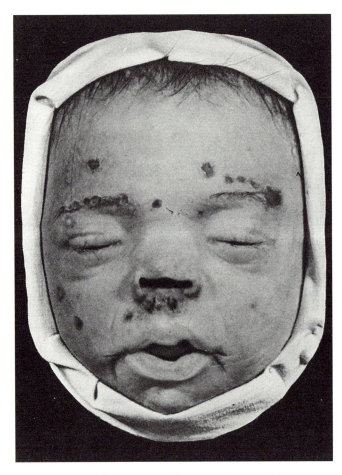

The noseless infant born with congenital syphilis.

fault, no matter what its cause, so as to allow the individual to "pass" as whole and healthy. By the end of the nineteenth century it was evident that surgeons were inclined to see all sunken noses as a single aesthetic error, "whether this has occurred from trauma or from the ravages of syphilitic disease."[15] Here the problem of the sunken nose such as Amy's remains trapped between moral condemnation and an accident in which no one really believes.

Theodor Billroth (1829–94), the famed nineteenth-century Viennese surgeon, often carried out "plastic operations with artis-

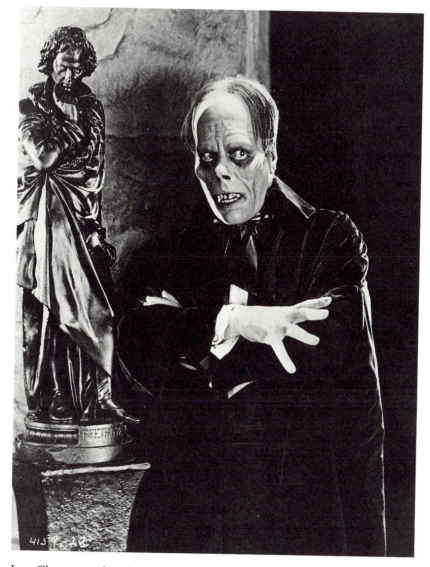

Lon Chaney as the Phantom in *The Phantom of the Opera*, 1925.

tic ability to correct defects of beauty [*Schönheitsgebrechen*]. . . . [O]ne could see his joy when he was able to successfully improve the appearance [*verschönern*] of a damaged person, so that that person was no longer the object of pity or horror."[16] Whatever the cause of their disfigurement, Billroth's Viennese patients struck their observers with the same pity and horror, the classical hall-marks of ancient tragedy, as did the victims of syphilis. One of his most distinguished students, Vincenz Czerny (1842–1916), pioneered the modern reconstruction of the saddle nose. Recounting a case in 1895, he stressed that the patient came from "a healthy family (without a history of rickets or lues) and had suffered a depression of the osseous nasal skeleton through a fall on his nose, when he was three years old."[17] Alcott too, opts to describe the origins of Amy's flattened nose as accidental, but as Dieffenbach stated, all of the claims that the too-small nose resulted from an accident will fall on deaf ears: we all know what such noses say about you and your parentage, whispers the gossip!

There has always been a moral dimension lurking in questions about the nose. One text certainly read by the characters in *Little Women* was the Bible, and there are numerous biblical prohibitions about the imperfect or diseased body. In *Leviticus* 21:18 men with "charum" are forbidden from becoming priests in the Temple. This term appears only in the passage in *Leviticus*. Exactly what constitutes "charum" is not clear, but Rashi defines it as "flat-nosed" in *Bechoroth* 7:3. In the rabbinical *Bechoroth* 7:4, there is another reference to disproportionate noses. The note to this in the *Mishna* states that the "nose is so flattened that the nostrils are exposed" and that the "nose between the eyes is so flat that it does not prevent the color running from one eye to the other." In other words, these are signs of physical anomalies, which are both unaesthetic and unhealthy. Later commentators observe that this injunction was aimed against those with leprosy who were seen as ritually unclean.[18] The unclean here is also the ugly.

Such a biblical view of the short nose is paralleled in Xenophon's *Banquet* when Critobolus notes that it is always the "handsomest old men" who undertake rituals at the Feast of Minerva. Religious purity and beauty are clearly linked. The ugliest old man at Xenophon's table is Socrates, who argues that his "short flat nose is more beautiful than another." He observes that a short flat nose has its nostrils turned up "to receive smells that come from every part, whether from above or below" and that "it never hinders the sight of both eyes at once; whereas a high nose parts the eyes so much by its rising, that it hinders their seeing both of them in a direct line."[19] It is a good thing to have an ugly nose!

Socrates' nose becomes proverbial for its ugliness. Michel de Montaigne (1533–92) wrote, for example, that "it grieves me that Socrates, who was a perfect pattern of all great qualities, should, as reports say, have had so ugly a face and body, so out of keeping with the beauty of his soul, seeing how deeply he was enamored of beauty, how infatuated by it! Nature did him an injustice."[20] In *The Symposium*, Plato, or at least Alcibiades, likens Socrates to an ugly Silenus. Images of the licentious, sexualized Silenus and Socrates merge by the eighteenth century into the physiognomy of one corrupt and corrupting figure, despite his melancholic genius.[21] The Enlightenment explained Socrates' ugliness by reference to Cicero's tale of Socrates' encounters with the physiognomist Zopyrus. Socrates' face struck Zopyrus as that of someone who was inwardly dull, brutish, sensual, and addicted to the vice of drunkenness. Socrates agreed with this assessment, Cicero noted, but stated that he was able to raise himself above it through the persistent pursuit of learning.[22] Ugliness and its internal parallel, bad character, can be checked by the autonomous individual's determined effort to change himself. By the early twentieth century one commentator saw Socrates' tooshort nose as a clinical sign of syphilis.[23] (This seems odd, since Socrates had his nose long before the illness was introduced into Europe in the fifteenth century—but this diagnosis was made by a scholar arguing against Columbus having "discovered" syphilis in the Americas and having carried it back to Europe.) The unclean nose embodies all of the horrors associated with the illness and the "bad" character of those who have it. The promise of change may be possible even for the syphilitic, but only through the active desire to transform oneself.

Johann Friedrich Dieffenbach had pioneered the sort of procedure that Klein undertook on the pauper. In the early nineteenth century Dieffenbach made the repair and replacement of missing body parts, such as the nose, a major part of his focus in reconstructive surgery. He developed a method of using external exci-

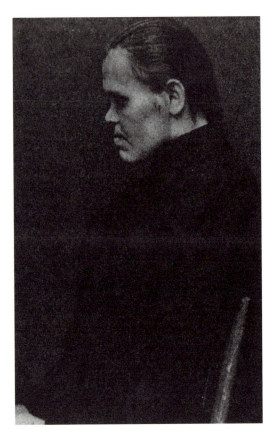

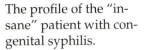

The profile of the "insane" patient with congenital syphilis.

sions to raise a flattened or depressed nasal tip as well as to reduce an overly large nose.[24] Dieffenbach proposed the total rebuilding of the nose both to restore function and to create a more human visage. He did not envision removing all traces of disease and treatment; visible scars would remain to alert healthy people against unwitting contact with carriers of venereal disease. But the syphilitic's extreme isolation and suffering would be lessened (1:334–35).

Dieffenbach also suggested the use of a gold bridge for a sunken nose (1:373). The case that Dieffenbach recounts, the only one in which he attempted to rebuild the bridge of the nose through the use of a gold insert, is that of a man who had lost the bridge of his nose through syphilis and the contemporary cures for syphilis, such as mercury. As with Dr. von Klein's operation on his pauper patient, Dieffenbach's attempt seemed to be successful. Even following the incision made on the exterior of the nose, "the appearance of the person was surprisingly natural." However, soon the bridge began to shift to one side and then to the other and eventually vanished into the nasal sinus. It had to be removed and a skin graft used to close the incision in the nose (1:374).

Dieffenbach explored the use of a nasal bridge to restructure the saddle nose between 1829 and 1832. This paralleled a long tradition of the use of materials such as rubber, celluloid, iron, copper, platinum, ivory, and gold as substitutes for the collapsed bridge of the nose.[25] Fifty years later, in 1892, the American aesthetic surgeon Robert F. Weir (1838–94) brought a live duck into the operating theater, killed and butchered it, and then used the duck's sternum (breastbone) to replace the nasal bridge of a "young man, about twenty-six years of age, with a history of syphilis and a sunken nose."[26] In 1896 James Israel, the leading surgeon at the Jewish Hospital in Berlin, performed the first bone grafts to repair the sunken, syphilitic nose.[27] Such procedures made the bearer of the "new nose" a member of the world of the "healthy-nosed" and employable. Returning individuals to the category of the employable meant that they were now visible members of the working class.

George H. Monks (1853–1933) operated in Boston in 1898 on "a young girl of sixteen, who as a result of inherited disease had a saddle-back nose of such an extreme degree that the bridge of the nose was sunken to nearly the level of the cheeks and was covered with a dense scar. The end of the nose was tipped up and the nostrils looked forward. On account of her deformity she could get no employment."[28] Monks commented that such procedures could make patients truly happy: "I have become convinced . . . that few patients suffer more of mental discomfort than the unfortunate possessors of some unsightly disfigurement on the face which attracts constant notice, few are more solicitous for any operation which promises relief, and none are more grateful for the slightest improvement in their condition." One presumes that the young patient on whom he operated was received by the world of work, which accepted her without excessive comment about her nose (and her parentage).

Yet the problem of style and visibility haunts the reconstruction of the syphilitic nose. What counted as aesthetic success in the 1890s turned out to be a sign of syphilitic repair a generation later. Harold Delf Gillies (1882–1960), one of the most important facial surgeons of the early twentieth century, noted in the 1920s that rebuilding the bridge of the syphilitic nose "would merely give the kind of result that had previously been given to the nose, and fail to remove the stigma of syphilis from the face."[29] He became aware that it was not only the loss of bone and cartilage that gave the nose its recognizable shape, but also the loss of substantial amounts of the mucous lining of the nose. He grafted a new epithelial lining into the new nose by freeing the entire nose from the face and adding the new lining of the nose to the inside of the stripped face. Thus the nose "lost its syphilitic character and resembled an ordinary depressed fracture of the nose, such as results from a septal abscess." Gillies created a nose that looked pathological but not syphilitic, and so enabled his patients to "pass."

At the same time, Charles H. Willi (c. 1882–1972), the London-based "beauty" surgeon, saw the sunken (read: syphilitic) nose also as a marker of class: "A patient may have had a broken-back plebeian nose which throughout his life has deprived him of self-confidence, giving him, quite naturally, an inferiority complex." An ivory implant gave him a "normal nose" and changed his life "for the better."[30] The use of endonasal ivory implants continued well into the twentieth century in Europe and, as we shall see, in Japan.[31]

The experiments to rebuild the syphilitic nose during the first half of the nineteenth century had their own risks. The overt rationale may have been to restore function, but one powerful impetus was to make patients happy. Dieffenbach rarely discusses the psychology of his reconstruction of the face and body in any detail. He writes of meeting an eighteen-year-old Polish woman whose face was the most horrible he had ever seen: "I trembled, for a death's head, of the sort I have never seen on a living body, stood before me." Her face had been eaten away by "scrofula" (tuberculosis). He undertook to restore her nose using a flap graft from her upper arm, and after a successful transplant, spent six months undertaking smaller corrective procedures to shape the nose. "The success of the operation gave this unhappiest of people her life again, so that she could boldly go among people, visited the theater with flowers in her hair and was able to leave Berlin with a happy heart" (1:386–89). The happy heart of his patient was paralleled by Dieffenbach's immense popularity in Berlin. The populace sang the following ditty:

> Who doesn't know Doctor Dieffenbach
> The Doctor of all the Doctors
> He takes from your arm and leg
> And makes you new noses and ears.[32]

Dieffenbach's popularity was tied not only to his abilities as a surgeon, which were evidently great, but to the specific types of procedures that he was seen to undertake.

Dieffenbach's Polish patient got off relatively well, given that patients regularly died from infection following such procedures. In a case reported by Jacques Lisfranc (1790–1847) in 1828, when a forehead skin flap graft was used in an attempt to reconstruct a destroyed syphilitic nose, the patient died of sepsis on the thirteenth day.[33] All of these operations, from Dr. von Klein's on the pauper to Lisfranc's on the patient who died, took place before the age of antisepsis and anesthesia. They were done in the most appalling conditions, done quickly, and done at great risk to body and spirit. It is a sign of the power of the stigma associated with the missing nose that patients were willing to risk such procedures for an almost human nose.

As in the case of Amy, the appearance of the nose leads to an internalized sense of unhappiness. The unhappiness here is not only linked to the diminished function of the nose but also to the social stigma associated with the collapsed nose—the reading of the saddle nose as a sign of licentiousness and disease, a sign of the sexualization of the patient as a sufferer from syphilis. Even in terms of nineteenth-century diagnostic categories, the saddle nose could "mean" a range of diagnoses from scrofula, lupus, leprosy, and yaws to syphilis. Yet it is clear that when the nineteenth-century physician and patient saw the collapsed or saddle nose, they saw before them the sufferer from syphilis. The need to rationalize the damaged nose as resulting from a childhood accident removes it, in Alcott's world, from the charge of syphilitic infection, not of the child but of her parents. In the diagnostic atlases of the day, such as that of Byrom Bramwell (1847–1931), the pug nose and the saddle nose represented heredity syphilis.[34] A literary trope linked this inheritance with unhappiness, illness, and, ugliness in complicated ways. At every stage it was also linked to the relationship of the missing or too-small nose to the world of cure represented by the physician.

THE STRANGE CASE OF TRISTRAM SHANDY

There is a history of aesthetic surgery before the nineteenth century. Its shadow lurks in the strange case of Tristram Shandy's missing nose. The story of Shandy's nose asks what the missing nose means, and what its absence implies about the individual. Can reconstituting the body with an intact nose restore the psyche? What makes the individual truly happy? Is it the invisibility of the body, looking like everyone else, or the masking of the body's difference from everyone else? Should the body be repaired and therefore reconstituted, even if the repair itself is noticeable and continues to mark the individual as different, or should one mask the deformity and create at least the illusion of social acceptability? What makes the person without a nose least unhappy?

The missing nose became a sign of uncleanness and immorality—of the syphilitic infection, which had appeared in Europe during the siege of Naples at the very close of the fifteenth century. When we turn to the world of medicine in the eighteenth century and before, its anxiety about sexuality, the erotic, and visibility is clear, although the diagnostic categories for sexually transmitted diseases were a bit less defined than later, so that scrofula and syphilis were not always understood as completely separate illnesses. All such illnesses were linked in being written on the skin, following the medieval understanding of leprosy as a sexually transmitted disease. They are always understood as deforming as well as making one's stigma visible.

Laurence Sterne's (1713–68) novel *Tristram Shandy* (1760–67) plays out an elaborate fantasy about the medicalization of the nose a hundred years before *Little Women.* It also leads readers (by their noses) to imagine the nose in what may seem quite a different context.[35] Sterne's claim is that the too-small nose of the eponymous hero was due to the fact that at birth the forceps used to deliver him crushed Tristram's nose. (This is analogous to Alcott's account of Amy's disfigurement.) It is the act of birth—not the act of conception—that forms the baby's nose. Chapter 27 of volume 3 of the novel reads in its entirety as follows:

> —This unfortunate draw-bridge of yours, quoth my father—God bless your honour, cried Trim, 'tis a bridge for master's nose.—In bringing him into the world with his vile instruments, he has crush'd his nose, Susannah says, as flat as a pancake to his face, and he is making a false bridge with a piece of cotton and a thin piece of whale-bone out of Susannah's stays, to raise it up. (p. 170)

Here the cause and the remedy of the too-short nose are linked— the forceps and the whale-bone bridge. Long noses are the mark of greatness for the world of Sterne's fancy. Tristram's nose is, however, one of a long series of short noses in the Shandy family: "he did not conceive how the greatest family in England could stand it out against an uninterrupted succession of six or seven short noses." The cause of the short nose of the youngest Shandy is either trauma (the forceps) or inheritance (syphilis). In either case, it is or will be a sign of character. Sterne raises this question when he comments, quoting imaginary medical authorities such as Prignitz, that "the excellency of the nose is in a direct arithmetical proportion to the excellency of the wearer's fancy." The counterargument of the fictional Andrea Scroderus, however, is that "on the contrary—the nose begat the fancy." Here the groundwork is being laid for aesthetic surgery. If all visible flaws are inherently moral, the physician seems to have a moral duty to fix them. Does the character determine the nose, or can the altered shape of the nose form the character? Sterne quotes one final authority, a dead physician named Ambroise Paré, to the effect that it is the "softness and flaccidity in the nurse's breast—as the flatness and shortness of puisne noses was to the firmness and elastic repulsion of the same organ of nutrition in the hale and lively" (p. 186). There is some type of universal nose, which is shaped by the nursing process and takes on qualities analogous to those of the breast. Here the question is raised as to the meaning of the nose and its relationship to the psyche and the happiness of the character. Is it an environmentally shaped nose, according to Sterne, or is it a pathological inheritance?

With his citation of Paré, Sterne turns to the real world of medical authority. The sixteenth-century French surgeon Ambroise Paré (c. 1510–90) wrote extensively on the reconstruction of the body, but not specifically on the rebuilding of the nose. According to Sterne, Paré was "chief surgeon and nose-mender to Francis the ninth of France, and in high credit with him and the two preceding, or succeeding kings (I know not which)—and that except in the slip he made in his story of Taliacotius' noses, and his manner of setting them on,—was esteemed by the whole college of physicians at that time, as more knowing in matters of noses, than any one who had ever taken them in hand" (p. 186). Paré suggested a prosthesis to mask the missing nose, of the type that many surgeons before and since have used. Indeed, he also suggested prostheses of the penis for sufferers whose syphilis had damaged that part.

Paré knew that remedies such as a prosthesis could only moderately well disguise the flaws of body and character. He tells of

a gentleman named the Cadet of Saint Thoan who, having lost his nose and having long worn one of silver, became angry at the remark that there was never a lack of laughing matter when he was present. And having heard that there was in Italy a master remaker of lost noses, he went to find him, and he made a new nose for him

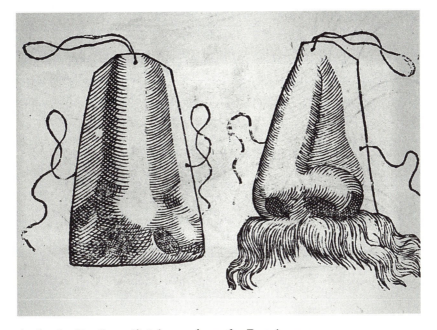

Ambroise Paré's artificial nose from the Renaissance.

..., as an infinite number of people have since seen him, not without the great marveling of those who had known him before with
a silver nose. Such a thing is not impossible; nevertheless it seems
to me very difficult and burdensome to the patient. . . . [I]n addition, this flesh is not the same quality nor similar to that of the nose,
and even when agglutinated and re-formed it can never be of the
same shape and color as that which was formerly in the place of
the lost nose: likewise the openings of the nostrils can never be as
they were originally.[36]

This is the next link in our tale of the too-small nose, the re-
creation of a new nose that is not quite a nose.

Shandy's nose is read within a world that already knows stories about how, once upon a time, surgeons were able to provide
new noses. When Sterne refers to "Taliacotius," he means Gaspare Tagliacozzi (1545–99), professor of surgery at the University
of Bologna. In the issue of Joseph Addison (1672–1719) and
Richard Steele's (1672–1729) *Tatler*, published on December 7,

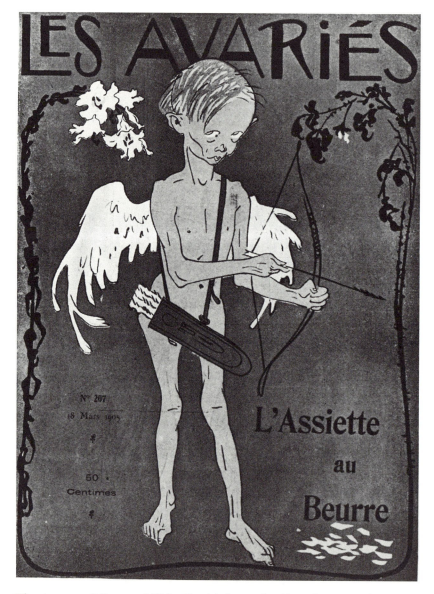

The image of the syphilitic Cupid from the French satirical journal
L'Assiette au Beurre, 1905.

1710, Addison evoked a myth about Tagliacozzi's by then lost work through a quotation from Samuel Butler's (1612–80) *Hudibras* (1663) also evoked later by Sterne.[37] Tagliacozzi, according to this legend, used not the patient's own skin for his grafts, but the skin off "the brawny Part of [the] Porter's bum," off the buttocks of the working poor. When they died, "off drop'd the Sympathetick Snout." A tale is then spun about the origin of syphilis, which led to these gentlemen needing their new noses—Cupid is born after the siege of Naples under the malevolent signs which (according to contemporary explanations) heralded the coming of the new epidemic. (Imported from the Americas, it was the Native Americans' return gift for Columbus's present of smallpox.) This Cupid "with a sickly look and crazy constitution" shot his poison-tipped arrows into the lovers' noses rather than into their hearts as was his brother's wont. He "dipped all his Arrows in Poison, that rottened every Thing they touched; and what was more particular, aimed all of his Shafts at the Nose." These gentlemen went to the porter for their substitute noses because of the activities of Cupid. This Cupid was sent to the "School of Mercury, who did all he could to hinder him from demolishing the Noses of Mankind." But this did not work, and he continued to "wound his Votaries oftner in the Nose than in the Heart." Syphilis is not controlled, in this tale, by mercury therapy, that is, by existing medicine; rather, Tagliacozzi evolved a means by which he "grafted a new [nose] on the remaining Part of the Grisle." The doctor, according to this account, was soon overrun by those seeking to remedy the affliction visited upon them by Cupid.

Note that Addison's comic tale ends with an "Admonition to the young Men of this Town." For today, he writes, there is no Tagliacozzi "to be met with at the Corner of every Street." The tale goes on to warn young male readers that Tagliacozzi's art has now been lost and that they should beware. "The general Precept therefore I shall leave with them is, to regard every Town-Woman as a particular Kind of Siren, that has a Design upon their Noses, and that, amidst her Flatteries and Allurements, they will fancy she speaks to 'em in that humorous Phrase of old Plautus: 'Keep

your Face out of my Way, or I'll bite off your Nose.'" It is from
this "distemper" that "mutilated and disfigured his species" that
Addison sees Tagliacozzi's art emerging. For "the nose is a very
becoming part of the face, and a man makes but a very silly figure without it." Such a man (and it is the man seduced by the
sirens of the town who is the *Tatler's* ideal reader) would be publicly marked by the loss of the nose. Here the erotic activities of
the "beautiful" but unclean "Town-Woman" can lead to the destruction of male beauty. The result is a face and a body marked
by syphilis.

The social stigma of the missing nose as a mark of difference
can be measured by the ironic inclusion of a "No Noses Club"
(and a "Big Noses Club") in Edward Ward's satiric list of *Compleat
and Humorous Account of Clubs* (1709). The club was open to members of both sexes who had sacrificed their noses to the God Pri-
apus:

> Why then should not one mighty nose
> With patience bear the scoffs of those
> Who hate to see a nose appear,
> Because themselves have none to wear,
> Since he is always made the jest,
> That is the most unlike the rest.[38]

No one without a nose could "pass" as whole and healthy. Such
clubs are clearly satirical because their ranks would have included only those whose very faces marked them as excludable.

RENAISSANCE NOSES

Gaspare Tagliacozzi (1545–99) introduced into early modern European surgery the flap graft procedures used to replace the nose
missing because of trauma or syphilis. Tagliacozzi is the other
"father" of plastic and aesthetic surgery in the historical literature.[39] According to this literature, this patrimony was lost in Europe at the time of Sterne—available only in part of the world of
the fictional text a century after his death. His surgical techniques

vanished, but his name and reputation survived as part of a mythic world in which doctors could actually build new noses.

What Sterne evokes in *Tristram Shandy* is not the repair of the flattened nose but its analogue, the replacement of the missing nose. Through notions of uncleanness and corruption he links the reconstructive tradition of flap surgery, which replaced missing noses, and the alteration of the sunken or flattened nose primarily for aesthetic reasons. In the sixteenth century Tagliacozzi introduced, or at least documented for the first time, the use of pedicle (attached) flap grafts for the reconstruction of the missing nose. Such flaps evidently had been used in the West in the early modern period. The Branca family in fifteenth-century Sicily employed such a technique. The father, Branca de' Branca, used a flap of skin taken from the cheek (*ex ore*) to rebuild the nose; his son, Antonie Branca, used a flap from the upper arm, which left less of a visible scar on the face. The son's procedure demanded that the flap, still attached to the arm, be joined to the now abraded stump of the nose for as long as twenty days. Unlike the much less cumbersome and much less complicated operation that took the flap graft from the cheek, it created no further scars on the face.[40]

Such surgery was a proprietary "trade secret," and was usually passed on from father to son. Heinrich von Pfalzpaint, a knight of the Teutonic Order, described the use of the connected arm flap to provide a graft with which to repair the nose as early as 1460.[41] According to his account he learned it from a "foreigner." and it enabled him to "earn very much money" (p. 487). It is, however, only with the work of Tagliacozzi that the relationship between the missing or flattened nose and the unhappiness of the patient is first articulated.

To trace this trope let us begin 137 years after the wealthy nose rebuilder Pfalzpaint, with Tagliacozzi, whose classic work on plastic surgery appeared in 1597.[42] Tagliacozzi's most important innovation was the development of a means of replacing the missing nose, for a person without a nose is bound to be "unhappy" and this unhappiness could well make him or her ill. It also marked that person as not only diseased but also infectious,

whether or not actual "infection," as we know it, was present. The
stigma was real enough. The noseless were polluted and polluting.

Here the problem of the relationship of reconstructive surgery
to aesthetic surgery appears at the very "origin" of aesthetic
surgery. It seems self-evident, that anyone without a nose will be
unhappy, and that the reconstruction of the nose will make that
person happier and therefore healthier. Tagliacozzi recognized
this. In chapter eleven of his book *De curtorum chirugia* (1597), he
discusses the means of replacing the missing nose by the use of a
pedicle flap graft.[43] Like the younger Branca, he chose to use the
skin from the arm. He made two parallel incisions over the bi-
ceps, loosened the skin between these two cuts, and placed linen
dressing under the skin. This he left untouched for four days and
then dressed the wound daily so as to encourage scar formation
under the loosened skin. On the fourteenth day he cut the flap at
one end. Two weeks later he abraded the stump of the nose and
grafted the attached flap onto the nose, holding the arm in place
with a strong halter. Twenty days later he cut the flap free from
the arm, and two weeks after this began to shape a nose and at-
tach this nose to the upper lip. Six procedures (at least) and more
than a month later, a rudimentary nose was present. The risks of
infection were great and the pain and discomfort excruciating.

In his written account Tagliacozzi stressed that such procedures are the duty of the surgeon and their primary purpose is
not cosmetic. Tagliacozzi's surgery aimed to re-create the original
or idealized form of the body. The surgeon's task is to "restore, repair, and make whole those parts of the face which nature has
given but which fortune has taken away, not so much that they
might delight the eye but that they may buoy up the spirits and
help the mind of the afflicted. . . . We do this . . . as becomes good
physicians and disciples of the great Hippocrates" (p. cvl). How
this task of recuperating the psyche is actually accomplished is
never discussed. It is simply assumed that not having a nose will
make one "unhappy" and that restoring it will "heal the spirit."

In his summary of his surgical techniques, Tagliacozzi evokes
the physiognomic theory that connects face and character, body
and spirit. This serious surgical textbook opens with ten chapters

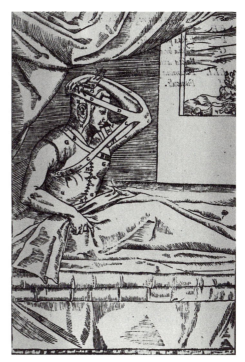

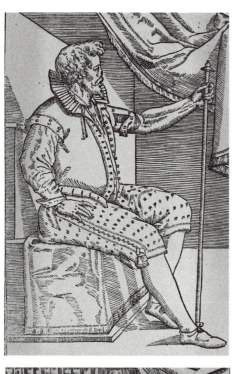

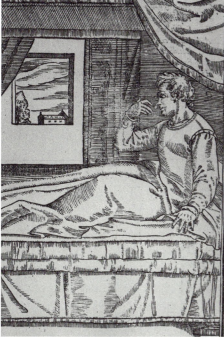

The missing nose, the operation,
and the nose restored.

recounting the meaning of the physiognomy. He argues (following Galen) that the face is the mirror of the soul, that its beauty or imperfections mirror the status of the soul. He provides a complex though in no way unusual catalogue of the meaning of the various "types" of faces and their anomalies. He shows how the face reflects the age, sex, and social status (free or slave) of the individual. He argues—still following Galen—that the placement of the face as the most visible part of the body reflects its meaning as the section of the body in which the temperaments that determine character and health can best be read. In this, Galen follows Hippocrates' view of the role of the physiognomy of illness. But Tagliacozzi, following the physiognomic guidelines in Pomponio Gaurico's (c. 1481–c. 1528) *De Sculptura* (1504), notes that symmetry is the measure of beauty of the face and, therefore, of health. All of this appears in preparation for a volume devoted to the rebuilding of aspects of the face to provide new character, new symmetry, and new happiness to the patient.

The ideology that underpinned Tagliacozzi's procedures was radical. It was linked to the claims of autonomy present in the high Renaissance. Anti-hierarchical thinkers such as Giovanni Francesco Pico della Mirandola (1463–94) presented individual autonomy as the central quality of the human being. These views surfaced again during the Enlightenment in its understanding of autonomy and difference. In opposition to views that saw illness or defect (and disfigurement) as a punishment from God for the transgressions of the individual or the parents, the view of autonomous self-remaking provided the basis and, indeed, the vocabulary for Tagliacozzi's surgical innovations. Pico has God say to Adam:

> "We have given you, Adam, no visage proper to yourself, nor endowment properly your own, in order that whatever place, whatever form, whatever gifts you may, with premeditation, select, these same you may have and possess through your own judgment and decision. The nature of all other creatures is defined and restricted within laws which We have laid down; you, by contrast,

impeded by no such restrictions, may, by your own free will, to whose custody We have assigned you, *trace for yourself the lineaments of your own nature.* I have placed you at the very center of the world. . . We have made you a creature neither of heaven nor of earth, neither mortal nor immortal, in order that you may, as the *free and proud shaper of your own being, fashion yourself in the form you may prefer. . . .* Who then will not look with awe upon this our *chameleon,* or who, at least, will look with greater admiration on any other being? This creature, man, whom Asclepius the Athenian, by reason of this very mutability, this nature capable of transforming itself, quite rightly said was symbolized in the mysteries by the figure of Proteus."[44]

Pico imagined in 1486 that he spoke of the transformation of the soul; a hundred years later Tagliacozzi realized the autonomy of individual choice in transforming the body. In Pico's view, God has given human beings a license for self-transformation. For Tagliacozzi, "passing," or "this nature capable of transforming itself," is the ability of individuals (now "chameleons") to transgress what are understood as "divine" taboos through the agency of the surgeon. Human autonomy is ceded to the physician, who now can remake man in his own image.

The problem was whether this new nose (and therefore the new character) allowed the individual to "pass" as "undiseased." Between Pico and Tagliacozzi lay the beginnings of the great syphilis epidemic, which gave the idea of self-transformation new and unexpected meaning. But Tagliacozzi's surgery did not answer the problem completely. Although facial scarring was avoided by taking the skin flap from the upper arm, the procedure still left a nose that was clearly reconstructed, as Paré noted. It was a "virtual nose," which its new owner could not entirely trust. When the weather turned cold it became livid, if one blew it too hard it might fall off. Young women with reconstructed noses were not exactly objects of desire.[45] Otto Hildebrand, writing in 1909 about Tagliacozzi's procedures, observed that canon law declared that the loss of the nose was grounds for the termination of a marital engagement. It is questionable, he remarked, whether having a new nose would be grounds for its reinstatement.[46] Such noses might restore function, but they would not allow one to "pass" as someone with a "real" nose.

This was equally true half a century later when John Bulwer, in his 1653 treatise *Anthropometamorphosis: Man Transform'd*, catalogued a wide range of cosmetic alterations of the body from a wide range of cultures. He approved of only those changes that repaired the "unnaturall and monstrous Incroachments upon the Humane forme" and returned the body to its "Naturall State." This natural state is "unblemished" and close to the ideal of beauty in its "original perfection."[47] For the physician Bulwer, only the doctor can undertake such procedures upon the diseased body; it is not the business of the patient or even the cosmetician to repair the body. It is solely the role of the physician or the surgeon. Of course, in the seventeenth century barber-surgeons not only groomed their clients but also undertook the "removal and mitigation of marks and blemishes."[48] In this context, the restoration of the erotic became the elimination of illness and disease.

For Bulwer as for so many others, the nose was the crucial site for the cosmetic reconstruction of the face: "certaine formes and strange shapes of the Nose, much affected and artificially contrived, as matters of singular beauty and ornament, to the esteem of some Nations." He cites "the Tartarian women [who in the court of the Tartar king] cut and pare their noses between their eyes, that they may be seen more flat and saddle-nosed, leaved themselves no nose at all in that place, anointing the very same place with a black ointment which sight seemed most ugly in the eyes of Fryar William de Rubraquis, a French Man, and his companions when they came to his court. . . . It is Impossible the adulterate wit of women should commit a fouler trespass against beauty and the majesty of nature, or introduce a more odious alteration in the Face, than is done by the contrivances of this Fashion." Bulwer saw such an alteration to create flattened noses as illogical and unaesthetic because of the illness and corruption ascribed to the flattened nose.[49]

A Cure from the Colonies

By the time Sterne sat down to create Tristram Shandy with his too-tiny nose, the actual surgical techniques of the Renaissance to create new noses had been lost. The age of Sterne still demanded a new way of replacing lost noses and disguising flattened noses (besides Paré's artificial noses). But they found the possible "cure" only in the lost and confused legend of the history of aesthetic surgery, which they read about in their libraries. By the time Tristram Shandy needed a new nose, the procedures associated with Tagliacozzi had already been lost to Western surgeons for a century and a half. The reason for this loss is not clear—it may have been the opposition of the Church which saw in the repair of the nose a means of disguising the immorality that led to its loss, or it may have been that banishing the ability to create a new nose was a powerful answer to the claims of individual autonomy that resurfaced after the Counter-Reformation. Could one really become something other than what one was intended or perceived to be? Was aesthetic surgery a victim of the shift in ideology of the day? Was it possible that having a functional nose (which did not fly off when you sneezed) was not sufficient for those long-suffering patients who underwent the procedure? Was it also necessary to have a nose that allowed you to "pass" as healthy? There certainly was a shift in surgical styles, which did not favor the painful and laborious types of surgery proposed by Tagliacozzi and the Bolognese tradition to which he belonged. Tagliacozzi's own teacher at Bologna may well have been the anatomist/surgeon Giulio Cesare Aranzio (1530–89), who is claimed to have replaced noses with flaps taken from the hand and lower arm.[50] Although such procedures were effective, they were also painful and very risky.

One can never be sure why the pedicle flap graft vanished from medical use. A rumor circulated after Tagliacozzi's death that his body was exhumed and the bones scattered by the orders of the Church. This did not happen, but the fact that generations

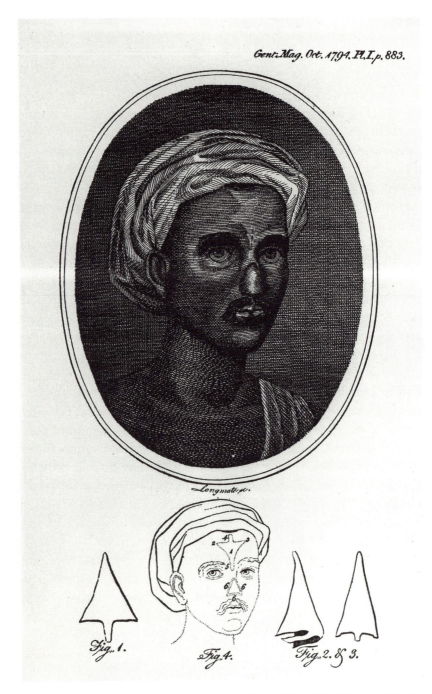

Longmate sc.

Fig. 1.   Fig. 4.   Fig. 2. & 3.

The image of Cowasjee in an article authored by "B.L." in the *Gentlemen's Magazine*, London, 1794. This article marked the reintroduction of rhinoplasty into Europe.

believed that it had is a sign of the danger that was associated with "passing." Indeed, Tagliacozzi's work continued to be cited by medical authorities such as Matthäus Gottfred Purmann (1648–1711) in 1684, even if his procedures were no longer used.[51] A statue of Tagliacozzi, holding a detached nose loosely in his hand, a nose in search of a patient, remained to grace the medical school at Bologna for centuries. His procedures vanished into the world of fiction.

It was from the expansion of British colonial power into the "Orient" that the "cure" for the missing nose, the technique of grafting used in seventeenth-century Europe, was reintroduced. The establishment of British colonial power in India brought with it, in 1794, the publication in the West of the first detailed account of the reconstruction of a nose since the disappearance of Tagliacozzi's procedures into literary legend.[52] Appearing under the initials B.L. in the *Gentlemen's Magazine* in London, the anonymous article (most probably written by the British surgeon Coly Lyon Lucas) documented "the ... very curious, and, in Europe, unknown chirurgical operation," the use of a connected skin-graft from the forehead to reconstruct or rather to replace the nose.[53] The patient, a Parsi "bullock-driver" named Cowasjee, had been in the service of the British when he was captured by the rebellious Tipu Sultan, Fath Ali, Nawab of Mysore (1753–99), who ordered the amputation of Cowasjee's nose and one hand.

When, twelve months later, Cowasjee minus his nose and hand rejoined the British army in Bombay, he went to a "member of the Brick maker caste" to replace his nose. The procedure began by tracing a replacement using a wax model onto Cowasjee's forehead and loosening the skin from the forehead. Leaving a connecting flap, the brick maker abraded the stump, twisted the graft around and formed the nose. Twenty-five days later, he cut the remaining bridge and Cowasjee had his new nose. This version of the pedicle skin-flap had the advantage over Tagliacozzi's arm flap that it did not encumber the patient with a brace for a long period, but it left an extensive scar on the forehead. An army surgeon who may well have read of it in the local Madras paper in March of 1794 reported this procedure. A portrait of Cowasjee by

James Wales appeared in the *Gentlemen's Magazine,* and was reprinted in all of the subsequent versions of this tale. This portrait shows a much diminished scar and a nose that appears aesthetically "normal."

The news of this procedure quickly spread throughout Europe and to America. The need for such a procedure was apparent in an age that saw itself as the age of syphilis. But Cowasjee never took his place beside Tagliacozzi and Dieffenbach in the pantheon of the heroes of aesthetic surgery. Patients rarely do; the anonymous brick maker who gave him his new nose also vanished, to be replaced in the concerns of the historians of aesthetic surgery by the question of who wrote the essay in the *Gentlemen's Magazine* for 1794. The focus remains on Western medicine and its heroes, for the world of the fabled "Orient" can only incidentally be of interest to the writing of modern medicine. This seems true from the Western perspective that sees the "East" as the place where modern medicine is imported, not exported.

The narrative of Cowasjee's nose is entirely dependent on the Western image of India and of the character of that culture. Thus, central to this story is the representation of the Indian ruler as the cruel and immoral figure needing the control of moral British authority. A century before Cowasjee's nose and Tipu Sultan's rebellion, in the British *Madras Government Consultation Book* of 1679, it was already observed that the Mysoreans' "custom is not to kill but to cut off the noses with the upper lips of the enemies, for which they carry an iron instrument with which they do it very dexterously, and carry away all the noses and lips they despoyle their enemies of, for which they are rewarded by the Naik of Mysore according to their number, and the reward is the greater, if the beard appear on the upper lip."[54] For the British, such mutilations were a sign of the primitiveness of their enemies and their own moral superiority.[55] Such "Oriental practice" came to be associated with cruelty and immorality. The "enemy" could do little more to show his barbarity than to remove the nose (as one sees in the warning about the "Babylonians and all the Chaldeans," who "shall cut off your noses and your ears," in *Ezekiel* 23:25).

However, according to the 1794 account in the British press, such "Oriental" and "barbaric" practices were the reason for the development of this aspect of traditional Indian medicine. In the early work on the surgery of the nose, this trope is repeated in the rationale for the "Indian" practice of rebuilding the nose. Following the British model, which he knew well, the German surgeon Eduard Zeis, writing in 1838, saw the "barbarism" of the East as the necessary impetus for the development of reconstructive rhinoplasty. It "owes its origin to the custom of punishing thieves, deserters, and, particularly, adulterers by cutting off their noses and ears, which was practiced in olden times, and is still practiced today. It is no wonder that the art of making noses developed much later in Europe, where such a grisly custom did not exist."[56] The barbarism of the "Orient" led to the development of reparative procedures, according to this narrative; but its adoption in England and then on the continent was also contingent on the meaning ascribed to "India" in the eighteenth century.

It was only because this procedure was "discovered" in the late eighteenth century that it had an impact on the British scene. During the late eighteenth century the assumption was that India "hid" great intellectual treasures under the debris of centuries of Mogul misrule. Thus the work of William Jones (1746–94) on Sanskrit, which laid the foundation for European historical linguistics, has the same cultural impetus as the "discovery" of aesthetic surgery in the case of Cowasjee.[57] By the mid nineteenth century, India could no longer be imagined as the source of medical knowledge; it was only the object of such knowledge.[58] The study of Sanskrit and the case of Cowasjee merge in discovering the hidden value of Indian culture. The image in the British press is that these procedures were a form of folk medicine or "sunken cultural traditions." But there is an extensive literature on the surgery of the nose in traditional Indian medicine. Within the Sanskrit writings of Susruta (900 B.C.E.) and the tradition of Ayurveda (classic) Indian aesthetic surgery, there is a detailed discussion of the use and development of grafts.[59] Susruta wrote chapters on reconstructive surgery of the split earlobe and of the nose. The repair of the nose that "has been cut off" necessitated the use of a pedicle (connected) flap of skin taken from the cheek.[60] This could be a successful restoration of the missing nose, even though it left an evident and nasty scar. The lost nose could be the result of trauma or of infection. Scrofula, yaws, and later even syphilis haunt the subcontinent of India as well as Europe.[61]

Joseph Constantine Carpue (1764–1846) introduced the Indian tradition of rebuilding the nose through the use of a connected graft into English medical practice in 1815.[62] The Cowasjee case provided Carpue with a complex rationale to avoid associating the reconstructed nose with the syphilitic's lost nose. Carpue presented the rebuilding of Cowasjee's nose as the treatment of a service wound. By stressing the nature of the patient rather than the source of the ailment, Carpue avoided being associated with the quack syphilis doctors whom he condemned. The loss of a nose at the hands of a brutal enemy was analogous to the loss of a limb on the battlefield, and its replacement was therefore not to be condemned by the social mores of the time. Indeed, Carpue's two reported cases included one of a soldier whose nose had been sliced off in battle during the Napoleonic peninsular wars. But Carpue's first case was that of a soldier whose lost nose was attributed to the effects of the mercurial treatment for syphilis, which could mimic the signs and symptoms of the disease.

Carpue doubted whether the patient had actually had a venereal disease at all, and thus makes the lost nose into an iatrogenic illness resulting from the treatment for a nonexistent disease. This is important for Carpue, for he does not want to equate his reconstructive procedures with the actions of the syphilis doctor, whom William Hogarth (1697–1764) had pilloried in his series *Marriage à la Mode.* Carpue presented his procedure as serious medicine for morally valuable individuals, such as the heroes of the Napoleonic Wars, not remedies to mask the consequences of immoral acts. This is important even in Carpue's writing of the history of this procedure. Acknowledging his own technique's Indian origins, Carpue stresses that the source of Tagliacozzi's earlier procedures had to have been independent of the introduction of syphilis into Europe in 1494. Indeed, he notes, the Branca family, which had undertaken similar procedures, flourished in the mid-fifteenth century (p. 53).

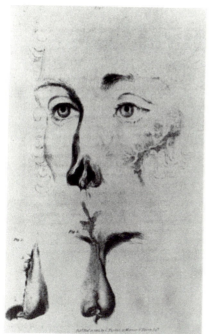

J. C. Carpue's second patient, Captain Latham, wounded in the Peninsular Wars, and the reconstruction of his nose.

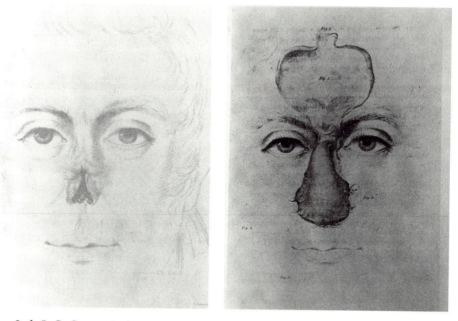

Left: J. C. Carpue's first patient, whose suspected venereal disease was treated with mercury, showing the "loss of the septum, all the anterior part of the cartilage, and in truth, the whole front of the nose." *Right:* The patient's nose replaced by the flap method, showing the progress of the reconstruction of the nose from the forehead flap to the adhesion of the graft.

Carpue's account of the early history of aesthetic surgery is paralleled by much of the later writing of the history of this medical specialty. Authors, usually surgeons themselves, defend the specialty against the accusation of immorality (whether in repairing the syphilitic nose or in creating a more "beautiful" face) by defining their actions as reconstructive rather than aesthetic surgery. This arbitrary distinction is made even when the stated intent of the procedure is a reconstitution of the happy psyche.

Other contemporaries of Carpue undertook similar procedures. In Germany, Carl Ferdinand von Graefe (1787–1840) published his book on the reconstruction of the nose in 1818, establishing *rhinoplasty* as the name for the procedure.[63] Graefe created a "German" school at the Charité Hospital in Berlin, according to his own account, by merging the "Italian" and the "Indian" methods of rebuilding the nose. Dieffenbach was of this "school." Graefe, like all of the early surgeons who used connected grafts as transplants, provided a long, detailed history of the origins of his techniques (pp. 16–25). Ranging from ancient India to the European Renaissance, Graefe stressed the continuity of the procedures and their loss during the eighteenth century. The reason asserted for that loss was the stigma associated with the noseless patient.

Graefe believed that the modern age understood the horrors experienced by the patient without a nose. Society was for the first time in centuries truly sympathetic to the individual patient's dilemma and did not see him or her as morally defective. "Those who should be pitied appear like grinning larva, which, if they are marked by the greatest degree of physical destruction even lose the purity of their voices. . . . They are quite aware of their situation, feel themselves oppressed a hundred fold, and believe themselves to be physically as well as morally branded. They scuttle quickly from one moment to another of their unhappy [*freudenlosen*] life" (p. vi). The new surgery is to "further individual happiness [*Glück*]." Those who have been "mocked through prejudice and vanity" now have "better hopes" (p. vii). Graefe established rhinoplasty as a serious part of modern surgery by giving it a classical name like those of other surgical procedures. This act of naming was a further gesture in the direction of making the rebuilding of the nose a medical rather than a moral problem.

The move to a medical model for understanding the lost nose spread relatively quickly. The reason for the explosion in popularity of the rebuilding of the nose, even in the age before antisepsis and anesthesia, is stated in Julius von Szymanowski's (1829–68) observation in 1857 that the leading causes for the possible need for the replacement of the nose in his experience was syphilis (thirty cases), followed by traumatic injury (twenty-five cases).[64] Syphilis haunts the image of the too-small nose. Julius von Szymanowski reported that in 1857, out of 243 rhinoplasties reported, 125 were performed in Germany, 39 in Russia, 34 in France, 21 in Britain, 12 in Italy, 3 in Switzerland, 2 in Belgium, 4 in America, and 3 in Asia. (This list sounds a bit like Leporello's aria recounting his master's sexual conquests in *Don Giovanni*!) The replacement of the nose meant being able to "pass" (even if scarred) as whole and healthy. This is a problem not only of the aesthetic of appearance but of the infection of the soul.

The tradition of rebuilding the nose was reimported from Europe into India following the establishment of the Raj. Within the Westernized tradition of Indian surgery in the nineteenth century there was a further development of this reception. Indian surgeons did indeed stress the idea of the "nose job" as an "original" Indian contribution to surgery. They read these origins quite differently from the way Europeans did. Tribhovandas Motichand Shah (1850–1904), writing in Junagadh in 1889, rationalized his clinical account of a hundred cases of rhinoplasty by labeling the Indian patients the victims of criminal activity: "The Makrani outlaws, who carried out depredations against the Jungadh State for a period of nearly three years, had not infrequently indulged in mutilating the noses of undefended and unarmed ryots [peasants] of villages."[65] Such activities are criminal, unsanctioned by the state. It is true that there is a tradition of vendettas in India, Motichand Shah continues, in which the nose is cut off, in contrast to the (much worse, he implies) Western tradition of vendettas in which "the chief modes of mortal revenge are homicide, either by poisoning, shooting, or wounding." It is true, of course, that the West, too, has a problem with lost noses: "In these countries loss of the nose is only a consequence of disease—chiefly syphilis." The rationale for the rebuilding of the Indian nose, on the other hand, is the reconstitution of "delicate feelings of honour" and the overcoming of "feelings of the greatest humiliation."

The end result of Motichand Shah's discourse on the Indian nose is to create a world quite the opposite of Zeis's; it is one in which defending the civilization of India, violated by criminals and acts of passion, demanded the medical intervention of the surgeon, as opposed to the use of similar interventions in the diseased and sexually corrupt West. Motichand Shah's India is a world without tyrants and syphilis. In England, the reading of "India" and the nose job shifted the meaning of the lost nose. Harold Delf Gillies wrote in 1934 that "in Ancient India the owner of a nose that had fallen to the ravages of syphilis or to the avenging knife of an outraged husband rose up and demanded a priest or barber surgeon to make a new one."[66] By the twentieth century it is syphilis and spousal abuse that defines the "Orient," not the "Oriental despot." This is the view of the British medical missionaries to India at the beginning of the twentieth century, such as T. L. Pennell (1867–1912).

According to Pennell, surgical procedures continued to be used to rebuild the nose of women who had been punished as "immoral."[67] Pennell comments that, as this is "a very old mutilation in India, the people centuries ago elaborated an operation for the removal of the deformity, whereby a portion of skin is brought down from the forehead and stitched on the raw surface where the nose had been cut off, and we still use this operation, with certain modifications, for the cases that come to us." He then tells of a woman whose husband had cut off her nose. Pennell could not use the forehead flap technique, as her forehead was too low. He suggested that an artificial nose be imported from England, and remarked ironically that the husband thought long about whether it was cheaper to buy a new nose or a new wife (p. 194)! Such anecdotes were recounted as signs of Indian "barbarism," and it is striking that the remedy for such an act is a nose "imported from England" rather than a "native" procedure.

Pennell also tells the tale of a man for whom he ordered an artificial nose. There arrived from England a "pale flesh-coloured nose," which was much lighter than his "dark olive" skin. The colonial nose is fine for the colonials, but is evidently a false nose when worn by the Indians. Pennell dyed the nose walnut, and when the man walked home the dye ran and he arrived home with a streaked nose to the laughter of his village (p. 195). From the discussion in the eighteenth century through texts such as Pennell's some hundred years later, it is clear that the repair of the nose in the Indian (colonial) context is a sign of the barbarism or primitivism of the "natives." The very act of repair or replacement is read as a comic comment on the barbaric nature of the exotic. This is a far cry from the awe in which eighteenth-century English physicians held the ability to rebuild the nose, which caused such prostheses to become rare in England.

In contemporary India the fashion of aesthetic surgery is part of the globalization of medicine. As elsewhere, the surgeon's anxiety about being seen as a vanity surgeon predominates, even (or perhaps especially) in a culture in which the "nose job" has had its longest uninterrupted history. Mathangi Ramakrishnan, who was trained at the Madras Medical College, took up plastic surgery during her medical education in the United Kingdom in the late 1950s.[68] In 1962 she created the burns and plastic surgery department at the Kilpauk Medical College, which became a unique center in the country. She was also the first woman president of the Association of Plastic Surgeons of India. She notes with a bit of hesitation that "about 10 percent of my work is cosmetic." Her favorite aesthetic work? "Nose correction," what else?

Fifteenth-century Europeans discovered the Americas, and contracted syphilis in the bargain, in the course of trying to reach the Indies. As syphilis epidemics spread throughout Europe and the rest of the world, they created a new class of patients among those who survived the worst effects of a usually fatal disease only to have their collapsed and missing noses—or those of their offspring—advertise their uncleanness. For a time in Renaissance Europe, Gaspare Tagliacozzi's surgical innovations promised at least partial restoration of the syphilitic nose and a chance for sufferers to "pass" as almost healthy. But after Tagliacozzi's techniques died with him in 1599, it was two hundred years before Europeans rediscovered them during a more successful round of efforts to colonize the Indies.

It would be another one hundred years and more before bacteriology and antibiotics could offer a real victory over syphilis. During that time, aesthetic surgery would continue its efforts to repair the syphilitic nose, and the syphilitic nose would take an ever larger place in European culture as the preeminent symbol of all that was unclean, inferior, and undesirable. As the nineteenth century wore on, and European culture continued to extract the profits of colonization, the symbolic locus of the too-small nose became inextricably associated with race.

CHAPTER THREE

The Racial Nose

ENLIGHTENMENT NOSES

𝒪N THE WORLD of nineteenth-century science, the great chain of being that was seen to stretch from the most human to the least human was also a chain of beauty, and beauty was measured by the nose. The tiny nose, the flattened nose, thus became part of the very definition of race. The difference of the too-short nose is a racial difference and racial differences are signs of character. Moreover, there was also the powerful idea in eighteenth- and early nineteenth-century anthropology that the noses of the black and the Jew were signs of their "primitive" nature. This was primarily because the too-flat nose came to be associated with the inherited syphilitic nose. In this view, flattened noses are nature's moral comment on the hygiene of a "race" in terms of both racial difference and dangerousness.

The widespread claim that the too small nose was the ugly mark of inferior races reflected the reception of the work, at the close of the eighteenth century, of the Dutch anatomist Petrus Camper (1722–89) who "discovered" the facial angle and the nasal index.[1] The nasal index was the line that connected the forehead via the nose to the upper lip; its reflex, the facial angle, was determined by connecting this line with a horizontal line coming from the jaw. This line came to be a means of distinguishing between the human being and the other higher anthropoids.

Camper's facial angle, which connected all the races of the human species and distinguished them from the ape, was also used by many of his contemporaries and successors, such as his

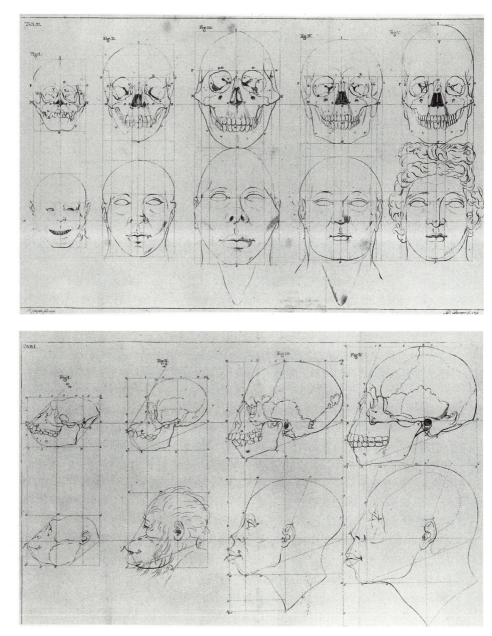

Classical models, facial angles, and the nasal index.

son-in-law, Theodor Soemmering, as a means of creating a hierarchy of the races. Camper defined the "beautiful face" as one in which the facial line creates an angle of 100 to the horizontal (p. 62). According to the contemporary reading of Camper, the African was the least beautiful (and therefore the least erotic) because he or she is closest to the ape in his or her physiognomy.

Too-short noses are pathological or primitive because they are disproportionate or asymmetrical even if they are functional. They are signs of the relationship between the unaesthetic and the corrupt. The shape of the nose is an essential element of that which defines the true human being. In 1811 Lorenz Oken (1779–1851), the German Romantic philosopher/naturalist, defined the notion of the beautiful face in terms clearly borrowed from Camper:

> The face is beautiful, when the nose is parallel to the spine. No face grows so, but every nose makes a sharp angle to the spine. The facial angle is known to be 80. What no one has yet observed, and what is also not observable without our understanding of the meaning of the skull, was evident to the ancient artists through their feeling. They not only made the facial angle correct, but also even exceeded it—the Romans to 96 and the Greeks, indeed, to 100. How is it that this unnatural face of the Greek work of art is even more beautiful than that of the Roman, even though the latter is closer to nature? The reason for this lies in the fact that Greek facial aesthetics represents even more the will of nature than those of the Roman; for there the nose is quite perpendicular, parallel to the spine, and thus returns from where it came. He who simply copies nature is a bungler, he is without inspiration and mimics no better than the bird, song, or the ape, gestures.[2]

Oken summarized not only the notion of the perfect face and nose, but also the way we measure and understand that face—through the Kantian idealization of high art as providing transcendent models for human beauty. For Oken, bodies are not to be judged against other real bodies but against the ideal forms of bodies in art.

The black nose is the key to an understanding of the aesthetics of facial deformity in the Enlightenment. Facial aesthetics is the aesthetics of race. Even among those thinkers who advocated a relativistic aesthetics (in which each people of the world has its own standard of beauty), the meaning of facial deformity remained constant. In his *Laocoön or On the Boundaries of Painting and Poetry* (1766), Gotthold Ephraim Lessing (1729–81) observed, "A scar in the face, a hare-lip, a flattened nose with prominent nostrils, an entire absence of eyebrows, are uglinesses which are not offensive either to smell, taste, or touch. At the same time it is certain that these things produce a sensation that certainly comes much nearer to disgust than what we feel at the sight of other deformities of body."[3] In his widely translated physiognomic study, Johann Caspar Lavater (1741–1801), who created the craze for physiognomy in the late eighteenth century, established the flattened nose as the icon of the black.[4] He cites Georges Louis Leclerc, comte de Buffon's (1707–88) *Histoire naturelle:* "All Hottentots have a very flat and broad nose, they would not have it but for the fact that the mothers feel it necessary shortly after birth to press the children's noses flat" (4:275). He also quotes Kant's essay on the "Various Races of Mankind" (1775): "The growth of the spongy parts of the body must increase in a hot and damp climate. Thick snub nose and sausage lips result. . . . [T]he black is appropriate to his climate, that is strong, fleshy, supple, but because of the rich provisions of his motherland, lazy, inactive, and slow." (4: 277) Aesthetics and character are linked to the shape of the nose. Indeed, Charles de Secondat, baron de Montesquieu (1689–1755), in *The Spirit of Laws* (1748) even weighs the appearance of the black as a justification for slavery.[5] In addition to the environmental explanation of the form of the black nose offered by Buffon and Kant, it also represents leprosy or yaws powerfully associated in European fantasy with the "tropics" and interchangeable with the idea and image of syphilis.[6]

THE JEWISH NOSE

The meaning read into the African's nose became interchangeable with that seen in the Jew's nose.[7] The noses of the African and the

Jew were equally ugly because the Jew's physiognomy was understood to be closer to that of the African than to that of the European. Johann Caspar Lavater quoted the Storm and Stress poet J. M. R. Lenz (1751–92) to the effect that: "It is evident to me that the Jews bear the sign of their fatherland, the orient, throughout the world. I mean their short, black, curly hair, their brown skin color. Their rapid speech, their brusque and precipitous actions also come from this source. I believe that the Jews have more gall than other people."[8] The character ascribed to the Jews is written on their skin. The Jews are black "Orientals." They bear the sign of the black, "the African character of the Jew, his muzzle-shaped mouth and face removing him from certain other races," as Robert Knox (1791–1862) noted in the mid nineteenth century.[9]

Camper also saw the physiognomy of the Jew as immutable: "There is no nation that is as clearly identifiable as the Jews: men, women, children, even when they are first born, bear the sign of their origin. I have often spoken about this with the famed painter of historical subjects [Benjamin] West, to whom I mentioned my difficulty in capturing the national essence of the Jews. He was of the opinion that this must be sought in the curvature of the nose."[10] The nose defines the Jewish face and links it to the African face. The African nose and the Jewish nose became abstract "racial" signs of the character and temperament ascribed to the Jew and the African.

The assumption of the Jews' close racial relationship to or intermixing with blacks becomes a commonplace of nineteenth-century ethnology. Both non-Jewish and Jewish anthropologists of the fin de siècle write of the "predominant mouth of some Jews being the result of the presence of black blood" and the "brown skin, thick lips and prognathism" of the Jew.[11] It is not only skin color that enables the scientist to label the Jew as "black," but also the associated anatomical signs, such as the shape of the nose. The Jews were quite literally seen as black. Adam Gurowski (1805–66), a Polish count, "took every light-colored mulatto for a Jew" when he first arrived in the United States in the 1850s.[12]

One of the central texts of the French Enlightenment, the *Encyclopedia* of Denis Diderot (1713–84) and Jean Le Rond d'Alembert (1717–83), argues against this source of the inherent difference in body and character of the black. The article on the "nose" contends that "most of the anatomists claim that this flatness comes from art and not from nature." Here the Encyclopedists place all of the deviant noses together: "the blacks, the Hottentots, and various peoples of Asia such as the Jews." Swaddling creates the flattened nose of the black, and the black is therefore no different from the European norm of beauty in his "natural" state.[13] The original nose, the normal nose, the healthy nose is that of the European, which may be altered through cultural interventions, but remains a sign of the universality of all human beings. This is quite different from the racial argument made in the German Enlightenment about the shape of the African nose. An echo of the Encyclopedists' argument surfaces a century later when Charles Darwin commented that the "Negroes rallied Mungo Park [the British explorer] on the whiteness of his skin and the prominence of his nose, both of which they considered as 'unsightly and unnatural conformations.'"[14] Darwin sees the response of the Africans as a natural one—to them, the British nose is as ugly and pathological as the African nose is to the British. The beautiful nose is specific to the culture in which one lives. Darwin's comment ironically links nose form and skin color as comic signs when they are articulated from the standpoint of the African. The nose becomes the site for such pseudo-scientific argument on both sides of the border of racial and cultural difference. This is indicative of some of the complex associations of the image of the sunken nose.

The nose comes to signify all that is static and immutable about the African and the Jew, whether natural or cultural. In 1926 the British novelist Robert Hichens (1864–1950), allowed one of his characters to recognize the Jew by his or her nose. "'You're right. He is a Jew. Directly I was able to look really at him, to examine his face, I knew it. Not the hook-nosed Jew—the other type, the blunt-featured type."[15] The flat-nosed Jew reappears in numerous guises, but always as the exemplar of capital. Thus Meyer Wolfshiem, in F. Scott Fitzgerald's (1896–1940) *The Great Gatsby* (1925) is described as "a small flat-nosed Jew [who] raised his large head and regarded me with two fine growths of hair, which luxuriated in either nostril. After a moment I discovered his tiny eyes in the half darkness." His nose is described as "expressive" and "tragic," capable of "flashing indignantly."[16] For ornament he wears human teeth as cufflinks, and he reduces everyone he sees to a similar commodity.

The German anthropologist Hans Günther (1891–1968) explained the competition between the "black Jews" and the "white Jews" as that of the blunt noses against the long noses. One of the sociologist Frances Macgregor's (1906–   ) American Jewish informants in the 1960s claimed that he wanted to show the Gentiles through his rhinoplasty that "there are nice Jews. I'll be a good-will ambassador. I can prove to people that I'm not only a 'white man' but a 'white Jew.'"[17] As we shall see, rhinoplasty in the twentieth century enabled Jews to imagine themselves as "passing" for "white." Here the model of the Jews as a mixed race is internalized as a quality of Jewish character. Becoming a "white Jew" is a psychic response to the image of the Jew in various aspects of the collective culture.[18]

Irish Noses

In the 1880s, John Orlando Roe (1849–1915) in Rochester, New York, performed an operation to "cure" the "pug nose."[19] The too-small nose he corrected was not the syphilitic nose; rather, he intervened to create new American noses out of the noses of Irish immigrants. Their new noses did not mask the sexual sins of their parents, but the fact that their parents came from elsewhere, in the case of the pug nose, from Ireland. Roe's innovation was not only to transform his patients from "Irish" into "Americans," but also to do so without the telltale scars that revealed the work of surgeons repairing or replacing syphilitic noses. They were no longer marked in terms of contemporary racial science as "Celts" but could truly "pass" as "Anglo-Saxons."

Aesthetic surgery of the nose as practiced by surgeons such as Johann Friedrich Dieffenbach before the introduction of anesthesia and antisepsis left scars and placed patients' lives at risk be-

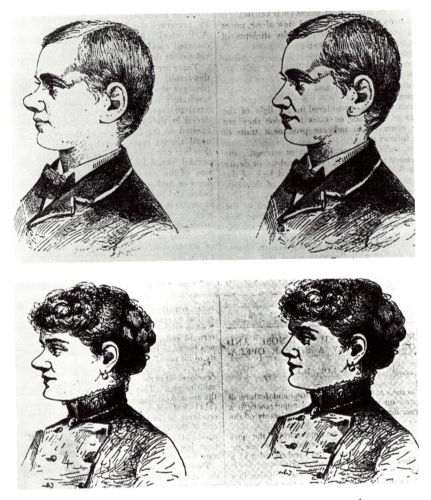

The "before and after" images of the "pug nose" in a man and a woman.

cause of the dangers of shock and infection. With the introduction of antisepsis and anesthesia, the scar itself remained the major "danger" for patients.[20] Scars showed that a medical intervention had taken place, and what patients came to fear most was having an operation, which revealed that they had had one. The vital difference in Roe's procedure was that he operated from within the nostrils, leaving no visible scar on the skin. This powerful innovation was to change the course of aesthetic surgery. Not only was his surgical procedure innovative in the United States, but so too was the nose on which he operated.

Roe provides us with substantial information about his theory of appearance and its meaning. Based on the profile, Roe divided the image of the nose into five categories: Roman, Greek, Jewish, Snub or Pug, and Celestial. Each type of nose indicated qualities of character, following Samuel Wells's (1820–75) phrenological/physiognomic theories: "The Roman indicates executiveness or strength; the Greek, refinement; the Jewish, commercialism or desire of gain; the Snub or Pug, weakness and lack of development; the Celestial, weakness, lack of development, and inquisitiveness" (p. 114). For Roe, the "snub-nose" is "proof of a degeneracy of the human race." Remarkably, he finds his rationale for this in *Tristram Shandy,* which he quotes on the problem of a "succession of short noses" in a family. Roe notes that Shandy's grandfather had little choice in his mate "owing to the brevity of his nose." Roe sees this as a sign of congenital pathology that must ultimately be racially based (as it is in many ways in Sterne's novel, too). The short nose announces the degenerate race.

Roe's sense of himself as an artist (as well as a physician) can be noted in a comment made in 1905. "In the correction of all facial defects the surgeon must be not only an artist but also more or less of a sculptor, with perception of symmetry as related to the different features."[21] Symmetry and balance are concepts of the "norm" as opposed to asymmetry, which is both "ugly" and "dangerous." Charles Bell (1774–1842), the author of the classic nineteenth-century anatomical handbook for artists and one of the great surgeons of his day, shared the "prevailing opinion that beauty of countenance consists in the capacity of expression, and in the harmony of features consenting to expression."[22] Harmony is the norm, which is disrupted by the too-small nose. Symmetry is the ideal that dominates the meaning of the healthy, beautiful face in the nineteenth century and is the wellspring of the normative ideals, which the too-small nose violated. Harmony and symmetry express the universal perfection of the human countenance. All variation from an idealized norm is thus given moral meaning. (In the course of the late nineteenth century,

James Shaw among others discovered that all adult faces are asymmetrical.[23])

But Roe was not only curing the "pug nose," he was also curing the psyche. His understanding of the relationship between mind and body was clear: "We are able to relieve patients of a condition which would remain a lifelong mark of disfigurement, constantly observed, forming a never ceasing source of embarrassment and mental distress to themselves, amounting, in many cases, to a positive torture, as well as often causing them to be objects of greater or lesser aversion to others. . . . The effect upon the mind of such physical defects is readily seen reflected in the face, which invariably conforms to the mental attitude, and leads after a time to a permanent distortion of the countenance."[24] This is very much in tune with Samuel Wells's basic understanding of physiognomy. If one can cure the anomaly, the attendant changes in physiognomy that represent psychological damage can be ameliorated. If you don't look different, you will act better and be happier. And that, in turn, will be reflected in your appearance.

What does the "pug nose" come to represent for Roe, and what sort of better and happier person would not have a "pug nose"? In the context of late nineteenth-century American physiognomy and popular caricatures, it is the Irish profile that is characterized by the snub-nose.[25] The racial anthropologists of the 1880s saw the Irish as derived directly from the big-eared Cro-Magnon man with a "nose, oftener concave than straight . . . [which is] a characteristic of the modern Gaels."[26] Irish character is "bad" character. "Though the head is large, the intelligence is low, and there is a great deal of cunning and suspicion." This is written on the face of "Bridget McBruiser" for all to see. She is contrasted in the physiognomies of the day with Florence Nightingale's "English" beauty (and moral value). The Irish physiognomy is servile, marking the Irish through animal analogies as doglike, which is why the nose itself was labeled "pug." The ultimate origin of this Irish type cannot be Ireland but Africa: "While Ireland is apparently its present centre, most of its lineaments are such as to lead us to think of Africa as its possible birthplace." The Irish nose is the African nose is the Jewish nose. All such noses represent difference and are alike.

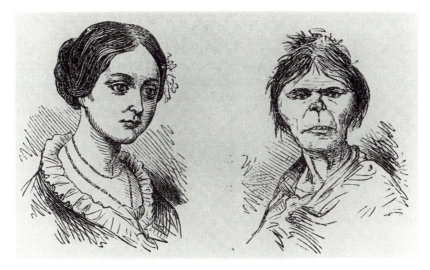

The English and Irish characters as revealed in English and Irish faces: Florence Nightingale versus Bridget McBruiser.

The "pug" nose defined the Irish as "black" in the racial climate of the United States.[27] This was not a social term—such as that distinguishing between the "black" (lower-class) and "lace curtain" (upper-class) groups of Irish immigrants. It is interesting, though, that the "lace curtain" Irish took this racial designation to distinguish themselves from the "dirty" Irish. Through projective identification they attempted to place themselves on the level of the aggressors and their long English noses. This idea of the blackness of the Irish did not originate as an American phenomenon. The notion of the Irish as a "black" race came from the vocabulary with which the English denigrated the Irish.[28] The constant and intense association of the Irish in Ireland and England with disease (especially diseases associated in the popular mind with dirt and sexuality) came to be defined in terms of the too-short nose. In England this was contrasted with the English nose; in the United States, with the German nose.[29] Such readings of Irish physiognomy lent power to the desire not to look Irish and to become (in)visible as English or German.

To cure the "pug" nose meant making the individual (in)visible, to allow the unregenerated "Celt" to "pass" as American. For,

as Samuel Wells had commented in the 1870s, the Americaniza-
tion of the Irish had caused a transformation of their character as
well as their bodies: "As proof of the fact that cultivation and external influences modify configuration, look at the Americanized
Celts—the Irish-Americans. The first generation born in this
country shows some of the finest faces we have among us. Causes
of 'arrested development' become more and more rare. Even
those born and brought up in Ireland often show a decided improvement in their physiognomy after having been here a few
years."[30] The modification of external signs of degeneration ("arrested development") is the goal of the surgeon. Roe's interventions were to be understood as forms of aesthetic surgery:
"mainly to improve the personal appearance of the individual"
(p. 116). Roe made better Americans by making the Irish (and the
syphilitic) look "American." By eliminating the scarring that attended cutting through the skin and by operating subcuta-
neously, from within the nasal passages, Roe made his new Americans (in)visible.

Roe later commented that the earlier operations resulted in "ex-
changing a deformity for an unsightly blemish" (p. 131). In an age
of "passing" novels, such as Mark Twain's (1835–1910) *Puddn'-
head Wilson* (1894), a genre in which mixed-race individuals were
"seen" as a social problem, the ability to "pass" as "normal" came
to be a function enhanced by the cosmetician or aesthetic surgeon.
Often it was the use of skin lighteners or surgery that enabled one
to cross the color bar or to believe that one could cross the constructed boundary between "white" and "black." But in the fantasy of the time it was believed that such acts of "passing" were
"natural" and not aided by external forces.[31] The puzzle at the
heart of Twain's liberal text hinges on the ability of a light-
skinned slave to exchange her child for the child of the house
without there being any possibility of distinguishing between
them. Neither skin color nor nose betrays the swapped children,
and the master's son is raised as the slave of the slave's son. But
there is, of course, a way of distinguishing the two—Twain has
his eponymous hero collect fingerprints, and since each human
being has different fingerprints, the confusion can be sorted out
and the guilty punished. It is not the Bertillon measures of ap-

pearance but the unique qualities of Francis Galton's simultaneous discovery of fingerprints that makes people identifiable—not as members of a class but only as individuals. Part of the fantasy of the culture of segregation in the United States was that skin color alone defined race, as the African-American commentator Walter White fantasized in 1949: "Supposed the skin of every Negro in America was suddenly turned to white. . . . Would not Negroes then be judged individually on their ability, energy, honesty, cleanliness as are whites?"[32] The answer was, at least in 1949, only if they have nose jobs.

Roe's procedures made it possible to be an "American" without any "blemish." Roe's procedure turned the Irish nose into "a thing of beauty."[33] Indeed, his patients began to look like their American surgeon! With the establishment of "beauty" the patient's happiness was restored. Looking Irish was one further category of difference that was written on the body and signified a poor character and bad temperament.

In contemporary Eire there has been a continued use of aesthetic surgery to remedy "Irishness." Not rhinoplasty but the ear pin-back is the operation of choice. Michael Earley, an aesthetic surgeon based in Temple Street Hospital, Dublin, says he treats a number of children for "what is called bat ears here, or Football Association Cup ears in England, [which] is a Celtic feature which some children get badly teased about."[34] This is also a permanent part of the Victorian representation of the "jug-eared Irish."[35] It is not surprising that it has maintained its importance in Ireland, while losing it in the United States, where the Irish became "white." Although "the removal of tattoos would not be considered medically necessary, for instance," and most aesthetic surgery is not covered by the Department of Health, "things like bat ears would be done on the medical card."[36] The other common procedure that is covered on the "health card" is breast reduction. As we shall see later, the very notion of breast reduction as aesthetic surgery comes about from the model of the racialized or "primitive" breast. Young women with large breasts are seen to be unhappy for reasons other than physical ones, as one prestigious Irish surgeon noted: "It can also be awkward for them to wear fashionable clothes or mix socially."[37] One can make people happy by reducing their breast size and correcting the visibility of their ears. In this way, they become less "Irish" and more "beautiful."

Between the writing of *Little Women* in the 1860s and Roe's development of his means of curing the unhappiness attendant on the pug nose comes the introduction of antisepsis and anesthesia. It is during this period that the movement of Amy's unhappiness to the operating room took place. This moment defines the differences between reconstructive and aesthetic surgery.

Thus the general question of how our society strives to "make the body beautiful" during the period from the close of the nineteenth century to our own fin de siècle is in large measure the story of how we turn to medicine to make us over and make us "happy" with our new faces and bodies. The general thesis of aesthetic surgery is that the conflict between the desire to be seen as "beautiful" or "handsome" and the difficulty in achieving that end leads to a general unhappiness with one's own body. The desired beauty has a moral dimension, for the beautiful is the good. If you understand your body as "ugly," you are bound to be "unhappy" with your bad character. In Western society, "unhappiness" with one's body comes to be understood as a form of mental illness. In its most radical form, it can be seen in the actions of psychotics who compulsively mutilate their bodies; another, milder form is the desire aesthetically to alter the body. Psychotics find themselves under the care of psychiatrists; those unhappy enough with specific aspects of their bodies seek help from aesthetic surgeons. Both the psychiatrists and the surgeons have, however, the same goals in their treatment—the amelioration of psychic "unhappiness" and the restoration (or creation) of a "happy" individual.

"Oriental" Noses — and Eyes

Ethnic difference among groups that are perceived as "ugly" and of "poor character" remains unacceptable even in a multiethnic society. One can look different, but not *too* different. Thus Asian-American men have been "stereotyped as being short people with flat faces and slanted eyes." To remedy this perception, some of them seek aesthetic surgery in order to "appear 'less Asian' and in the extreme to appear 'more Caucasian,'" and, one might add, to appear more erotic, as Asian men are generally imagined to be unerotic in American society. The most commonly sought aesthetic procedures, which are thought to accomplish this, are nose jobs (rhinoplasty) and eyelid surgery (blepharoplasty).[38] Asian-American women, whose "blank" look is equated in American society with "dullness, passivity, and lack of emotion," have "their eyelids restructured, their nose bridges heightened, and the tips of their noses altered."[39] (One might add that the reading of the Jewish eyelid in the early twentieth century was that it gave the Jewish face "often the expression of one who is tired, sleepy, relaxed, threatening." Therefore the Jewish glance was also seen as "conspiratorial."[40]) The shrunken nose coupled with the revealing eye take on yet other meanings as a sign of difference and visibility.

In ancient China, as in Pharonic Egypt and classical Greece, there are early records, such as the bone oracles (1334 B.C.E.), which mention illnesses of the nose.[41] The physician Bian Qiu (407–310 B.C.E.) wrote texts in which he described how he treated the ears and eyes of patients. Likewise the physician Hua Tuo (110–207 C.E.) documented his treatment of the eyes and ears. The traditional Chinese prohibition against opening the body limited all forms of surgical intervention until fairly recently. It is only in the northern T'ang and Gin dynasty in the late 900s C.E. that medical texts begin to record the reconstructive surgery of the harelip. Aesthetic surgery is a development of "modern" China, and "modern" China can be defined as the world where Western and traditional models of treatment clash.[42] There "modern" medicine is in many ways Western medicine with a traditional inflection. As in Japan, which replaced traditional Chinese medicine (*kanpo*) with Western medicine at the end of the nineteenth century, aesthetic surgery of the eye and nose became one of the markers of the modern and the new in medicine.

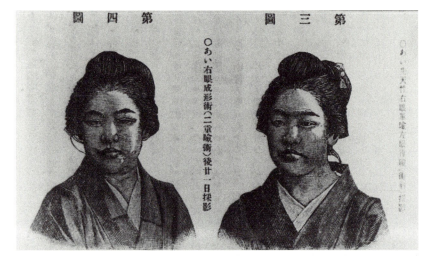

Mikamo's procedure to create a double eyelid in the right eye of a woman with a natural double eyelid on the left, 1896.

In Japan as early as 1896, under the domination of Western medicine, K. Mikamo introduced a nonincision procedure to create a double eyelid, mimicking that of the Western eye.[43] His procedure was developed to create symmetry in a patient who had a single double eyelid. Its impetus was "reconstructive," though evidently its import and influence were aesthetic. From 1896 to the present, some thirty-two different procedures were developed in Japan for purely aesthetic surgery of the eyelid. The desire, well before the defeat of Japan in 1945 and the occupation of the country by the Americans, was "to have a well-defined nose; a clear-cut, double eyelid fold; and larger, more attractive breasts." One must add that plastic surgery was recognized as a medical subspecialty in Japan only in 1975, and aesthetic surgery only in 1978. All of these procedures existed on the boundaries of official medical practice.[44] This was quite similar to the situation of aesthetic surgeons in Europe and North America.

The procedures to alter the look of the eye did not change the total image of the Japanese visage. During this period the ideal form of the face as captured in Japanese traditional portraiture shifted. Traditional portraiture had emphasized the "straight eyes and nose, flat, single eyelids, and receding chin."[45] There are specific meanings associated with the "Oriental" eye and nose in binary opposition to that of the "Occidental" eye and nose. The rather wide variations in the "Japanese" visage, running from the ethnic "Japanese" to the Ainu, was evidently idealized as a pan-Japanese face in traditional portraiture. Japanese physician/anthropologists, such as Yoshikiyo Koganei (1858–1944), the head of anatomy at the Tokyo Medical School at the end of the nineteenth century, were obsessed with distinguishing "real" Japanese faces from those of the "primitive" Ainu.[46] Central to their concern were the long noses and round eyes of the Ainu (features that had virtually vanished through intermarriage by the late nineteenth century). They needed to construct the Ainu's "primitive" visage as "different" from that of the Japanese.

The emphasis on the special nature of the Japanese (and also the Chinese) face rests on the dominant theories of physiognomy that defined health and beauty in terms of the face. Charles Darwin commented that the

> obliquity of the eye, which is proper to the Chinese and Japanese, is exaggerated in their pictures for the purpose, as it seems, of exhibiting its beauty, as contrasted "with the eye of the red-haired barbarians." It is well known, as Huc repeatedly remarks, that the Chinese of the interior think Europeans hideous, with their white skins and prominent noses. The nose is far from being too prominent, according to our ideas, in the natives of Ceylon; yet Chinese in the seventh century, accustomed to the flat features of the Mongol races, were surprised at the prominent noses of the Cingalese."[47]

While "Western" scientific medicine was determining the "true" nature of the "Japanese" visage, Western surgical techniques were making that visage not *too* Japanese.

In 1923 Nishihata and Yoshida presented the first study of augmentation rhinoplasty using ivory implants to alter the shape of the Japanese "sunken" nose.[48] Indeed, as traditional, nonsurgical medicine was transformed into a subordinate form of Western medicine in Meiji Japan, surgery of the eyelid and nose became commonplace signs of the advantages of Western clinical practice. The constitution of a new aesthetic ideal, that of Western art representing the Western face, meant the alteration of the eyelids in order to add the superior palpebral fold between the eyelid and brow (which is absent or indistinct in about half the population of Asia) and the introduction of augmentation rhinoplasty, innovations that radically change the morphological characteristics of the "Japanese" face. Following the lines of the Chinese creation of a unified "Han" racial typology in the course of the nineteenth century, the Japanese created and then reconstituted idealized faces and bodies.[49]

However, it was also believed that such aesthetic surgery had quite different meanings when applied to men than it did when applied to women. The belief was that aesthetic surgery could help enhance a man's masculinity by making him a better soldier. The American surgeon Henry Junius Schireson wrote in the late 1930s that

> the effect of this [shape of the eyelid] is not only esthetically unpleasant; it is also a definite impediment to good vision. That is why the Japanese are reputedly such poor marksmen, why this highly intelligent race has so high a percentage of airplane crashes. Japanese women were the first to seek correction of this defect, for esthetic reasons. Today in military Japan the functional objective is the moving motive and thousands of Japanese men are having this correction made. . . . It is estimated that more than twenty thousand persons . . . have recently undergone this operation.[50]

The claim that the eyelid form has a negative impact on sight is nonsense, but it was evidently believed that aesthetic surgery would make more efficient soldiers and more beautiful women.

The introduction of aesthetic surgery was likewise in Japan an attempt to cure unhappiness, *jibyo,* that amorphous sense of being unwell that haunts the Japanese medical world.[51] The traditional conception of the individual in *kanpo* (traditional) Japanese medicine was one who possessed *taishitsu,* an inborn constitution. Certain constitutions manifested various forms of *jibyo.* Can one alter one's *taishitsu?* Certainly one can intervene through tonics and medicines, but changing one's constitution through aesthetic surgery became possible only when another model, that of Westernized medicine, superseded the traditional categories of *kanpo* medicine after the Meiji Restoration of 1868. Unable to open the body, traditional medicine was relegated to second-class status with the Medical Act of 1874, which demanded that all new physicians be trained in Western medicine.[52] Western medicine and surgery were given privileged status to alter and open the body and its *taishitsu*.

Following World War II and the American occupation of Japan, a resurgence of interest in creating "Western" eyes and bodies in Japan led to further developments of such procedures as well as breast augmentation using silicone injections.[53] This responded to the introduction of the Western notion of the larger breast as a sign of the erotic. Traditional Chinese and Japanese portrayals of the female breast, even such as in Kitagawa Utamaro's nineteenth-century images of nursing mothers, stress the flat-chested look, which "carried the implication that a woman should be modest in her appearance."[54] As late as 1952 paraffin injections, and then silicone injections in 1958, were used for breast augmentation, with devastating results. Akiyama actually produced a silicone breast prosthesis as early as 1949.[55]

In today's Japan the explosion of interest in aesthetic surgery is related closely to the argument about whether aesthetic surgery can indeed create "happiness" in banishing the negative *jibyo*. As elsewhere in Asia, the search is not limited to the world of authorized medicine. Thus there are now "aesthetic salons [that] cater to Japanese women seeking a new look, a new face or a new body. . . . Yet unlike in the past, women who pay for services at these controversial places are not afraid to talk about it if only anonymously. Most seem to believe that cosmetic surgery will open career doors and put a sparkle into their social life."[56] One case report can suffice:

> One 22-year-old woman, who asked to be identified only as Mariko, said she had cosmetic surgery six months ago to widen her eyes, lift her nose and chin, and slim her cheeks. She explained

that since she was a teenager, she had 'hated' her own face and had been working to save money for cosmetic surgery. She put ¥1 million toward the ¥1.5 million operation and is paying off the rest in installments. Her decision to go under the knife was also prompted partly by a desire to land a job as a receptionist, and she thought having better looks would improve her chances. After the operation, she promptly got a job. A photograph of her before surgery showed a different woman, at least from the chin up. Some friends complimented her on her new look, but others pointed out the inevitable: beneath the surface, she had not changed. Her father, she claims, did not even notice that she had had surgery.

But are such patients really happy? Can you really change your *taishitsu*?

Dr. Ichiro Kamoshita, a physician who is the director of the Hibiya Kokusai Clinic, believes that women patients "are being duped by cosmetic surgery and aesthetic salon advertising that appeals to a woman's inferiority complex about her looks. Many women believe that if they improve their looks their personal relations with other people will also improve. . . . They are seeking a sense of social achievement while wishing to be lovely as a woman." Nachiko Morikawa, director of another medical clinic, noted that "they don't have a clear vision of what happiness is." The skeptical attitude of the medical profession mirrors a generation shift of attitude toward aesthetic surgery in Japan.

The changes are mirrored to a great extent in not only cultural presuppositions but in the new gender politics.[57] The ongoing popularity of aesthetic surgery in Japan has led "an increasing number of Japanese mothers [to] take their straight-A 15-year-old daughters to a cosmetic surgeon."[58] There is now a pattern of presenting procedures as gifts from parents to children, especially those seen to be "hindered by small eyes, a flat nose or a big face." In April and May, at the beginning of the school year, there is a run on aesthetic surgery for teenagers. "It was just amazing to see this many young girls at my clinic all of a sudden. I felt there was something funny going on around mid-March, so I asked my assistant to go through the files. The number [of customers], by the

end of the month, had tripled [in 1997] compared with the previous year," said Fumihiko Umezawa, president of Jujin Hospital
and chair of the International Cosmetic Surgery Association.
"And what surprised me even more was the fact that they were
the graduates of those prestigious top-ranking junior-high
schools. They weren't girls dreaming of becoming a TV star or a
magazine model. They were serious, innocent-looking girls with
their mothers." The mother of a fifteen-year-old girl told the
weekly magazine *Focus:* "Well, I did feel psychological resistance
[in myself], but she really wanted it and I couldn't tell her no.
After all, pretty women have a better time in this world, don't
they? I asked my husband to stop smoking to cover the amount
necessary for her operation."[59] The daughter, on the other hand,
insists that such operations are nothing special for her generation.
"It's like piercing your ears. Everyone is doing it now. I cannot
understand why some people make a big fuss out of it." The actual number of patients is relatively large. Forty-five fifteen-year-
olds came to Jujin in March 1997, compared to fifteen in March
1996. And twenty-nine girls were treated during the holiday
week in May, but there was a waiting list of an additional eighty-
one. The assumption of vanity as the basis for desiring procedures is still present in Japanese medicine, but the patients are
now understanding such procedures as truly "cosmetic" and not
a sign of class identity.[60]

Body imagery follows the lines of political and cultural power.
In Vietnam, after the American withdrawal and the reunification
of the country, a detailed physiognomic study determined the relative facial dimensions of the Vietnamese so as to provide an adequate, non-Westernizing model for the relationship among the
features, including the form and shape of the eyes, for aesthetic
surgeons.[61] This was clearly in response to the explosion in aesthetic surgery, which remade the faces and breasts of the young
women of Vietnam into "Western" faces and bodies. Although
there was a lively aesthetic surgery industry in Saigon until 1975,
it virtually vanished after the end of the war.

In contemporary Vietnam, the function of aesthetic surgery has
become "normalized." Indeed, reports from Hanoi claim that

even the criminals undergo aesthetic surgery.[62] The nose and the eye remain at the center of concern with the reconstitution of the face in today's Vietnam. "It is the opposite of the Europeans," Nguyen Huy Phan, one of the leading aesthetic surgeons in Hanoi stated to an interviewer. "Here plastic surgery increases the size of the nose, Europeanizing it. We make a superior double eyelid, with a groove, to give a livelier appearance and to awaken the glance."[63] The costs of such procedures are quite low. To have a nose rebuilt in Hanoi costs about one hundred dollars, "Westernizing" the eyelids, forty dollars. Such procedures, however, do not assure successful transformation of the psyche. "We only operate when it's reasonable, otherwise we have to send them to the psychiatrist," Nguyen Huy Phan said. Today in Ho Chi Minh City (formerly Saigon) there are a dozen mini-clinics, sometimes masquerading as barber shops and staffed by lay surgeons. Their patrons are most often men. Clinic owners say that the most popular operations are for the nose, the chin, the eyes, and the buttocks. One man even asked surgeons to bulk up his chest, which he believed would make him more attractive to women. A popular operation in southern Vietnam, too, is to have the eyes widened by creating the Western eyelid (the superior palpebral fold). Such procedures are especially popular with male stage performers. Nguyen Thu Huong, who owns one of the "beauty salons," claimed that 80 percent of the young performers of a popular drama style known as "cai luong" and some singers have paid her a visit for Westernizing procedures.[64]

The function aesthetic surgery serves as a marker of the shift to a market economy, with its claims of individual autonomy (as opposed to state control), can also be measured in the People's Republic of China with the liberalization after the death of Mao Tsetung. Ruyao Song, president of the Chinese Plastic Surgery Society, noted in 1994 that "altering eyelids is the most popular cosmetic surgery practiced at [my] Institute of Plastic Surgery in Peking, which with 400 beds is among the largest plastic surgery hospitals in the world."[65] The explosion of interest in aesthetic surgery in the People's Republic is to no little degree a sign of the increasing affluence of the general population. It has fueled an explosion of "beauty parlors [that] offer cheap cosmetic surgery promising miraculous outcomes but often mutilating their customers."[66] Ten cosmetic surgery parlors were set up in Shanghai in the early months of 1996, but when eight hundred beauty parlors opened within one year in Sichuan province's capital city, Chengdu, the municipality began to try to regulate them after numerous patient complaints.[67] In the southeastern city of Shenzhen, a "quack" named Hu Jinsong performed breast augmentation surgery in 1995 and 1996.[68] According to his account, he used a "sophisticated and top-quality" procedure, which removed body fat by liposuction and injected it into the breasts. This was supposed to reduce obesity while enhancing breast size. "The operation is simple," the ads said. "There is no hospitalization or scars and the surgery does not affect normal life and work afterwards." His patients wound up hospitalized when the procedures went horribly awry. Hu had gone to university but had no medical credentials. The most popular aesthetic surgical procedures in these new clinics are the "double-eyelid operation" and nose-bridge surgery, in which a bone graft is shaved from a patient's hip or rib to augment the existing nose. Unlike at the Institute of Plastic Surgery, aesthetic surgery in these establishments is undertaken by marginally qualified or unqualified practitioners. Even though recently China's cabinet-level State Council has put beauty parlors under the management of public health departments, abuses continue to mount. Local hospitals also participate in the beauty business, and hospital beauty centers do not need to even register with local industry and commerce administrative departments.

Aesthetic surgical procedures to modify the "Chinese" eye had been widely carried out elsewhere among Chinese communities in Asia. Khoo Boo-Chai is the Singaporean surgeon who developed the modern double eyelid modification about forty years ago in the midst of the American occupation of Japan and the Korean War. He stitched along the eyelid to create a fine line of scars, which provided the appearance of a supratarsal fold. He wrote in 1963, "Our Eastern sisters put on Western apparel, use western make-up, see Western movies and read Western literature. Nowadays, there even exists a demand for the face and especially the eyes to be Westernized."[69] The specific reason for such aesthetic surgical procedures was the ability to increase one's income or marriageability by looking more Western and thus to ensure "personal happiness."[70]

The "Asian" development of aesthetic surgery as a sign of the modern is paralleled by the focus on the alteration of the body among the new immigrants labeled by American census law as "Asian Americans." Thus, Vietnamese in the United States show a similar fascination with the newest and latest developments in aesthetic surgery. The fascination with skin lightening, nose lengthening, and eye reshaping in Japan and Vietnam today reflects the globalization of standards of beauty rooted in Euro-American stereotypes. In the case of the youth of Japan and Vietnam, the ideal is not to be "too Asian." In the United States, this desire is more directly shaped by the notion of fitting into a niche of an acceptable "American" physiognomy. As with many of the "ethnic"-specific procedures, they are undertaken by ethnic, here Vietnamese-American, surgeons. One such case, in the large Vietnamese-American community in Houston, has now made it to the courts.[71] The forty-eight-year-old Chau Truong claimed that Ho Tan Phuoc's insertion of a plastic nasal bridge caused massive infections and scarring. Her goal was to look like Dr. Phuoc's wife, "with her Vietnamese slenderness, Anglo features, and miraculously round breasts," whose image graced the Phuocs' large ad in a Vietnamese-language newspaper. "The thought of a Vietnamese-speaking doctor encouraged her. Even more alluring, there was a photo of Victoria Phuoc, bounteous in a tight pearl-colored gown, wide eyes glowing over a razor-straight, divinely symmetrical nose." The result of the surgery was the opposite: massive infection and, when the implant was removed, "a grisly, vertical dent in its place." This case and others have become the focus of debates about the politics of the Vietnamese-American community more than about medical malpractice, yet it is not accidental that keyed to a politics of appearance all of this remains linked to the ability to "pass" as not *too* Vietnamese.

A parallel development can be found in the Republic of Korea

(South Korea) which has the largest single group (430) of aesthetic surgeons to be found in Asia in the 1990s.[72] The alterations of the nose and eyelid have become a major source of income for the physicians of the new economies of Asia. With the movement of Korea onto the global stage during the 1980s, the globalization of Korean advertising brought images of the Western face into the culture as part of the new middle-class ideal. In the United States, Korean Americans, like other groups of new immigrants, began to offer eyelid surgery to their teenage children "to make their eyes look 'more American.'"[73] Such ideals seem less present in Korea (or Vietnam or Japan) among the middle class. There, aesthetic surgery is a sign of middle-class rather than "American" identity, though one could argue that there is a fatal parallelism between these two ideas of imagining oneself as different. Thus, among Asian Americans in California, double-eyelid surgery has become "the gift that parents offer their daughters when they graduate from high school or college."[74] This parallels the experience of Jewish Americans in the 1960s. For the Vietnamese and Koreans in America, aesthetic surgery becomes a means of defining the flexibility of identity as opposed to its permanence.

The most striking recent literary representation of the anxiety about the composite "Asian" body in an American context is to be found in Gish Jen's novel *Mona in the Promised Land* (1996).[75] Jen ironically comments on the American construction of a "pan-Asian" body out of the varied and "different" bodies present in China and Japan. But this is possible only because the inherent comparison in the novel reflects on the function of aesthetic surgery in the acculturation of "Jews" and "Asians." Set in suburban Scarsdale in 1968, the novel chronicles the adolescence of a Chinese-American woman whose family moves into a "Jewish" neighborhood in its quest for upward social mobility. The protagonist identifies strongly with the Jews in her peer group and sees her body in terms of their anxiety about their own physical visibility. One day she and her friends sit around and discuss aesthetic surgery. "'Do Chinese have operations to make their noses bigger?' someone asks" (p. 92). Yes, Mona replies: "She too envies the aquiline line . . . in fact she envies even their preoperative noses. . . . 'You can't mean like this schnozz here?' somebody says, exhibiting his profile. . . . She nods politely. 'And your eyes too.'" She continues to explain about "operations to make single-fold eyelids into double-folds." In this course of this discussion, Gish Jen supplies an ironic environmental explanation of how and why "Oriental" eyes have their specific form, but concludes with one of the Jewish boys commenting about Mona's eyes: "You look like straight out of the Twilight Zone" (p. 93). The exoticism of the "too-small" nose and the "too-Oriental" eyes for the Jews is a clear marker of their sense of their own difference.

It is no surprise in this world as seen from Gish Jen's perspective that it is not Mona who gets the new nose or Western eyes: "Barbara Gugelstein is sporting a fine new nose. Straight, this is, and most diminutive, not to say painstakingly fashioned as a baby-grand tchotchke" (p. 124). Although Mona "admires her friend's nostrils, which are a triumph of judiciousness and taste," she herself is not moved to have aesthetic surgery. What Mona does is to convert to Judaism. But becoming a Jew in religion but not physicality, as one of the African-American characters disparagingly comments, is difficult in her world. For in order to be a "real" Jew "that nose of yours has got to grow out so big you've got to sneeze in a dish towel" (p. 137). Jewishness means belonging to a visible outsider group. For Mona this has become an insider group, which defines her sense of her own body. The role of aesthetic surgery is to reshape the external visibility of that group. Yet, as the novel shows, it is a sign of false acculturation. Barbara's nose job is faulty; it "runs extraordinarily when she cries" (p. 237). Jews with short noses remain marked as Jews in this seemingly hostile world, and the Chinese, such as Mona's physician-sister, acculturate with the rise of multiculturalism by becoming "Asian-American," a form of the alteration of identity without the alteration of the body. Happiness is becoming something else, something identifiable as "Asian" that is not too "Chinese." It is fitting in—and having a nose that enables you to do so. In the fictional world representing the imaginary body of the American Jew, the retroussé "Oriental" nose comes to be an ideal. But for the Chinese American, according to Gish Jen's portrait, it is a sign of the new "Asian" identity. One nose *does* fit all.

BLACK INTO WHITE

Disguising of the African nose becomes a concern of American aesthetic surgeons at the close of the nineteenth century. Black was not beautiful, and those whose skin was light enough to "pass" often attempted to do so. In the United States, there was an explosion of hair straightening and skin lightening among African Americans at the beginning of the twentieth century. The drive to look less black put cosmetology, but not necessarily aesthetic surgery, at the command of those who desired to acquire happiness by approximating a "white" appearance. The cosmetologist Madame C. J. Walker (1867–1919), with her hair straighteners and skin lighteners, became the first African-American millionaire.[76] (Today in Hong Kong and Taiwan, aesthetic surgeons undertake skin lightening using methods similar to Madame Walker's.) The gradual introduction of procedures to enable individuals to "pass" as white came to play a role in the shaping of aesthetic surgery. At the end of the twentieth century, it is no longer the intent to be (in)visible but rather not to be too visible— one should not look too black or too ethnic (however that is defined).[77] Here one can apply Werner Sollors's view that self-avowed ethnic identity in the United States became possible only with acculturation.[78] Once the stigma of ethnic identity (however defined) was removed from a group, that group could begin to think of itself as ethnically distinct, but not too distinct.

Anxiety about changing the shape of the nose was rooted in notions of the permanence of racial markers. In early twentieth-century discussions of "mixed races," it was often the "impure" physiognomy that gave a clue to the decline of the pure races through miscegenation. Thus M. L. Ettler commented in 1904 that the "lack of physical beauty in Central Europe has its roots in unnecessary racial mixing."[79] This can be seen in "disharmonies of various types" such as a "long face with a short nose." He demands "psychical and aesthetic racial selection." For racial selection is also the perpetuation of "good" character and "appropriate" noses. In the United States and in Germany, where "racial mixing" had resulted in "mixed-race" individuals with perceived qualities of both races, there was a constant anxiety about having "black" or "Jewish" features. To be seen as "mixed race" was to be seen as being of lower moral character.

The origin of the "correction" of the black nose is masked within the medical literature. No reputable surgeon in the United States wanted to be seen as facilitating crossing the color bar in the age of post-Reconstruction "Jim Crow" and "miscegenation" laws. This is very different from the situation, which we shall discuss later, of the Jews in Germany, whose civil emancipation and legal status had been clarified (if not accepted) by the same period. In 1892, the New York surgeon Robert F. Weir proposed a procedure for the restoration of "sunken noses without scarring the face."[80] This procedure altered the sunken nose through the introduction of an implant, and dealt quite explicitly with syphilitic noses. Weir also discussed the alteration of the nasal alae (wings). The operation resulted in a "parrot nose," which made his patient look "black." A further surgical intervention to shave the nostrils remedied this problem. When the Berlin Jewish surgeon Jacques Joseph (1865–1934) in 1931 reported on Weir's paper, he described it as a "method of correcting abnormally-flared nasal alae (Negroid nose) by means of sickle-shaped vertical excisions."[81] Weir's procedure to reconstruct the syphilitic nose was thus also seen as an intervention to enable black noses to "pass."[82]

The history of the racial nose and early aesthetic surgery in the United States is one of understatement and dissimulation. In 1934 Jacques W. Maliniak (1889–1976) noted that "the nose has strong and easily discernible racial characteristics. In an alien environment these may be highly detrimental to its possessor. A negroid nose is a distinct social and economic handicap to a dark-skinned Caucasian."[83] Or, one might add, to someone desiring to cross the color bar. The counter-case was also true. Henry Schireson noted

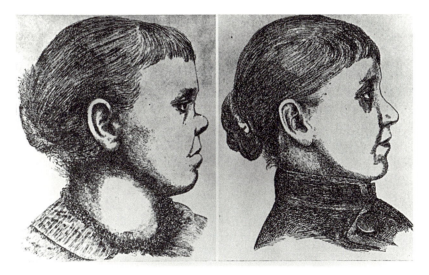

Robert F. Weir and the rebuilding of the saddle nose using the "Martin's nasal supporter," 1892.

that one of his patients, a nurse, had massive freckles. She wished to have her freckles removed: "the excess pigmentation in the lower layers of her otherwise perfect skin was interfering with her work. In a dim light she looked to some of her patients like a mulatto."[84] Perhaps she was indeed someone trying to cross the color bar.

The discourse on "passing" in the age after the introduction of aesthetic surgery is notable in its demand for ever more strictly identifiable and immutable physical characteristics of mixed-race individuals. Thus, in a letter dated September 26, 1935 from the eugenicist Harry Laughlin (1880–1943) to Madison Grant (1865–1937), the author of *The Passing of the Great Race; or, The Racial Basis of European History* (1916), Laughlin informed him that "Stanton D. Wicks, an animal breeder from Syracuse, New York," was going to Virginia to "make some field studies on the determination or identification of 'pass-for-white individuals.' At present the Virginia law which defines a colored person as 'any one of whose ancestors are colored' has to depend in its diagnosis of pass-for-whites mainly on definite negro signs among the near blood-kin; upon associates and reputation; and lastly upon personal qualities."[85] What Wicks intends to search for are "signs of colored blood whether the criterion be anatomical, chemical, mental or temperamental—but mainly physical and chemical." Tracing the "black within" would be "applicable to other races beside the negro." If, however, the physical body can be disguised through surgery, then the identification of those "passing" can only be made through either circumstantial or "chemical" means. The need for a litmus test for race was made more urgent by the ability to alter the body surgically.

The notion of permanent racial markers becomes vital in societies that desire to impose racial classifications as social norms. Thus in South Africa under apartheid, the flair of a nostril could brand one as "black." Jack Penn (who has developed the first modern decircumcision procedure, as we shall discuss later) recounted the story of a patient who came to him with the request that he narrow her nostrils.[86] "Her nose was small and her nostrils slightly flared, but I felt it suited her face, and said so. Under the circumstances, therefore, there was no point in performing an operation which I felt was unnecessary." The young woman "burst into tears." When she had decided to marry, her abusive father shouted at her that "today no white man would marry a coloured girl." In stunned amazement, the young lass asked her father what he meant. The answer was "Ask your mother, and look at your nose, and you will see what I mean." Her mother informed her that she was "coloured." The operation was undertaken, her "overwhelming fixation" on her nose was remedied, and the surgeon received "a letter from the Eastern Province to say that this couple was happily married." "Passing" was now possible—by a nose.

When "black became beautiful," in the 1970s, there was also a change in the meaning ascribed to aesthetic surgery for the African American. The shift to the "ethnic-specific" aesthetic surgery of the 1980s introduced procedures such as lip-thinning that were clearly attempts to approximate "white" categories of beauty. Although other black-skin-specific procedures, such as removal of the upper layer of the skin (dermabrasion) for disfiguring skin bumps (pseudofollicultitis barbae) were introduced for men, the majority of ethnic-specific procedures remained aesthetic. Rhinoplasty is still the procedure of choice. African-American clients in the 1990s (like Penn's patient in the 1960s) complain that "the base of their nose is excessively wide, particularly with regard to the rest of the face."[87] In one paper that presented the preoperative complaints of 134 "non-Caucasian" individuals seeking rhinoplasties over a period of sixteen years, the "black" noses were labeled as "wide and flat nasal dorsum, flared ala, increased interalar distance and a nasal tip with little projection and definition."[88] Thus, according to such patient observations, there seems to be the need for "tip defattening" as well as a resectioning of the base of the nose. The risk of a poor outcome of aesthetic surgery is heightened among Africans and African Americans because many have a tendency to develop raised and obvious scars (keloids).

Still, such operations are regularly undertaken, often against the objection of the families. The Jewish aesthetic surgeon Robert Goldwyn recounts the case of a "twenty-one-year-old black aspiring model" who wanted her "nose less Negroid."[89] Her family strenuously objected, as "they felt she was abandoning her heritage, in particular the family nose." Goldwyn commented that "they object to Sara for wanting a nose that is not typically black. Why deny their inalienable right to inconsistency?" The notion of a consistent racial type haunts a world obsessed with "passing." In today's America the anxiety about being seen as trying to "pass" is tied to the notion of consistency. Like the earlier risk of being scarred and thus revealing to the world one's desire to "pass," the inconsistent nose marks one as different.

Such a position can pose a true dilemma. One of the leading spokespeople for the New Critical Race theory, Patricia J. Williams, professor of law at Columbia University, notes that she is anxious about the "morality" in the "morass" of African Americans who turn to aesthetic surgery: "What made it 'the very worst kind' of assimilationism was that it was also assimilation out of the very right to coexist in the world with that most basic legacy of our own bodies. What made it so bad was the unselfconscious denial of those violent social pressures that make so irresistible the 'choice' to cut off that perfect replica of one's grandmother's nose in favor of a trendier, more 'acceptable' model."[90] She condemns the autonomy ("self-assertion") preached by the "eager plastic surgeon" who advocated "the choice to go under the knife. 'Just say yes to yourself,' he glowed repeatedly." For her this is merely false consciousness, which is the result of the "call to conform . . . that is the perpetual risk of any socializing collective, whether family or polis." This drive to "pass" is not only the desire to "pass" as white, but to "pass" as "black." For with the emphasis on a unitary idea of "blackness" within African-American culture, the onus is not to look too "white" or too "black." Indeed "grandmother's nose" may well have been a "white" nose as well as a "black" nose, given the history of miscegenation in America. Here the problem of inconsistency turns out to be purely ideological. Goldwyn and Williams have their norms of "blackness" and do not recognize how culturally determined they are.

With the rise of a multicultural model in the United States, the meaning of the "black" nose also shifted. "New thinking on cosmetic surgery," the title of a popular essay in 1992 proclaimed, "keeps your ethnic identity."[91] Ethnic identity has value in this new world. Clients should not "have their cultural heritage erased from their faces by the wrong surgery," writes W. Earle Matory Jr., a plastic surgeon at the University of Massachusetts Medical Center. Or, as a *Living Section* essay in the *New York Times* put it in 1991, "Surgeons are learning to put the right nose on the right face."[92] The meaning of the "right face" has shifted over the past three decades.

African Americans who undertook aesthetic surgery in the 1940s and 1950s did so in order to "pass": "I don't find it advantageous," said one young African-American woman, "to have decisive Negro features. The less you look like a Negro, the less you have to fight. I would pass for anything so long as I'm not taken for a Negro. With a straight nose I could do costume work and pose as an Indian, Egyptian, or even a Balinese."[93] Such views began to shift by the 1970s, for example in the writing of the

African-American surgeon Harold E. Pierce, writing in the
(African-American) *Journal of the National Medical Association*
about the importance of "race" as a factor in "cosmetic surgery."
He found that "there are but a few required modifications in [fa-
cial cosmetic surgery]. The major difference concerns rhinoplasty."[94] Rhinoplasty, which in the past twenty years has become
the aesthetic surgical procedure most frequently performed on
African Americans, is usually used to correct patients' complaints
of "flared nostrils, prominent tip, and/or a depressed and low
nasal bridge."[95] When such perceived unaesthetic qualities are
removed, "the surgeon must be careful to avoid overcorrection
and creation of a nose that is racially incongruent."[96] The movement in the post-1970s period to an ethnic-specific cosmetic
surgery presupposed the existence of aesthetic boundaries by
which each group was defined as beautiful. Now the "black" look
has become the referent.

Thomas Rees, who claimed in 1968 that the question of African
Americans' wanting to "pass" had to do with Caucasian ideals of
beauty, came in 1986 to observe that many patients wanted to look
like other "black" role models who had come to alter their appearance: "Patients are mightily impressed with the Caucasian-
like transformation of the previously Negroid features of Michael
Jackson, the noted entertainer."[97] One "passed" now by looking
like a socially more acceptable (read: white) version of the black
nose. In 1996 African Americans accounted for 6 percent, Asian
Americans 7 percent, and Hispanics 9 percent of aesthetic surgeries. However, ethnic-specific aesthetic surgery among African
Americans is increasing—by 2 percent from 1994 to 1997.[98] One
can be "black," but "black" turns out (like "Irish" and "Jewish")
to be in the eye of the beholder and the hand of the surgeon.

Whether black, Irish, or Asian, the nose that is too small or too
flat has been altered by the aesthetic surgeon because of its "otherness" in relation to Western ideals. These ideals are not just concerned with beauty and attractiveness, but with markers of who
is and is not acceptably human, who can and cannot be trusted.
The "primitiveness" of the flat nose represents groups who are
not only fit to be kept down, but who must be so treated lest they

infect the dominant group. The danger of infection is always present, among other reasons, because the too-small, too-flat nose is the sign of the syphilis carried by those whose undisciplined sexual behavior is said to have crossed all appropriate boundaries.

Such beliefs and attitudes, continually propagated and strengthened by the relations of power and economic advantage among the world's peoples, create an ideal arena for aesthetic surgery, with its promise to help people "pass" as whoever they wish to be. The aesthetic surgeon operates in a world in which everyone's appearance is charged with meaning, most profoundly the meaning of who can and cannot be honored with acceptance as an equal. Let's now look at how questions of honor, especially the honor of full citizenship in the modern nation-state, have centered around another sort of "abnormal" nose, one that is not too small but entirely too big.

CHAPTER FOUR

Marks of Honor and Dishonor

CHARACTER INSCRIBED ON THE FACE

BEFORE WE EXPLORE the surgi-
cal history of the too-long nose, let's explore one of our most en-
during collective beliefs in our ability to read character in the face:
the moral weakness written on the noses of "topers" and Jews;
the manliness and moral worthiness inscribed in the dueling scar.
No pathology of the "too-big nose" has a clearer reading in the
nineteenth and early twentieth century as a sign of "dishonorable" character than rhinophyma, the growth of tumors on the
nose.[1] This too-big nose, called "red-nose" or "toper's nose," has
been long associated with heavy drinking and "bad" character.
Although W. C. Fields (1879–1946) found it a winning visual
trademark in films of the 1930s and 1940s, the banker J. Pierpont
Morgan (1837–1913) was caricatured with it as a sign of his moral
weakness.[2] The "red bulbous nose" is actually a symptom of the
skin disorder rosacea.[3] But the persistent popular association of
it with moral decay ensures that a confidence man is described by
his nose: "short, squat, cigar-smoking man with a heavy Southern drawl, thinning gray hair, a red, bulbous nose like W. C.
Fields' and a fondness for light orange sports jackets."[4] Even the
president of the United States can be criticized in this way. "Also,
what's with President Clinton's nose? He looks like W. C. Fields.
It's—I don't know; study it."[5] If Bill Clinton has the nose of W. C.
Fields, the epitome of the leering, self-indulgent drunkard, then
clearly he must have just as dishonorable a character.

Beginning in the 1840s surgeons recognized that such tumors

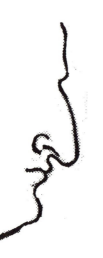

George Jabet, writing as Eden Warwick, characterized the "Jewish, or Hawknose" as "very convex, and preserves its convexity like a bow, throughout the whole length from the eyes to the tip. It is thin and sharp." Shape also carried here a specific meaning: "It indicates considerable Shrewdness in worldly matters; a deep insight into character, and facility of turning that insight to profitable account."

could be "shaved" and that the nose could be reshaped with skin flaps carefully preserved from the skin of the side of the nose. The American surgeon John Orlando Roe (1849–1915) discovered that such flaps were superfluous and that shaving the tumors sufficed to change the face of a drunkard into one of a good family man. One could disguise the drunkard—but could one change his character? The implicit analogy was powerful, and it resonated with similar queries about racial difference.

Could racial difference, which was understood as indelibly written on the body, be altered? Could one actually change the Jewish character by changing the Jewish nose? In the late nine-

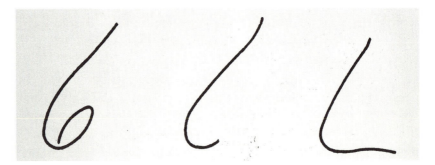

The creation of the "nostrility" of the Jew, and its unmaking, at least in caricature.

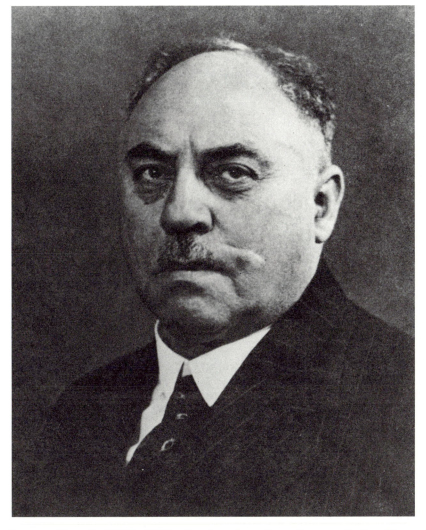

Jacques Joseph (1865–1934), the founder of modern aesthetic rhino-plasty. Note the dueling scars in the formal portrait.

teenth century the too-long nose was often read as the natural sign of the Jew. John Orlando Roe characterized the "Jewish nose" as the sign of "commercialism or desire of gain."[6] The material-ism of the Jew was the impetus for the development of a second set of surgical interventions to change the character, or at least the appearance, of the nose. It was undertaken on Jews or those who looked "too Jewish," whether or not they were Jews. The key visual stereotype of the Jew that had to be unmade was the feature nineteenth-century scientists labeled "nostrility." At the close of the nineteenth century, the size and shape of the Jew's nose were signs that everyone, including Jewish physicians, associated with the Jew's character and permanent visibility within society.[7]

The means to change the nose, and perhaps the character, was supplied by Jacques Joseph (1865–1934), a highly acculturated young German Jewish surgeon practicing in fin de siècle Berlin. Born Jakob Joseph, he had altered his too-Jewish name when he studied medicine in Berlin and Leipzig. Joseph was a typical acculturated Jew of the period, and he understood the cultural signification of marks of honor and of dishonor. At the university he, like many Jewish students, had joined a conservative dueling fraternity, and he bore the scars of his saber dueling with pride. (Jews were at that time admitted to the general fraternity systems in Germany.) Indeed, he must have appeared much like Kunz, the oldest Jewish sibling in Thomas Mann's (1875–1955) vaguely anti-Semitic novella "The Blood of the Walsungs" (1905), "a stunning tanned creature with curling lips and a killing scar."[8] As Mann describes him, he remains essentially Jewish in spite of his scar.

Like many acculturated Jews, such as the founder of Zionism, Theodor Herzl (1860–1904), Joseph "relished the test and adventure of the duel, the so-called *Mensur,* which was considered manly and edifying."[9] The scars (*Schmisse*) from the *Mensur* were intentionally created. Students challenged each other to duels as a matter of course, without any real need for insults to be exchanged. Being challenged was a process of social selection. "Without exclusivity—no corporation," was the code of the fraternities as late as 1912.[10] The duelists had their eyes and throat protected, but their faces were purposely exposed to the blade of the saber. When a cut was made, it was treated so as to maximize the resulting scar. The scar that Joseph bore his entire life marked him as someone who was *satisfaktionsfähig* (worthy of satisfaction), someone who had been seen as an honorable equal and thus had been challenged to a duel. Marked on the duelist's face was his integration into German culture.

The more marginal you were the more you wanted to be scarred. In 1874 William Osler (1849–1919), then a young Canadian medical student visiting Berlin, described "one hopeful young Spanish American of my acquaintance [who] has one half of his face—they are usually on the left half—laid out in the most irregular manner, the cicatrices running in all directions, enclosing areas of all shapes,—the relics of fourteen duels!"[11] Such scarring was not extreme among the medical students of the day. The scar marked the individual, even within the medical faculty, as a hardy member of the body politic. This was the context in which the Jewish fraternities (most of which did not duel) sought to reconstitute the sickly Jewish body into what the early Zionist Max Nordau (1849–1923) called the "new muscle Jew." The Jewish fraternity organization stated in 1902 that "it desires the physical education of its members in order to collaborate in the physical regeneration of the Jewish people."[12] For some Jews, a dueling scar marked the socially healthy individual.

At the very close of the nineteenth century, after Joseph and Herzl left the university, Jewish men were strenuously excluded from the Christian dueling fraternities. Being a member of a fraternity, like being an officer in the army, was a sign of truly belonging to the in-group in the society. It was a sign of being a German. With the expulsion of the Jews from the dueling fraternities, this sign of belonging was denied to Jewish men at the close of the nineteenth century. In 1896 the Christian dueling fraternities had accepted the following proposal: "In full appreciation of the fact that there exists between Aryans and Jews such a deep moral and psychic difference, and that our qualities have suffered so much through Jewish mischief, in full consideration of the many proofs which the Jewish student has also given of his lack of honor and character and since he is completely void of honor according to our German concepts, today's conference . . . resolves: 'No satisfaction is to be given to a Jew with any weapon, as he is unworthy of it.'"[13] Jews are different and thus dishonorable; they are unworthy of satisfaction, even if those with facial scars look just like "real" Germans. The visible scar advertises and guarantees the purity of the group. Because Jews cannot be pure, they must be denied the right to scar and to be scarred in duels. For a Jew to bear a facial scar is to hide his sickly essence from the mainstream. This duplicity is what is meant by Jewish "mischief."

By the 1920s such seemingly "false" scarring came to be part of the German discourse on aesthetic surgery. The aesthetic surgeon Ludwig Lévy-Lenz tells the tale of a young man who came to him after having won money in the lottery, and wanted him to create artificial dueling scars through a "cosmetic" procedure.[14] In this way, he could "pass" as someone who was worthy of being challenged to a duel. Lévy-Lenz refused to do the surgery and the young man went to a barber who scarred him with a straight razor and in doing so severely damaged his salivary glands. The visible scar enabled the young man to "pass" as a man of honor. But was it an authentic mark of honor or merely cosmetic? Can the essentially "dishonorable" character be changed by changing the nose or the face in which society reads character inscribed?

Too-Jewish Ears and Noses

The scarred Jacques Joseph was trained as an orthopedic surgeon under Julius Wolff (1836–1902), one of the leaders in the field. In 1893 Julius Wolff developed a surgical procedure to correct the "saddle nose," which followed up James Israel's (1848–1926) earlier work repairing the syphilitic nose in the mid 1880s. Wolff's major surgical innovation was not cutting the graft from the forehead, thus avoiding a telltale scar.[15] More important, he established the "law of the transformation of the skeleton," which stated that every function of the skeleton could be described through the laws of mechanics and that any change in the relationship between single components of the skeleton would lead to a functional and physiological change of the external form of the entire skeleton.[16] Wolff's wide-ranging contributions to the practices of his day included developing a therapeutic procedure for correcting a club foot with the use of a specialized dressing

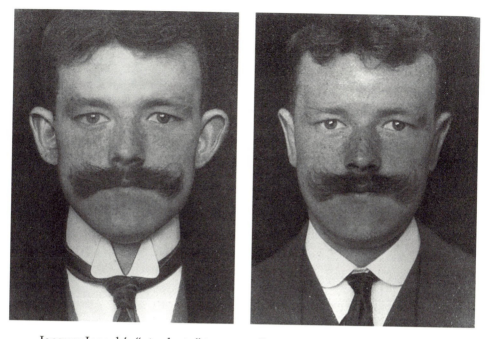

Jacques Joseph's "otoplasty" to correct "otopostasis," the abnormal projection of the ears, so-called donkey-ears.

that altered the very shape of the foot.[17] Orthopedics, more than any other medical specialty of the period, presented the challenge of altering the visible errors of development so as to restore a "normal" function.

Joseph's interests did not lie with the foot (even though it was another sign of Jewish inferiority), but with other parts of the anatomy. In 1896 he undertook a corrective procedure on a young child with protruding ears, which, although successful, caused him to be dismissed as Wolff's assistant. Joseph's procedure was his own, but it paralleled the work of the American otorhinolaryngologist Edward Talbot Ely (1850–85) who had corrected a "bat ear deformity" on a twelve-year-old boy in 1881. Ely undertook the procedure because the child had been "ridiculed by his companions."[18] In Berlin in the 1890s this sort of operation was seen as "beauty" rather than "real" surgery.[19] When Joseph was dismissed, he was told by his Jewish supervisor, Julius Wolff, that

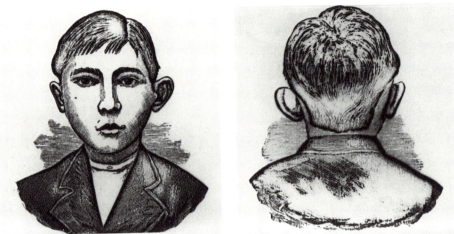

Fig. 1. Front view, after first operation to set back right ear   Fig. 2. Rear view, after first operation to set back right ear

The correction of the "bat ear," by Edward T. Ely.

one simply did not undertake surgical procedures for vanity's sake. Correcting a child's protruding ears was not in the same class as correcting a functional disability, such as a club foot, or reconstructing the external ear, which had been a major problem for surgeons from the earliest written accounts.[20] (The congenital absence of the external ear, the microtia, was often attributed to hereditary syphilis. This would have been grounds to operate!)

Yet according to the child's mother, he had suffered from humiliation in school because of his protruding ears. It was the child's unhappiness with being different that Joseph was correcting. Abnormally big and protruding ears alone might account for the child's "unhappiness." But it was the specific cultural meaning of protruding ears at the close of the nineteenth century that added insult to injury.

An old European trope about the shape of the Jew's ears can be found throughout the anti-Semitic literature of the fin de siècle. The racial anthropologist Hans Günther summarized the turn-of-the-century view that Jews, especially the males, have "fleshy ear lobes" and "large, red ears" more frequently than other peoples do. They have "prominent ears that stick out." According to Günther, prominent ears are especially prevalent among "Jewish children; one refers to them in Austria as 'Moritz ears.'"[21] Moritz (Morris) was a typical Jewish name of the day. "Moritz ears" are "elongated ears" that appear as "ill-shapen ears of great size like those of a bat," according to an English-language anti-Semitic text of 1888.[22]

In his major paper of 1910 on the correction of "prominent ears," William H. Luckett of New York comments obliquely about the "odium attached to these ears."[23] In the American context, these may have been the jug-ears that dominated the caricatures of the Irish in American culture (and which, as we have seen, Irish aesthetic surgeons continue to treat aggressively in modern Eire). They may also have been the ears of the Jewish immigrants on New York's lower East Side. They were a visible and repugnant sign of difference; a difference ascribed to the character as well as to the body. Luckett reports that one of his patients suffered "the constant harassing by classmates [that] frequently is the cause of so much distress as to produce a very bad mental condition in the child as well as in the parents, and to warrant our surgical interference." The strife that a big-eared child sows among his classmates spreads so much unhappiness in the world that the surgeon's larger duty, as well as the needs of his patient, demands that he operate.

The "scientific" belief in the visibility of the ear as a racial marker is also a major subtheme of one of the major works satirizing the world of turn-of-the-century Prussia, Heinrich Mann's (1871–1950) *Man of Straw* (1918).[24] In that novel, Mann's self-serving convert, Jadassohn (Judas's son?) "looks so Jewish" (p. 85) because of his "huge, red, prominent ears" (p. 86) which he eventually has cosmetically reduced. He goes to Paris to have this procedure done. Mann clearly intends the ugly ears to be read as a sign of the Jew's lack of good character. They give the lie to any claim of conversion away from Jewishness. They mirror the shallow characterlessness of the Jewish parvenu. Jadassohn is put down as merely "witty" (p. 87), just as other Jews in the novel are "too clever" (p. 57). The Jew's ears are signs of his superficiality, a sign recognized by the other characters in the novel as a reason to mock and taunt him.

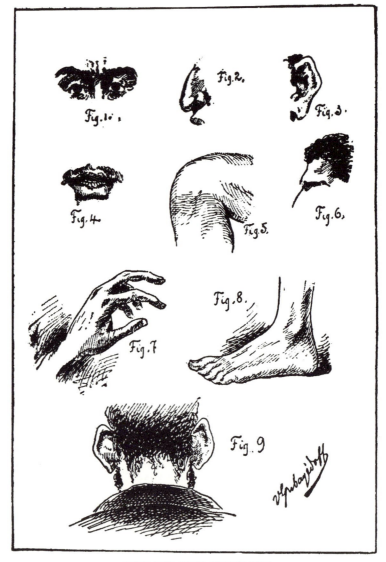

HOW WE MAY KNOW HIM.

Fig. 1. Restless suspicious eyes.	**Fig. 5.** Round knees.
Fig. 2. Curved nose and nostrils.	**Fig. 6.** Low brow.
Fig. 3. Ill-shapen ears of great size like those of a bat.	**Fig. 7.** Long clammy fingers.
	Fig. 8. Flat feet.
Fig. 4. Thick lips and sharp rat's teeth.	**Fig 9.** Repulsive rear view.

The "ill-shapen ears of great size like those of a bat" and the "repulsive rear view" as well as other body parts of the Jew.

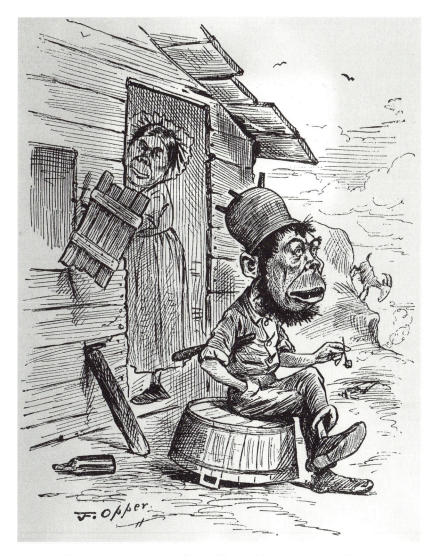

Frederick B. Opper's image of "Paddy and his wife" as "The King of A-Shantee." The pun represents the "prognathism" of the Irish as a mark of character identical to that of the "primitive" African. Note the large, projecting ears.

Heinrich Mann sends his character to France rather than Berlin for surgery. He saw the difference represented by Jadassohn as physical and identified it with the "foreign," which during World War I meant "France." "Like cures like," to follow the homeopathic model evoked in the novel. Mann also uses the name of one of the most prominent German Jewish dermatologist/ syphilologists, Josef Jadassohn (1863–1936), for the name of his character. The association of Jews with syphilis was not merely a fantasy of anti-Semitic rhetoric, which depicted Jews either as carriers of the illness or as being immune to it, but also reflected disapproval of notable *Jewish* scientists such as Adolf von Wassermann (1866–1925) and Jadassohn for choosing to study and treat such a disreputable disease.

This image of the "Jewish" ear flourished into the twentieth century. Adolf Hitler (1889–1945) was convinced that Joseph Stalin (1879–1953) was Jewish (as he claimed all Bolsheviks were), and he arranged to have photographs analyzed to see whether his earlobes were "ingrown and Jewish, or separate and Aryan."[25] Race is written clearly on the body—especially on the ear. As late as in the 1970s, in Central Europe "men request plastic operations of the ears more frequently than do women."[26] No wonder. A standard textbook on physical anthropology published in 1974 still listed the ear as a sign of Jewish racial identity: "The ear is large, wide in its upper part, and provided with a large lob."[27] From its inception, the operation on the ear has been a deracializing operation that is gendered in complex ways. It has taken on the same significance for Jewish males as the Jewish nose and the circumcised penis. It is a sign of the male child's humiliation, which comes to be coded in complex ways. The desire to "pass" as "normal," which is the result of the felt need to be completely "male," created the need for a new specialty, which would dispel psychic pain by intervening in the body of the male child. For Jewish women and girls with big ears, long hair obviated surgery and allowed them to "pass."

After being dismissed from Wolff's clinic, Joseph opened a private surgical practice in Berlin. In January 1898, a twenty-eight-year-old man came to him, having heard of the successful opera-

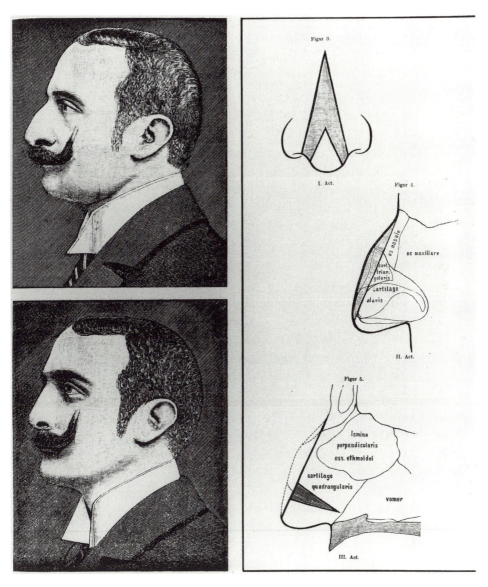

Jacques Joseph's first nose job. "Before and after" photographs and the outline of the surgical procedure.

tion on the child's ears. He complained that "his nose was the source of considerable annoyance. Wherever he went, everybody stared at him; often, he was the target of remarks or ridiculing gestures. On account of this he became melancholic, withdrew almost completely from social life, and had the earnest desire to be relieved of this deformity."[28] The symptoms were analogous to those of the young boy whose ears Joseph had repaired.

Joseph took the young man's case and performed his first reduction rhinoplasty, cutting through the skin of the nose to reduce its size and alter its shape by chipping away the bone and removing the cartilage. On May 11, 1898 he reported on this operation before the Berlin Medical Society. In that report Joseph provided a detailed "scientific" rationale for performing a medical procedure on an otherwise completely healthy individual: "The psychological effect of the operation is of utmost importance. The depressed attitude of the patient subsided completely. He is happy to move around unnoticed. His happiness in life has increased, his wife was glad to report; the patient who formerly avoided social contact now wishes to attend and give parties. In other words, he is happy over the results."[29] The patient no longer felt himself marked by the form of his nose. He was cured of the "disease" of "nostrility." In his own eyes, he looked less different from the group he desired to join—the non-Jews. Joseph had undertaken a surgical procedure that had cured his patient's psychological disorder. Yet he had left scars, which pointed to the procedure itself, and this became a major concern to Joseph. He warned his colleagues that "disclosure to the patient on the problem of scarring is very important. Many patients, however, will consider even simple scars too conspicuous."[30] He raised the specter of a court case in which the "unsightly scar might represent a greater degree of disfigurement than the enlarged cartilage [of the nose] presented previously" (p. 35). More important, surgical scars, unlike dueling scars, reveal the inauthencity of the body and the effort to "pass" through medical intervention.

On April 19, 1904 Joseph undertook his removal of a hump from within the nose using cartilaginous incisions. He retrospectively commented that in 1898 he had used the extranasal proce-

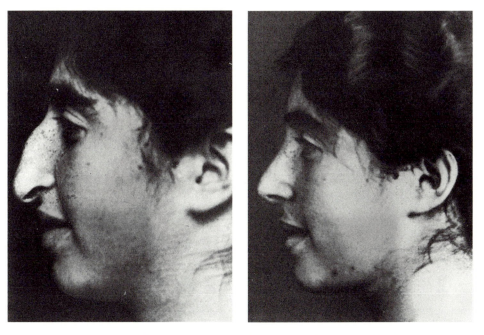

Jacques Joseph's "hanging septum of moderate degree (with abnormal length of the lateral walls, and hump nose) corrected" following bilateral segment resection ("total" shortening and hump removal).

dure, which "caused a scar, but this scar will be hardly visible after a short time, assuming that the incision is sutured exactly."[31] But "hardly visible" was not sufficient. Even the slightest scar was enough to evoke a visual memory of the too-big nose. The invisibility of the patient hinged on the elimination of the scar. Both patients needed to become (in)visible to "pass." And Joseph had learned that only (in)visibility left his patients "happy."

Joseph's claim to fame was his solution of the problem of the visible scar. His procedure to remove the bone and cartilage from within the patient's nose is still used today, as are the surgical tools he used to carry out the procedure. But others also claimed to have recognized this failing earlier and to have corrected it. His priority as the first surgeon to reduce the size of the nose by removing excess bone intranasally (from within the nose) was challenged in 1923 by Berlin surgeon Friedrich Trendelenburg

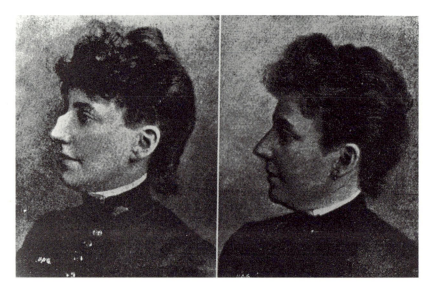

John Orlando Roe's reduction of a nasal hump through an intranasal procedure, 1891.

(1844–1924), who described undertaking (and documenting) such a procedure in 1889.[32] Joseph's procedure also paralleled one developed by John Orlando Roe (1849–1915) in upstate New York. In 1891, Roe's patient, a Miss C—— , came to him for a "winter cough," but used this apparent excuse to complain to him about the "angular, bony projection of the top" of her nose. Roe developed a procedure to shorten the nose intranasally and corrected the source of her perceived ill health and present unhappiness.[33] Roe's procedure, like Trendelenburg's, did not leave scars; this was a major difference from Joseph's initial attempts at reduction rhinoplasty. In his 1892 paper on "sunken noses," Robert F. Weir (1838–94) presented a case of "monomania" focusing on the too-large nose and his attempts to cure it by the reduction of the size of the nose.[34] But Joseph's procedure dominated the field because his patient population among the Jews in Central Europe was extensive, exposed, and anxious about their "nostrility." Large numbers of Central European Jewish patients needed to become invisible to become happy. But the men and women among them had different visions of happiness.

In his summary paper on the reduction of the size of the nose published in 1904, Joseph commented on the psychology of his male patients: "The patients were embarrassed and self-conscious in their dealings with their fellow men, often shy and unsociable, and had the urgent desire to become free and unconstrained. Several complained of sensitive drawbacks in the exercise of their profession. As executives they could hardly enforce their authority; in their business connections (as salesmen, for example), they often suffered material losses. . . . The operative nasal reduction—this is my firm conviction—will also in the future restore the joy of living to many a wretched creature and, if his deformity has been hindering him in his career, it will allow him the full exercise of his aptitudes."[35] According to Joseph, the patient "is happy to move around unnoticed." The visibility of the Jew (often defined in the nineteenth century in terms of his mercantile ability) made it impossible for him to compete equally with the non-Jew in the economic world at the turn of the century. Only vanishing into the visual norm and "passing" as non-Jewish in appearance enabled the young Jewish male to become part of the general society. "Passing" thus meant functioning more fully as a male, because masculinity was defined in economic terms.

Such a transition became possible in late nineteenth-century Germany when the legal restrictions that limited the Jew (and especially the Jewish male) were lifted. Jewish women were still bound by the limitations applied to women in late nineteenth-century Europe, but Jewish males generally could enter into the world of masculine endeavors as long as they were not too evidently Jewish. No law bound them (unlike African-American males in the United States at the same moment) from becoming officers, doctors, lawyers, or businessmen in the general society, but the powerful social stigma associated with the Jews continued in spite of civil emancipation. Thus one did not want to appear Jewish—one needed to be able to "pass" as "German." A contemporary commentator notes about Joseph's procedures, "Even today, 70 years later, one often hears the erroneous remark that rhinoplasty is an operation for vanity's sake. That is not true. Vanity is the desire to excel. The average rhinoplasty patient

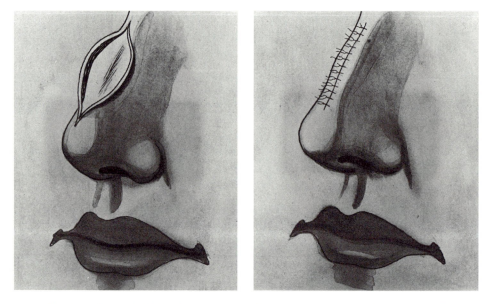

Charles Conrad Miller's image of the correction of a "hump nose" through an external incision.

wishes to be relieved of a real or imagined conspicuousness of his nose."[36] The route to happiness lay not in standing out but in blending into the dominant group whose silently taking no notice of one was the key sign of one's acceptance. Being (in)visible is being intensely visible, but as a member of a group that defines itself as the "norm," as "beautiful" and "healthy." Friedrich Nietzsche noted that we are only aware of our bodies when we become ill. This is the boundary Joseph's patients desired to cross. They wished to forget their bodies, to become one with those they imagined had no worries about the acceptability of their bodies. This is the essence of "passing," and it set the model for all aesthetic surgery for the future. In order for such a model even to appear efficacious, all awareness must be on the level of consciousness; no unconscious desire or hidden goals can influence the individual. Physical change must alter consciousness. But the male Jew's hope of "passing," of vanishing into the world of the "German," depended not just on the alteration of all-too-visible ears and noses, but on the surgeon's ability to alter the most hidden and secret aspect of the male body.

THE TELLTALE FORESKIN

The anxiety about the visibility of the Jewish nose paralleled an anxiety about the intact penis within medical discourse at the beginning of the century.[37] The nose and its surgical repair seemed a natural analogy to myths about Jewish sexuality, which haunted the medical literature of Europe.[38] Jewish sexuality, as represented by the practice of infant male circumcision, became the touchstone for the belief that Jewish social practices were the cause of the biological differences of the Jew.[39] (Circumcision is a religious, not a medical, practice for traditional Jews. Indeed, the theological understanding is that had not God commanded its practice, it would not be sanctioned under Jewish law, which prohibits *chavalah* [wounding]. The religious rationale is that circumcision "completes" the body much as grinding makes wheat usable as flour.)[40] The act of circumcision is seen by Europeans as most setting the Jews apart from Gentiles.[41] Because of this, the botched nose job became a symbolic site for the displacement of fear and unhappiness about the circumcised penis, which defined the Jewish male as the "Jew" at the turn of the century.

This cultural anxiety was but the continuation of an older response to the Western critique of circumcision as a sign of Jewish self-isolation and resulting feminization. The circumcision of the penis became the outward sign of the immutability of the Jew within. It marked the Jewish body as inherently different. Even the Jewish philosopher Benedictus de Spinoza (1632–77), in a passage often cited and commented on in the nineteenth century, labeled circumcision as the primary reason for the survival of the Jews, as "they have incurred universal hatred by cutting themselves off completely from all other peoples." It also made them "effeminate" and, like women, unlikely to assume a political role in the future.[42]

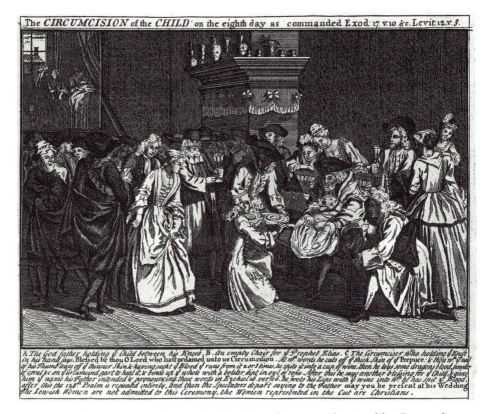

The CIRCUMCISION of the CHILD on the eighth day as commanded Exod: 17. v.10 &c. Levit 12.v.3.

A ritual circumcision in the Sephardi tradition, as depicted by Bernard Picart, 1722. Already here the image of the visibility of the male Jew's genitalia becomes part of the visual tradition of Western European art.

The repair of such a damaged and dishonorable masculinity could only be undertaken through the institution of medicine. The response was to operate. The operation to restore the foreskin and, hence, masculinity, clearly had aesthetic implications for the Jewish body. The nose job had its origin in the desire to "pass"; the complementary practice of foreskin restoration (also known as posthioplasty, epispasm, decircumcision, or preputioplasty) reappeared during the nineteenth century and responded to a similar desire.[43] Foreskin restoration can be understood as "reconstructive," as it rebuilds the prepuce, which had been removed from the infant shortly after birth; it can be understood as "aesthetic," as it restores the beauty of the body. In either case, it remedies the "unhappiness" of the patient. Indeed, such questions are even raised in the total reconstruction of the penis after it is amputated. Maxwell Maltz (1899–1975) described his procedure for the construction of a new penis (phalloplasty) out of a tubed-pedicle graft. After two or three weeks, the new penis was detached from the wall of the abdomen and "a cosmetic procedure is carried out to the tip of the 'new' penis" to make it look like—a circumcised or an uncircumcised penis?[44] That Maltz does not tell us.

Jews have practiced foreskin reconstitution for almost as long as they have practiced circumcision. Thus, there was a classical model that was evoked at the turn of the nineteenth century. The Roman physician Aulus Cornelius Celsus (25 B.C.E.–50 C.E.) recorded two surgical procedures for elongating or replicating the male foreskin. The first stretches the foreskin, incises the skin at the root of the penis, and holds it with a band until it remains in this form; the second, intended for men who had been circumcised, separates the skin at the corona of the penis from the corpora cavernose, pulls it over the glans, and fixes it in place.[45] (Celsus's concern for the beautiful body also led him to suggest procedures to correct the misshapen nose.)[46] Following the aesthetic demands of the Greek athletic games, in which circumcised men were not permitted to take part, the Hellenized Jews of the Roman Empire began to "pass" through aesthetic surgical intervention. The cultural demand was that the Jews give up their individual traditions in favor of one universal and enlightened culture. For the Jewish male, this meant masking, among other cherished traditions, his unique sign and seal of the covenant. This Greek idealization of the "natural" male form reappeared in the eighteenth century in the writings of the art critic Johann Joachim Winckelmann (1717–68). As one can see in the works of neoclassical anatomists such as Ernst Brücke (1819–92), the uncircumcised body is represented as the beautiful (read: healthy) male body in the age of aesthetic surgery. In Germany and Austria decircumcision became a means of restoring that beautiful and healthy male body.[47]

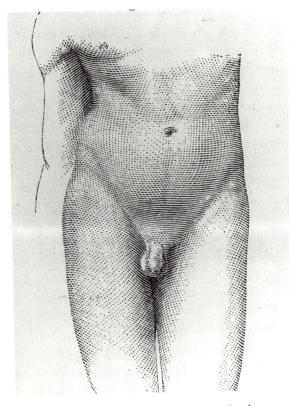

The perfect male torso, uncircumcised, of course.

Decircumcision procedures were in circulation at the close of
the nineteenth century in Germany, just as infant male circumcision became commonplace in the United States as a sign of "hygiene."[48] The text that had made the reconstitution of the prepuce
the boundary between "reconstructive" and "aesthetic" surgery
in the nineteenth century was Johann Friedrich Dieffenbach's
classic *Operative Surgery* (1845).[49] Dieffenbach's text remained the
touchstone for reconstructive surgeons well into the twentieth
century, at least as the major historical landmark of their subspecialty.[50] His was the classic discussion for his own time.[51] Indeed,
a paper from 1908 simply and authoritatively summarizes Dieffenbach's views on decircumcision as the state of the art.[52]

Dieffenbach began by noting that such a reconstruction can

have medical significance or it can be a "beauty operation" (*Schönheitsoperation*) (p. 515). This seems to be the beginning of the modern distinction between reconstructive surgery (as "real" medicine) and aesthetic surgery (labeled as dealing with vanity and hypocrisy). Citing Celsus as his authority, as did all of the commentators following Celsus, from the Roman physician Galen (129–99) and Paulus of Aegina (fl. 640) to the Renaissance anatomist Gabriele Fallopio (1523–62), Dieffenbach described how the prepuce can be restored either by stretching or by surgery in those who had been circumcised. Dieffenbach suggested certain elaborations of the procedures in order to make the foreskin look more authentic, as he claimed that the classical procedures did not create a foreskin that looked like a "real" foreskin. But then he stopped and addressed his readers directly:

> One must understand me correctly. I present such methods only for their physiological-surgical principles and to illustrate Celsus' idea of the extension of the prepuce out of luxury, belief, shame, or politics. It would be a denigration of the art [of surgery] if in this manner bachelors are created like virgins through the reconstitution of the hymen, about which one writer so pointedly said: "a fine operation!" Both are a morbid mockery of humanity from the practice of the oriental slave trader. (p. 517)

Dieffenbach had already contrasted the reconstruction of the scrotum (oscheoplasty), because of disease or burns, with the reconstitution of the prepuce (pp. 512–15). His further clinical indicators for the reconstruction of the prepuce were cases of hypospadia and phimosis, and if the prepuce is not clearly separate from the penis. His prime clinical example here was of the young man who had such incredible sensitivity of the exposed penis that he had to wear a sack full of cotton to protect it. But, except for such cases of extreme discomfort, one can exist without a foreskin, as another text on reconstructive surgery from the 1840s stated. One can live without a foreskin, "as the Jews' common ritual of circumcision shows," but what sort of a life would that be?[53] What is one without a foreskin, but a Jew waiting to be exposed?

Medical procedures made Jewish males marriageable in the

world of Christian brides by giving them foreskins. The commonly held view in the eighteenth and nineteenth century was that Jewish males were more often than not born circumcised. Such procedures meant that the constitution of a foreskin (for those inherently marked by its absence) enabled Jewish males to "pass" as Gentiles in spite of their "natural" circumcised state.[54] Such men should no more be able to "pass" as Gentiles than the sexually promiscuous woman should be able to "pass" as a virgin. This is the view of the period when Jewish males were beginning to enter the broader social network, converting to Christianity and marrying non-Jewish women.

Dieffenbach's anxiety about decircumcision is that Jews will "pass" as Christians. When Gabriel Groddeck wrote on decircumcision in 1690, he repeated the classic charge of Jewish hypersexuality and immorality. He evoked St. Paul of *Corinthians* 7:19 ("Circumcision is nothing, and uncircumcision is nothing.").[55] Groddeck commented that Paul wrote in a time when Jews had their foreskins reconstituted "because they imagined their fleshly desires could be fulfilled by greater stimulation if they were provided with that little bit of skin, and they believed also that they would give pleasure to their harlots and sweethearts, who broadcast in a depraved manner their very great pleasure if they have slept with a man who either never had the foreskin removed or had it restored." Groddeck noted that it was very rare for Jews in his own day to undertake such a procedure because of the "severity of the laws concerning circumcision."[56] In the seventeenth century it was other circumcised groups, such as the Turks, who seemed to desire decircumcision in Germany.

Given the surgeon's ability to rebuild the foreskin, to restore the wholeness and (in)visibility of the Jewish male, why does a fixation on castration remain central to the representation of circumcision? Even in the age of Dieffenbach, Karl Julius Weber (1767–1832) in his *Demokritos* (1833–36) made one of his characters jokingly exclaim: "'By God,' cried an Italian, when he heard of Tagliacotto's art, 'He could even restore the parts of poor Abelard!'"[57] Castration and, by extension, circumcision remove the essence of masculinity; a reconstruction of the penis, of the scrotum, or of the foreskin is no more real than the artificial penises that Paré proposed for his patients. In the making of "real" men, no simulacrum will do, because what defines masculinity in this culture can never be restored once it is lost. A reconstructed penis remains always a poor copy, no matter how accurate the reproduction. In this modern age of technical reproduction, the copy never has the same value as the original, because it is understood as "inauthentic."

There are pathological conditions that constrict the penis, such as phimosis, balanitis, and posthitis; in surgical practice today, these conditions seem to require circumcision. All of the other medical rationales for circumcision are unsupported claims about potential prophylaxis—the "prevention" of sexually transmitted diseases, AIDS, and penile and (in one's female partner) cervical cancer.[58] Yet Dieffenbach saw the reconstitution of the foreskin as necessary to correct congenital errors of the penis. The clash of cultures here is evident. By the middle of the twentieth century, with the rise of the Nazis in Germany, circumcision of the male became the symbolic sign of inherent male difference and danger. When male Jews in Germany imagined the act of disrobing, of revealing the body, which reveals the nature of the Jew, they imagined revealing their circumcision. It is notable that Jacques Joseph did not touch this question in his summary work of 1931.

The Parisian psychotherapist Susann Heenen-Wolff, in her interviews with Jews who remained in Germany after 1945, uncovered the continuing power of this anxiety about the male body. Hans Radziewski, a Berlin Jew, told her of his capture at the beginning of 1943 on the streets of Berlin.[59] She asked him how he was recognized: "Well, you had to tell your name. They asked about the [Yellow] Jewish Star, and if everything else failed, one had to drop one's pants." When she asked him how the Germans could tell a Jew from a Moslem, he remarked that because of their Arab specialists, the SS could tell whether the cut was made on the eighth day after birth (Jew) or on the twenty-eighth day (Moslem).

The powerful fantasy about the immediate visibility of the Jewish body was shaped by the sense that the male Jew's body was indeed inherently different. The marker of circumcision remains a powerful sign of identity for Jews in Germany. This theme is reflected in the film *Hitlerjunge Salomon* (1991) (released in English as *Europa, Europa*), in which the circumcised penis of the Jewish protagonist can never be revealed, as it would betray him to the Nazis among whom he is hiding. The failed procedure for the reconstruction of the prepuce represented in this film, drawing the foreskin forward and tying it so that it will stretch, is a version of one of the procedures that Celsus suggested. It is the nonsurgical procedure (using a special ring) most often suggested today by anticircumcision activists. The Polish-Jewish director Agnieszka Holland deftly dealt in the film with this theme taken from the actual experiences of Solomon Perel, a survivor of the Shoah. And this theme has become a leitmotif in contemporary Jewish writing in Germany.[60] In the nineteenth century Jewish men turned to aesthetic surgeons to restore their bodies to an intact and healthy state and to enable them to "pass" as whole and happy. The fantasy about the hidden yet revealing aspect of the male body is, as we shall see later, a continuing anxiety in Western culture, even today.

GREEK IDEALS

Jacques Joseph's task was to cure the psyche of his patients by making them "(in)visible," and the result, for him, was happy patients. What type of bodies and faces, however, would make the patient (in)visible? When Joseph sought out models that would make his patients happy and, therefore, healthy, he turned to classical models of the body similar to those used by the Viennese anatomist and physiologist Ernst Brücke. A lecturer in anatomy at the Berlin Academy of Arts before coming to Vienna to become one of Sigmund Freud's favorite teachers, Brücke published his handbook of the anatomical "beauty" of the body in 1891. He presented a normative body based on classic aesthetics: he used Michelangelo's sculptures of the female breast as the model for the perfect breast and the classical Greek sculpture known as the Diadumenos for the perfect male torso. The perfect female body is pubescent, unmarked by childbirth but prepared for it; the perfect male body is also unmarked, here by circumcision.

Brücke's image of the beautiful drew on Kantian notions of "classical" perfection, but used them to stress the values of his contemporary society. The aesthetics of high art were, according to Brücke's assumption, rooted in an idea of art as imitation. Works of art imitated the most beautiful human beings, rather than creating ideal types. Brücke's ideal body was that of Greek sculpture. He imagined the body as symmetrical, according to the guidelines extrapolated from classical models by nineteenth-century art history, which stressed a perfect, symmetrical physique for both men and women. Brücke presented the "real" image of the beautiful foot and leg. The beautiful foot is not the flat foot, at least according to Brücke.[61] The flat foot, as I have shown in detail elsewhere, was the foot of the black and the Jew in fin de siècle European medicine, a foot that disqualified its possessor from ever being a full citizen of the modern European state.[62] The idealized image of the beautiful also represents the healthy and the good.

Joseph, too, based his sense of the ideal body on images taken from the cutting edge of the racial aesthetics of his day.[63] He found his mathematical formulas for beauty and deformity in Albrecht Dürer (1471–1528): the beautiful is the symmetrical, the regular, and the proportioned. Beginning in the latter half of the nineteenth century, German nationalist advocates of a true German art used Dürer as the essential creator of "Germanic" types.[64] Dürer's visions of the people of his time were made into modern national symbols of beauty and ugliness. Whether of the nose or the breast, balance and proportion were the hallmarks of the beautiful and therefore healthy "German" body. The unhealthy, ugly bodies were those of the syphilitic and the Jew.

Joseph's ideal female face had a "greco-roman profile with a 33 facial angle" (p. 23). What is striking is that he chose a portrait of his (non-Jewish) wife to illustrate the ideal female face. His "proof" of his wife's beauty was the similarity of her profile (and nasal

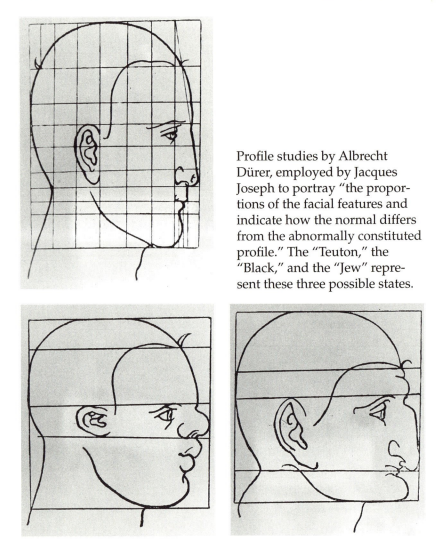

Profile studies by Albrecht Dürer, employed by Jacques Joseph to portray "the proportions of the facial features and indicate how the normal differs from the abnormally constituted profile." The "Teuton," the "Black," and the "Jew" represent these three possible states.

angle) to a drawing, which he reproduced, by Leonardo da Vinci (1452–1519). The international universal of the Renaissance represented by da Vinci was thus grafted onto the national local as a model for beauty, as sanctioned by the aesthetic politics of the turn of the century. The norms for Joseph's ideal beauty were taken from high art, with all of its status for the educated German of the age. Thus he reproduced an image of the Venus de Milo's profile (p. 23) and noted that "when the correction of an abnor-

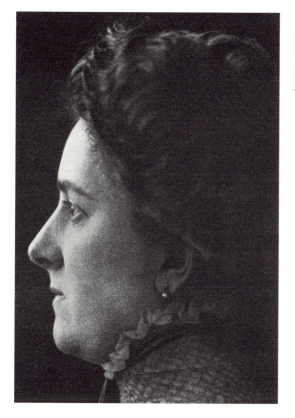

"The ideal female profile actualized," actually a photograph of Jacques Joseph's wife.

mal (ugly) profile is desired, a Greek nose is usually requested since it is well recognized as being normal and beautiful" (p. 24). And, one can add, (in)visible.

Joseph's models animate more than elite academic notions of "art." They also illustrate the handbooks on the "beautiful" that typified the libraries of educated German middle-class readers. These handbooks provided a canon of the beautiful through the merger of reproductions of "classical" works of art with contemporary (often erotic) photographs presented as modern parallels to the classical world.[65] Such books cemented the relationship between social status and the beautiful. You can acquire a new nose just as you can acquire objects such as the illustrated book. Joseph's wife is beautiful because she resembles a work of high art reproduced in the illustrated book.[66] High art becomes his and

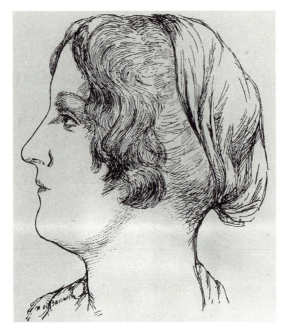

"The ideal female profile," taken from a sketch by Leonardo da Vinci.

his patients' ideal of the healthy. Such art is, however, an ideal that can be purchased: it is available as a commodity on the market either in the bookstore or on the surgeon's table. It is infinitely reproducible, like the images in the book. There are no longer any "authentic" works of art or noses that cannot be copied. Jews who do not look like the aesthetic norms of European artistic "beauty" are sick, but they can remedy this and become like the cultural ideal. However, there is a double bind for Jewish consumers of aesthetic surgery: in purchasing the new nose and healthy (read: [in]visible) visage, they are acting "just like Jews," purchasing a false mask of honor through material means.

To answer this charge and repudiate the accusation of contemporary thinkers such as Otto Weininger that the Jewish physician was simply mired in the material world, Joseph and his fellow Jewish aesthetic surgeons saw that they must become artists. As Joseph put it, the aesthetic surgeon must "possess a certain degree of artistic aptitude in order that he may fashion with certainty the exact form determined for the specific case . . . and also that he may know the shapes of individual facial parts, and their

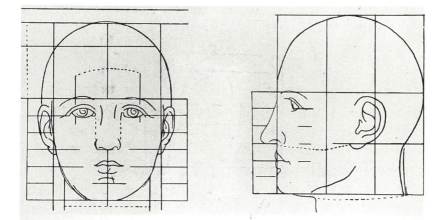

Jacques Joseph employed, along with Dürer, the German classicist Gott-fried Schadow's "canon of beauty." Schadow divided the face into six parts, and designated the nose as covering only three of these segments. The relative nature of this scale provided an "imprecise" but "useful" canon of symmetry for the aesthetic surgeon.

harmonious grouping. In a word, the plastic surgeon must have something of the artist in him" (p. 30). This was a commonplace of nineteenth- and early twentieth-century medicine. It echoes the claim of the influential early twentieth-century Canadian physician Sir William Osler that medicine is an art rather than a science. Yet there is a concrete sense here that is lacking in the metaphoric world of the physician-philosopher of the time. For Joseph, the aesthetic surgeon is really a sculptor: he uses hammers and chisels and shapes an object—just like an artist. This also answers the charges of materialism against the surgeon. If he is an artist in terms of post-Romantic imagery, he is an honorable man of the "spirit" rather than of the material world. The surgeon has become "a 'creator,' a magical word that can be used once one has defined the artistic operation as a magical, that is, typically social operation," to quote Pierre Bourdieu.[67] Thus the choice of models and the self-definition of the surgeon complement one an-other and enable the physician to become one with the culture in which he lives.

The surgeon as sculptor, a theme omnipresent in the reflections of the aesthetic surgeons before and after Joseph, also implies the problem of period and style. Harold Delf Gillies stated in 1934 that this was a problem of reconstructive as well as aesthetic surgery:

> For it is [the aesthetic surgeon's] aim and object in life not only to restore beauty to the human form, but also to change for the better such portions of human bodies that are now considered in the present trend of thought to be of an ugly or non-aesthetic character. Still further do some of us go, and whole groups of people are turned out through the plastic mill, bearing the unmistakable stamp of the hand that molded them. Even in the early days of the Great War, when there were ten of us making new faces to replace those that had been left behind in the trenches in Flanders, it was possible to say, "Oh, that one is so-and-so's nose . . . that's another's lip . . . there goes a typical so-and-so's eyelid," mentioning the names of individual surgeons. The same habit of style that in an artist enables the expert to say that a certain picture is that of a Rembrandt or Constable, is at work in the plastic surgeon's make-up and his results tend to run to type. There is even a certain element of impressionism that is justifiable, and there is also, unfortunately, in our poor results an element of cubism.[68]

Much of the "correction" for ethnic difference dealt with Western notions of aesthetic symmetry and balance. Although it is clear that certain ideas of symmetry may be universal (a crudely drawn "smiley face" is recognized by infants in all cultures), the ideology that defines the beautiful and healthy as symmetrical is espoused by European, post-Enlightenment aesthetics. Here again, notions of an aesthetic ideal are imposed on images of difference. It is all right to look "ethnic" (defined clearly by the culture in which one lives), but there must be balance and symmetry within that notion of difference. Thus, in a late twentieth-century study of the appropriate nose, investigators measured "the noses of 34 attractive young North American Caucasian women."[69] (The study offers no definition of what "attractive" means.) The measurements echoed those of Oken and Joseph, but were even more extensive, using "19 nasal measurements (6 single and 7 paired linear measurements, 3 angles, and 3 inclinations) and 15 craniofacial measurements (10 linear measurements and 5 inclinations)." The more detailed the measurement, according to such views, the more "scientific" the findings. These "beautiful" faces (or "happy" people?) were compared to "21 women with below-average faces." The investigators located their subjective response (which constructed the contrast between "beautiful" and "ugly") in the absence of symmetry in the faces of the "below-average" faces: "Two types of facial harmony disruption were identified: disharmony, a normal index with a visually apparent failure of proportionality, and disproportion, an index value outside of the normal range. The percentage of disharmonies and disproportions was significantly higher in the group of 21 women with below-average faces." What the investigators labeled as "symmetrical" and "disharmonious" came to be the criteria for ideal beauty. In these distinctions the nose carried disproportionate weight. "The greatest disproportion in the attractive face was the moderately short columella in relation to the tip protrusion and in the below-average face the long nasal bridge related to the upper-lip height." To translate: Irish noses are cute, Jewish noses aren't, and a cute nose makes a cute face.

Indeed, the study showed that an "analysis of ethnic and racial differences showed the . . . nose as the main feature of the most characteristic differences. The study revealed that the key to the restoration of facial harmony was the renewal of the uniformity of proportion index qualities by eliminating disharmonies and/or disproportionate relationships." The emphasis on proportion, from Joseph via Oken and Joseph's own sources to Dürer and other theories of the proportionate face in art, is a reading of ideal types. How does one want to "pass"? Well, art does provide idealizations that one can imagine as one's own body, but these idealizations are based on mathematical and structural principals perhaps better suited to architecture than to aesthetic surgery.

For we are confronted with François Xavier Bichat's (1771–1802) paradox, as paraphrased by Charles Darwin: "if every one were cast in the same mould, there would be no such

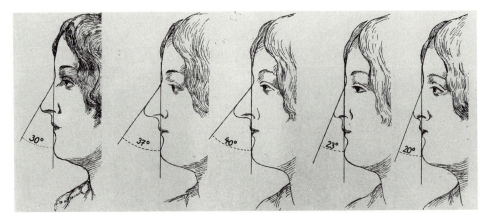

Jacques Joseph's scale of the nose. *Left to right:* The ideal nose, the maximum normal aesthetic profile, the too-large nose, the minimum aesthetic profile, and the too-small nose.

thing as beauty. If all our women were to become as beautiful as the Venus de' Medici [*sic*], we should for a time be charmed; but we should soon wish for variety; and as soon as we had obtained variety, we should wish to see certain characters a little exaggerated beyond the then existing common standard."[70] If we all look like works of art, will the works of art still be our idealized type?

Joseph's fantasy about high art as the appropriate model for aesthetic surgery never truly vanished. One extension of this will be discussed at the close of this book. In 1988 Xavier de Callatay, then the Director of Studies at the New York Academy of Art, spoke at a "Symposium on Beauty" sponsored by the American Academy of Cosmetic Surgery. "They are making too many cute, bland faces, with small turned-up noses, like the women on soap operas.... The prototype should be the Greek gods, like Aphrodite and Apollo, whose faces in sculpture had a classical structure, characterized by a prominent forehead and a straight nose.... The Greeks were beautiful, healthy and youthful—and that's exactly what people want to look like today."[71] Symmetry is equal to beauty is equal to health is equal to happiness.

Such analyses construct a set of mutually reinforcing value systems—"above"- and "below"-average appearance based on the aesthetic norms of the general culture. These are defined in terms of the importance of symmetry for Western culture as a model of defining beauty *and* health. It is striking that the "discovery" of the asymmetrical face (all adults have asymmetrical faces) was first done in a study of the inhabitants of nineteenth-century asylums, when it was discovered that the inmates all had asymmetrical faces. This was taken as a sign of the fixed physiognomy of the mentally ill.[72] One wonders how long it took the nineteenth-century investigators to discover that their own faces were asymmetrical. By the early twentieth century, human asymmetry was established as the norm.

Symmetry defined dental aesthetics in the same period, as dentists came to value the symmetrical form of the smile as a cultural asset. No greater marker for happiness can be found in Western culture than the smile. A beautiful face is a happy smile! A review of the orthodontic literature reveals that many of the writers believed that different "races" have standard facial shapes or "cephalometric norms." This belief has had great implications in the aesthetics associated with the placement and arrangement of teeth and in the construction of the "beautiful smile" in people of dissimilar ethnic origins. A "black" smile is different from a "Jewish" smile. Prosthodontists and restorative dentists are concerned with the "phylogenetic characteristics of their patients" because they believe that "the resultant esthetic differences can have significant importance in the function and design" of the smile and, therefore, the perceived happiness of their patients.[73] These "types" are static and are always understood within the context of the extremes of the beautiful permitted within any given category. Thus having a beautiful smile is specific to the notions of symmetry and balance within the various ethnic categories. No one can look too Jewish or too black and have a perfect smile.

The impossibility of beauty (and therefore true health and happiness) existing within the extremes of any constructed ethnic category has an older history within aesthetic surgery. One of Jacques Joseph's self-proclaimed "students," the Swiss "beauty surgeon," Charles Willi, commented in 1926 that "the Semitic nose is hooked, and in its extreme and exaggerated form is not beautiful."[74] It is not beautiful because it is not symmetrical from any angle. And for Willi "health and beauty are as closely related on the physical side as truth and beauty on the spiritual side, and both medicine and surgery in working for health work for beauty" (p. v). In moderation, the Semitic nose, according to Willi, who corrected such noses in London, "bespeaks intelligence and practical sagacity." All of the older physiognomic associations were retained within the world of aesthetic surgery during the 1920s. The implicit question was whether Jews could be cured of their "practical sagacity" (read: materialism) through an operation on their noses and thus be restored to social health, like the woman with a "saddle nose" that "stamps a face as plebeian": "A lady with a saddle nose can never ride a high horse as Lady Clara Vere de Vere" (p. 98). Class and race are the two spaces out of which and into which one desires to "pass," and they are closely related.

Like Joseph's initial patients, his subsequent patients were so glad about their new status that they danced with joy! Joseph reproduced images of their "spontaneous" dancing in his textbook of cosmetic surgery as proof of their psychic cure. A "misshapen" body inevitably results in an unhappy mind; making the body beautiful makes the mind happy. Joseph's patients have become beautiful people, because the blemish on their character, their racial identity, is no longer written on their face. They, like Joseph's first rhinoplasty patient, become newly socialized and eroticized.

We do not know whether Joseph's first rhinoplasty patient was Jewish, but the depiction of his psychological sense of social isolation due to the form of his nose certainly mirrors the meaning associated with anti-Semitic bias at the fin de siècle. Subsequently, Joseph's clientele was heavily Jewish, and he regularly reduced "Jewish noses" to "gentile contours." Many of his patients underwent the operation "to conceal their origins."[75] In justifying the procedure, Joseph called upon the rationale of the psychological damage done by the nose's shape. He cured his patients' sense of inferiority by changing the shapes of their noses. His primary cure was to make them less visible in their

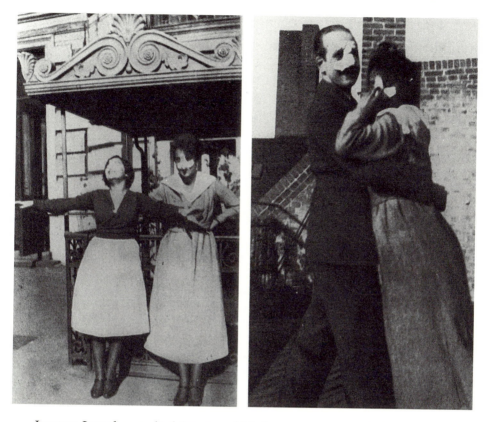

Jacques Joseph supplied images of his happy patients in his comprehensive textbook of rhinoplasty.

world. This was one of the rationales cited by the other German-Jewish aesthetic surgeons of the period, such as the art historian-physician Eugen Holländer (1867–1932).[76] Joseph's orthopedic training served him well. He could holistically cure the ailments of the entire patient, including the patient's psyche, by operating on the patient's nose. Change the shape of the ear or the nose and you have altered the psyche. He thus extended the "law" of his teacher, Julius Wolff, that changing one aspect of the body alters the entire body, into the realm of the psychological.

In treating those whose appearance denied them the honor of being accepted as equals in a society that promised them equality, and as full citizens of a modern state whose laws guaranteed their citizenship, the aesthetic surgeon also laid claim to his own status as an honorable practitioner of an honorable medical specialty. Such efforts are bound to be contested by the dominant culture at any time, but never more so than during periods of war and social upheaval. For German Jewish patients and physicians, the first half of the twentieth century would turn questions of "passing" into matters of life and death.

CHAPTER FIVE

Noses at War

FIXING SHATTERED FACES

*H*APPINESS AND BEAUTY were never easy to come by. For the surgeon, happiness was often tied to status, and the practice of aesthetic surgery remained relatively low status in the beginning of the twentieth century. The tension between reconstructive (serious) and aesthetic (frivolous) surgery continued to haunt Jacques Joseph's career. During World War I the "racial" question seemed to be suppressed as the focus shifted from aesthetic procedures to reconstructive surgery. Joseph eagerly joined the world of military medicine, taking a key role in founding and running the division for reconstructive surgery in the Charité, the major Berlin public hospital. He founded the division in June 1916 to deal with the extraordinary range of facial wounds being suffered on the front lines of the war. It was dissolved on January 1, 1922, having completed its task.[1]

Whole bodies and all parts of bodies were being shattered in the war, but the facial wounds were often the worst, because in the trenches the face was the most exposed part of the body, as the soldiers peeped over the embankments at the enemy. On the Allied side the New Zealander Harold Delf Gillies (1882–1960) and the French surgeon Hippolyte Morestin (1869–1919) undertook similar work. Like Joseph, both had chafed at the marginal status the medical establishment gave them before the war and they welcomed the opportunity to show the world how necessary and noble and redemptive their kind of medicine could be. Morestin, the most innovative reconstructive surgeon on the

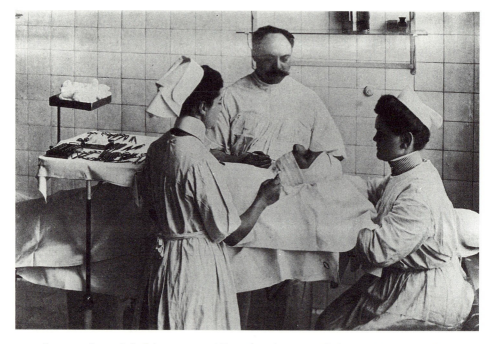

Jacques Joseph in his surgery. Note the absence of gloves. He was only marginally convinced of the germ theory of infection, though in this image the sponge tray and T-bar are sterilized along with the instruments.

Western front, was himself "seen" as different. Gillies wrote of his impression of visiting Morestin during the war: "He was a strange and moody octoroon, whose dagger-like sharpness was accentuated by his pointed mustache and tapering beard as well as the agility of his long thin hands. In the space of a moment he could reveal the gentleness of a kitten and the savagery of a tiger."[2] It is striking that many of the major figures in European reconstructive (as well as aesthetic) surgery in the generations from 1880 to World War I were themselves perceived as "marginal" to the cultures in which they worked. They were colonials or Jews or people of mixed race or women—for whom the problem of "passing" was and remained a central feature in their psychic lives. Their new roles as aesthetic surgeons gave them the "neutral" status of physicians, and yet their social status was heavily dependent on their racial, ethnic, or colonial status. As aesthetic surgeons they were as marginal to the medical profession as they were to European society.

Gillies came to the front from England and worked with Charles Auguste Valadier, a dental specialist to the officers of the imperial staff, who repaired jaw defects by using tissue, such as bone, from other parts of the body.[3] Gillies also worked with Hippolyte Morestin. Like Joseph, Gillies persuaded the medical authorities of the need for special centers for treating faciomaxillary injuries. In 1916 the Cambridge Hospital at Aldershot was opened and Gillies was assigned special duties as head surgeon. To assure that soldiers with facial injuries were sent to his new unit, Gillies bought ten pounds' worth of labels reading "Faciomaxillary injury—Cambridge Hospital, Aldershot," and sent them to the field hospitals in France to be pinned to the casualties' chests. In January 1916 the first naval casualties arrived, followed shortly afterward by two thousand injured soldiers from the battle of the Somme.

The most horrendous facial wounds came to the clinics of the Allies and the Central powers. Faces were literally blown away, jaws ripped off, skulls crushed, and soldiers with such wounds lived. Those thus wounded were so marked that their photographs assumed a major function in the immediate postwar iconography of European pacifism. No more horrible result of war could be represented in the public sphere than the mutilation of the face. In perhaps the best-known Weimar pacifist text, Ernst Friedrich's *War against War* (1924), twenty-four photos from Joseph's clinic were used to represent the "visage of war."[4] These images of the reconstructive surgical patient as the representation of what war means evoked the stench and horror of the trenches.[5] The images used were those of the *reconstructed* faces, the horror of which became the horror of war.[6] Even the rebuilt faces were understood as so grotesque as to mirror the anxieties about the impact of the war on everyone's humanity. There were exhibitions of casts of these faces at the Val-de-Grâce military hospital in Paris, at the Charité in Berlin, and at King's Hospital in London, where "thousands of people visit on holidays, to look with

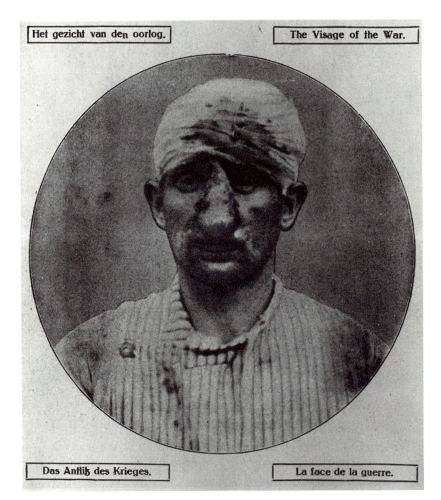

Het gezicht van den oorlog. | The Visage of the War.

Das Antlitz des Krieges. | La face de la guerre.

"The Visage of War."

awed horror on the authentic reproduction of the suffering and mutilation of war."[7] They came and looked to see what horrors war had created and how the hand of the surgeon as artist was able to restore these faces to the semblance of humanity. One can see the powerful representation of this as a comment on both the war and Weimar Germany in the world of Weimar art from Georg Grosz's (1893–1959) postwar work, especially his *Ecce Homo* (1922), to August Sander's (1876–1964) project to record the face of the "citizen of the twentieth century" in thousands of physiognomic portraits.

It is fascinating to compare the use of the photographs as images of destruction in Europe after World War I with their use in Reconstruction America.[8] During the Gilded Age, with its obsessive focus on racial "passing," the wounded of the Civil War were rarely described in terms of their facial wounds. The work of Gurdon Buck on facial reconstruction during the war and after provided a set of photographs and engravings that could have fulfilled this function and yet did not. Despite the great interest in the photograph as part of the ongoing memorialization of the Civil War during Reconstruction, the representation of the wounded face did not achieve iconic significance.[9] Hundreds of photographic histories of the war and its various aspects were compiled for general consumption, but the damaged face rarely appeared as part of this visual memory of the war. The ability to rebuild the face in an age that already understood surgery as the road to transformation meant that the world of the 1920s was better able to deal with the facial wounds, if only as antiwar propaganda.

Decades after World War I, Ernest Hemingway (1899–1961) remembered having observed the French veterans, *les gueules cassées* (the broken faces), with their "*Croix de Guerre* ribbons in their lapels and others also had the yellow and green of the *Médaille militaire,* and I watched how well they were overcoming the handicap of the loss of limbs, and saw the quality of their artificial eyes and the degree of skill with which their faces had been reconstructed. There was always an almost iridescent shiny cast about the considerably reconstructed face, rather like that of a well-packed ski run, and we respected these clients."[10] These were clearly reconstructed faces, as Harold Delf Gillies noted twenty years after the war: "the old gibe of the French that 'before' the patient was horrible, and 'afterwards' ridiculous, held only too true."[11] Yet when Hemingway imagined the wounded soldier after the "war to end all wars" it was certainly not with a missing face. In *A Farewell to Arms* (1929), his autobiographical novel of the Great War, his protagonist suffers a wounded knee, which makes him all the more a figure of erotic attachment in the fiction. In Frank Borzage's 1932 film of the novel, Gary Cooper's Lt. Frederick Henry is certainly not unattractive. In Hemingway's *The Sun Also Rises* (1926), Jake Barnes, like Hinkemann in Ernst Toller's Expressionist drama of the same name (1924), is impotent or castrated because of war-wounds. Their faces are unmarred, though their bodies are no longer those of "real" men.[12] They remain, each in his own way, an erotic figure. Heroes remain erotic figures; men without faces are not imagined as erotic objects. The popularity of the Phantom of the Opera in the film of the 1920s rested to little degree on this theme.

In the Weimar Republic there is an explosion of images of the war-wounded as examples of the pointlessness and meaninglessness of war. On the political right, the "noble" war-wounded were represented by those with missing limbs, a sign of valor; the missing face could only be understood as a loss of humanity.[13] Already in 1818 Carl Ferdinand von Graefe had commented, "We have compassion when we see people on crutches; being crippled does not stop them from being happy and pleasant in society. . . . [But those] who have suffered a deformation of the face, even if it is partially disguised by a mask, create disgust in our imagination."[14] These patients' mangled, half-reconstructed faces represent the visible results of war and empire. In this regard it should not be overlooked that the young soldiers, the best and the brightest of their generation, were also the "handsomest" of their generation. Both sides rejected from service "men who were badly disfigured for the reason that the psychologic effect on other soldiers interfered with discipline."[15] Thus the wounded represented the transgression of the boundary between the "handsome" and the "badly disfigured." Everyone in uniform came to be seen as "attractive."

During World War II, Harold Delf Gillies's younger cousin replaced him as the leading reconstructive surgeon for the Allies. The New Zealander Archibald McIndoe (1900–1960) founded the celebrated wartime Royal Air Force reconstructive surgery unit at the Queen Victoria Hospital, East Grinstead.[16] There he created the "Guinea Pig Club," which reconstructed burn patients both physically and psychologically. Indeed, the intent was to get wounded airmen back into the air as soon as possible, no matter how bad their wounds were. McIndoe used both text and film to make public his case for the importance of his undertaking, and for him the reconstructed face became a badge of honor. The social acceptance of the burnt face of the soldier had been substantially impaired by the use of such images from World War I as antiwar propaganda. Among McIndoe's first "Guinea Pig" patients was the pilot Tom Gleave, who had been shot down in flames over Kent at the height of the Battle of Britain in the summer of 1940. He arrived suffering from "standard Hurricane [airplane] burns," to his face, hands, arms, and legs, and he went back into combat after treatment. To return to the war was the new standard of happiness, actually developed in World War I but made explicit at East Grinstead, where the ability to take a recognizably "human" face back into the fighting had a clearly defined eroticism. McIndoe made a special effort to arrange for "fraternization" for his patients, believing that erotic attraction would prove to them their restored physical and emotional state. The aim of it all, as in the treatment of shell shock, was to get the rebuilt faces and bodies back into combat. This apparently made both the patients and the surgeons happy, to a degree that is almost shocking in a post–*Catch-22* world.

The most famous member of the "Guinea Pig Club" was Richard Hillary. Hillary's best-selling autobiographical novel *The Last Enemy* (1942) was made into a BBC-TV series in the 1980s.[17] Hillary was badly burned on his face and hands (his fingers "clawed and curled down into his palms" and his eyelids melted away) after being shot down over the North Sea in 1940. After surgery Hillary toured the United Kingdom and the United States. In 1942, at age twenty-three, he convinced the Royal Air Force to allow him to fly again—an unwise decision on its part, as his vision and manual dexterity were limited—to "finish the job" that others who had since died had started. He was killed in 1943, not in action, but during training maneuvers. Was happiness the outcome of his surgery?

Michael Ondaatje (1943–   ) evokes precisely this problem of the visualization of the war in the body of the scarred victim/ hero in his novel of World War II, *The English Patient* (1992).[18] Ondaatje's character follows in the literary footsteps of Hemingway's erotic wounded warriors, but even more so of Dalton Trumbo's (1905–76) rigorously left-wing critique of war in *Johnny Got His Gun* (1939). There the reader identifies with the dismembered and faceless veteran because of the use of the first-person narrative. In *The English Patient*, Ondaatje defines the horribly burned face and figure of the eponymous hero as the sign that defines all opposition to war.[19]

How powerful this image is can be judged in the visualization of the eponymous figure of Count Laszlo Almasy (played by Ralph Fiennes) in Anthony Minghella's Academy Award–winning 1996 film of the novel. The makeup of the burned patient emphasizes his own line: "I am a just a bit of toast, my friend." The reading of this body as representing the impossibility of love in time of war rather than "bravery" is never left in doubt, all the more so because Almasy is an archaeologist/spy, not a soldier. Almasy is given the line: "I once heard of a captain who wore a patch over a good eye. The men fought harder for him." Ondaatje, who was also coauthor of the script, did not want any false sentiment lost on the "heroic." In the film and the novel, the mutilated hands of the pickpocket Caravaggio, maimed by the Gestapo, become the hidden sign of betrayal in the novel. They are the sign of true valor, for they represent Almasy's betrayal of the British agent Caravaggio to the Germans. Caravaggio's thumbless hands remain a powerful yet unseen comment on the surface of burns. He is unable to be the thief as artist because of Almasy's perfidy. The "English patient's" burned body represents a world gone mad in war; it is not that far from the function of the mangled faces in the iconography of Weimar Germany. The reconstructive surgeon's morbid fantasy remains in both these cases—if the body cannot be reconstituted, the soul must remain in torment, incapable of happiness.

In the United States by the 1920s the very presence of reconstructed faces of veterans was used to claim a greater tolerance for aesthetic surgery. J. Howard Crum (1888–c. 1970), in his 1928

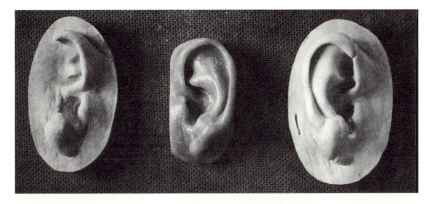

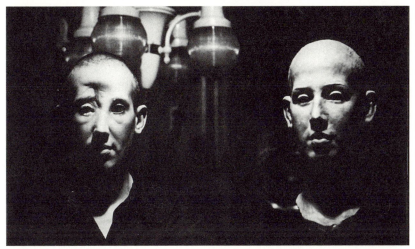

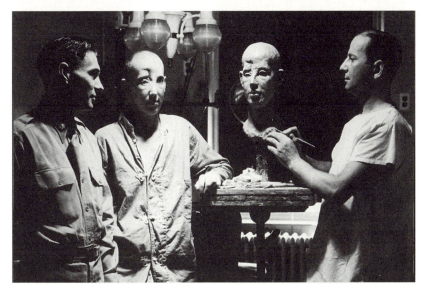

The creation of rubber prostheses of the face during World War II.

volume advocating face-lifts, noted that "the world felt that horrible disfigurement of face was too great a price for one to pay for his patriotism. . . . The modern man and woman are more sensitive to facial beauty, and, unlike the ancients, can not stoically look at faces disfigured by war and other causes. The prospect of a considerable number of war-mutilated men being let loose upon the streets seemed appalling."[20] According to Crum, aesthetic surgery came to the rescue of postwar society, and the horrors of war provided an environment in which aesthetic surgery could be undertaken without the charge of vanity. (But the techniques, which were popularized and improved between 1914 and 1919, had been developed with very different patients in mind in the surgical theaters of Berlin, Paris, and New York in the 1890s.) The war-wounded were all men who had evident physical deformities—which is true in Ondaatje's novel, as well. After the war this masculinization of reconstructive surgery out of the cauldron of battle provided a new status for aesthetic surgery and newer satisfaction for its practitioners. There is a parallelism between the argument for reconstruction (based on the heightened aesthetic sensibility of the modern viewer) and the alteration of that viewer's own physiognomy to make it more beautiful.

Joseph's reputation after the War to End All Wars was extraordinary. Indeed, even though he may not be have been the first ever to develop the procedures for reduction rhinoplasty and facial reconstruction commonly used today, he evolved a series of brilliant variations and the instruments to carry out these procedures. Like Tagliacozzi in the seventeenth century and Dieffenbach in the nineteenth century, he became the signature figure of the early twentieth century that defines and is defined by aesthetic surgery. His myth overshadowed all of his predecessors. He became the most influential aesthetic surgeon of his day.

Joseph's contemporaries flocked to Berlin to learn the newest techniques of aesthetic surgery from him. Robert Alan Franklyn from the United States "followed the good methods of Berlin's late Professor Jacques Joseph."[21] The aesthetic surgeon to the stars in the 1920s, Henry Schireson, dedicated his book to "Jacques Joseph, M.D., of Berlin, Germany, . . . my friend and my inspiration as well as my teacher."[22] Maxwell Maltz, physician and historian, evoked Jacques Joseph, with whom he had studied in Berlin, as his model: "the great Jacques Joseph—the ardent, stocky, irascible Joseph, the first man to prove that it was possible to reconstruct and reshape the nose by operating inside rather than outside the nostrils, so that no visible scar was left."[23] For those who could not go to Berlin to study with Joseph, his comprehensive handbook of aesthetic surgery of 1931 provided the basic outline for many of the procedures that were the basis of modern aesthetic surgery. The British surgeon Leslie E. Gardiner noted this after he found Joseph's work on the shelves at the Royal Society of Medicine and appropriated his procedures to shape unhealthy noses and unhappy psyches in the London of the 1930s.[24]

All of these physicians became psychologists in their practice. Gardiner, for example, was first confronted with the issue of whether or not to cosmetically alter the nose of a patient who had come to him for what she claimed was a deviated septum. "Orthodoxy called upon me first to restore function. I would meet this prime requirement when I corrected the deflection in her septum. Was there any reason why I should not look further to appearance, and still further even to the psychological realities beyond appearance? If the surgeon has it in his power to promote the mental comfort of a patient, should he refrain simply because of a strict and narrow interpretation of his duties?" (pp. 40–41). This is the model of the treatment of the psyche through the body that was advocated by Joseph and other nineteenth-century aesthetic surgeons. This was all taking place during the explosion of growth in another arena—that of psychoanalysis—which also had its roots in the context of racialized medicine in the 1890s. It is little wonder that aesthetic surgery dips into the vocabulary of psychoanalysis to articulate its means of treating the psyche.

In Jean Boivin's account of his own career as an aesthetic surgeon in Paris during the 1930s and 1940s, and in George Sava's (1903–) accounts of the history of French aesthetic surgery,[25] in which Boivin plays the role of hero, there is an analogous argument. "A changed physical appearance often leads to a metamorphosis of the personality and the character. . . . Aesthetic surgery is also a surgery of complexes. The knife not only delivers you from a physical disfigurement but from an obsession at the same time."[26] Boivin recounted the result of a rhinoplasty in which he altered the nose of a young woman: "It plunged downwards so that it reached her upper lip, it had several bumps on it, one nostril was bigger than the other; in short, that nose constituted a catastrophe in itself" (p. 176). He operated on her, and two years later met her again. She greeted him with the salutation: " 'I am the happiest of women. At last I'm fully alive!" (p. 177). The healthy psyche became the goal of the aesthetic surgeon; but the meaning associated with the reconstructed face, the visible face, as opposed to the (in)visible face, underwent a shift after World War I.

The question of "passing" is not raised with the faces reconstructed by the surgeons following the battles of World War I. There is never any doubt that the only cadre into which they could "silently" pass would be that of the war-wounded. This cohort was visible because their bodies and faces were read as signs of war. After the war such images were full of horror, having lost any vestige of the myth of war as a time of masculine testing. Yet the restoration of the psyche remained paramount. With the restoration of function and the return of the visage to a "somewhat human" form, the "happiness" of the patient became central. Thus Joseph noted, at the conclusion of his first annual report (1917) as the director of the department for "facial-plasty" at the Charité, that "the discharged patients have all been cured of their psychic depression which the consciousness of bodily deformity always involves."[27] These were patients horribly maimed in the war who, Joseph claimed, were made whole, both physically and psychologically. How equally true of his private patients. When these same surgeons turned to their aesthetic surgical patients after the war, both the power of their new status and their clear need to see their undertakings as psychological dominated the self-presentations of both surgeons and patients. The postwar era also presented aesthetic surgeons with a professional opportunity to expand the patient pool.

Patriotic Noses and Weimar Surgery

The faces of the war-wounded also shifted the meaning attached to aesthetic surgery during the Weimar Republic. War surgery and the reconstructive undertaking of Joseph and his colleagues at the Charité had major repercussions for the definition of visibility within Weimar culture. In the 1920s Martin Gumpert (1897–1955), another Jewish reconstructive surgeon and well-known writer, proposed the creation of a public clinic for aesthetic surgery in Berlin.[28] Gumpert advocated the creation of a publicly funded center for *Entstellungsfürsorge* (care of the mutilated) as part of the social network in the capital that already included clinics for occupational medicine, sport, marriage counseling, the war-wounded and children.[29] After much argument in the city council, the Berlin authorities authorized a department of "social cosmetics" at the Institute for Dermatology at the University of Berlin (p. 206). The idea of the institute was supported by the leading French aesthetic surgeon Dr. Suzanne Noël, an early advocate of eyelid surgery and face-lifting, and her appearance before the public health committee of the German parliament was, according to Gumpert, the first appearance of a French national there after World War I (p. 210). In 1926 Noël had published a detailed study of the socio-psychological impact of aesthetic surgery.[30]

That the tale of a social tradition of aesthetic surgery in the Weimar Republic leads back to a Jewish surgeon in Berlin is not surprising. Marginal figures, as we noted, have a disproportionate role in the history of aesthetic surgery. And they were seen as playing such a role. Enabling others to "pass" was understood as a reflex of the marginal physician's own desire to be accepted. Indeed, a Jewish identity in this context comes to be defined as a marginal identity. Gumpert's understanding of his Jewish identity seems parallel to that of Jacques Joseph. His Jewish identity was subsumed in his sense of belonging to the German cultural sphere. He claimed to have "never found it an advantage or a disadvantage being a Jew" (p. 37). Gumpert accepted the notion of racial difference and advocated racial mixing as the solution to anti-Semitism. He dismissed the image of the Jew evolved by the anti-Semite as "unreal." He describes it as a "Jew with Negro lips, giant nose, bloody eyes, and side locks" (p. 38). According to his own estimation, he could not have looked *that* different, but his occupation was allowing people who did look *that* different to merge seamlessly with the "faceless" crowd.

These views were not limited to Weimar Germany. Here one can note from contemporary accounts that Morestin, a man of mixed race from Martinique, was understood as being highly sensitive about "his racial admixture [which] might have left him with a feeling of being a minority who perhaps could not enter as fully into French society as he might have wished."[31] The marginality of the surgeons (whether colonial, mixed-race, or Jewish) was a central part of the tale of constructing the world in which the unacceptable could become (in)visible (or at least less visible). Certainly the autobiographies of aesthetic surgeons, such as the Hungarian Jew Max Thorek (1880–1960), whose career was made in Chicago, stressed their own racial visibility and the fear that such visibility created in them.[32] In remembering the pogroms in Hungary, Thorek bleakly noted: "[That] any minority can escape its dark destiny is unthinkable. Let them accept it with stoicism. There is no other hope—not here. Not in this land" (p. 43). For Thorek the escape to America became a mode of his own transformation, an escape to a place where invisibility can be acquired and one is not fixed in terms of one's physical nature and identity.[33]

Such views are not simply an artifact of late nineteenth-century Europe. The most articulate aesthetic surgeon of our day, Robert Goldwyn, stresses his Jewish identity over and over again in his autobiography. He tells of looking for a surgical residence in the 1950s: "That a Semitic background could be an obstacle soon became evident. . . . I applied for plastic surgical residencies away from Boston. . . . Two chiefs of service wanted to know my religion, and though I responded, I resolved not to go to either of them because I felt their query was degrading."[34] A sense of his own marginality haunts this autobiography by an aesthetic surgeon and professor at Harvard University who acknowledges that he is "successful" (p. 219). It is not only that Jews and other marginal figures shaped the field of aesthetic surgery in the nineteenth century, but that the stigma of marginalization continues to haunt the entire profession. Marginal figures entered into the profession because it was of low enough status to be open to them; its questionable status makes even successful, mainstream, late twentieth-century American surgeons who happen to be Jewish aware of their own marginality. This tradition of the marginality of the aesthetic surgeon is most evident in the world of Weimar Germany. Marginal physicians improved the lot of marginal patients, both defined by how society imagined they looked.

To remedy visible signs of difference meant returning the patient (and the physician) to the world of the unseen. According to Gumpert, his patients came to him to be turned into useful "workers" and therefore into contributing members of Germany society: "No one would hire a girl with a birthmark on her face; a businessman with a large, unformed nose or a teacher with large, protruding ears cannot acquire authority because they are always the butt of jokes" (p. 208). The cases he highlights were all ones of economic difficulties resulting from physical appearance. They revealed psychological difficulty at the core of the economic problem: "a lack of self reliance, inferiority complex, destruction of erotic relationships, anxiety about aging, professional failure" (p. 206). The Nazis closed the Gumpert clinic in 1933, only to reopen it in 1938.

The visibility of the war-wounded was understood as socially parallel to that of the racially visible. As we have seen, Weimar Germany had an intense concern with images of the war-wounded. It is fascinating that the spectrum of unacceptable appearances ran the gamut from the war-wounded to the racially unacceptable—because of their visibility. The notion of Gumpert's institute for *Entstellungsfürsorge* (care of the mutilated, a term that applies far more to horrific wounds than to anxiety about a too-large or too-small nose) reflects the contradictory meaning of being visible in modern Europe. But Gumpert's institute was created as a parallel structure to the public clinic for the war-wounded, so there was clearly a need for a different center for aesthetic surgery in the Weimar Republic. Such a clinic did not deal with the mutilated former soldier, but with the "normal" members of Weimar society set apart from the new state by their appearance.

The parallel question of gender was also raised in Gumpert's clinic, because one important category for the acknowledgment of one's successful "passing" was the erotic. Was one seen as a member of the desirable class and did that class silently acquiesce to one's membership in it? The erotic came to be racialized in the course of the nineteenth and early twentieth centuries because the erotic was linked to healthy reproduction and to productive attraction (cornerstones of the pronatalist movement). In a world in which sexuality and the erotic were no more stable than the ability to read race in the shape of the (new) nose, a new role of aesthetic surgery was to enhance the individual's erotic potential, even to enable one successfully to "pass" as a member of the other sex. Among Gumpert's patients were "transvestites whose male forehead lines spoiled their pleasure at wearing women's clothes." Male transvestites in Weimar Germany were given police photo-identity cards that legally permitted them to "disguise" themselves as "women." Their ability to do so was a reflex of the quality of their appearance and their ability to "pass" as "female" (but not as a racially marked female) (p. 212). Gumpert's comments lead us to the other strand in the Weimar social history of aesthetic surgery: the role that aesthetic surgery played in the Institute for Sexual Science, founded by Magnus Hirschfeld (1868–1935). One of Hirschfeld's longtime associates at the Institute was Ludwig Lévy-Lenz, whose role at the Institute, according to a contemporary French source, was the "castration of certain exhibitionists, the improvement of the skin," and "plastic surgery."[35] He studied aesthetic surgery with Noël in Paris and with Joseph in Berlin.[36] In addition to his surgical activities, Lévy-Lenz was a prolific writer on aesthetic surgery and its implications for sexual health in the 1920s. Indeed, his was one of the voices that made aesthetic surgery most acceptable among liberal circles in Weimar Berlin.

However, it was not in the realm of reconstituting the racial body in order to make the Jewish psyche "happy" that Lévy-Lenz worked. He was primarily a gynecologist who worked with transgendered males to alter their genitalia and create artificial vaginas and labia (p. 454). (These procedures shall be more closely examined later.) One of his transgendered patients complained, "Doctor, now I am a woman, but even when I wear women's clothes people say to me: Mrs. Schulze, you have the nose of a man." "Passing" means not being seen by others as inappropriately gendered, even in the form of the nose, but again "Jewishness" is what being marked with a "male" nose comes to mean in such circumstances. The construction of the feminine meant the elimination of racial typology through surgery. Jewish transsexuals were new women (and later new men); their Jewishness seemed to vanish under the knife. Lévy-Lenz understood his aesthetic surgery as an art form, unlike other forms of surgery (p. 459), but, like Gumpert (and many American surgeons of the 1920s), he also saw aesthetic surgery as a form of psychotherapy that should not be limited to the wealthy (p. 455). He argued against those surgeons who thought that surgery should only be undertaken when a life is in danger, and noted that many of the procedures they were pleased to do (such as the repair of a club foot or of a cleft palate) are also aesthetic procedures. He stressed the role that aesthetic surgery played with the war-wounded, where scars define the patient, but even more the role that aesthetic surgery could play in operations that leave no scars (such as rhinoplasty) (p. 456). Such rhinoplasties, Lévy-Lenz noted, were the most common operation that he performed, "whether on snub noses or Semitic noses or wide or long or potato or hanging noses" (p. 461). Turning men into women meant eliminating the source of their featural as well as their sexual difference.

Lévy-Lenz followed the psychological ideas of the Italian Jewish forensic psychiatrist Cesare Lombroso that underlay Magnus Hirschfeld's Institute for Sexual Science. Lombroso believed in the fixity of types but also in the ability of these types to change by acquiring new characteristics, such as those created through surgery. The racial model, even for the Jewish members of Hirschfeld's institute who distanced themselves from discussion of race, became paramount. Hirschfeld, who like Lévy-Lenz was Jewish, dismissed the very notion of race as a peripheral phenomenon in contrast with the reality of sexuality.[37] Ideas of race shaped his understanding of the mutability of the body (and thus of the psyche). Like Gumpert, Lévy-Lenz strongly believed in racial mixing as the solution to the "Jewish problem," and was himself married to a non-Jew. His views were clearly selectionist: "From a drunken Zulu black and a degenerate white whore you cannot expect a Goethe—not because the father is black and the mother white, but because both are humanly worthless" (p. 213). According to Lévy-Lenz, one must start with good stock, but one can improve the stock. At this point in time, he wrote, Jews are weaker than most because of the "exaggeration of certain spiritual qualities from incest [*Inzucht*]." Incest (another way of speaking about inbreeding) is the reason why the Jews have no "heroes" in "the realms of physical or sports activities" (p. 216). Racial biology and the alteration of constitution must be understood as part of the rationale for aesthetic surgery in Weimar Germany.

In a 1933 piece in Hirschfeld's popular journal *Marriage* (*Die Ehe*), Lévy-Lenz's collaborator, Friedrich Pruss von Zglinicki, suggested to the reader that it was now "normal" to use cosmetic surgery.[38] Zglinicki, like Lévy-Lenz, had been involved in the film industry in Berlin during the 1920s, and much of the popular reputation of both surgeons came from this association.[39] Zglinicki's argument is interesting because it defends the legitimacy of aesthetic surgery by connecting it to the rise of the modern and locating it in those cities associated with the emergence of the modern. So, for example, he tied contemporary aesthetic surgery to the high status of Viennese medicine. He noted also that aesthetic surgery is "modern" because it is now most widely practiced in the United States. For writers in Berlin (where Jacques Joseph practiced), New York and Vienna were the central sites of modernism, while New Yorkers saw Vienna as the hub of modernism. As the American novelist Gertrude Atherton (1857–1948) ironically observed in 1923 about the popularity of rejuvenation: "When it was discovered that New York actually held a practicing physician who had studied with the great endocrinologists of Vienna, the street in front of his house looked as if some ambitious hostess were holding a continual reception."[40] The modern is located wherever one is not and must be sought there or among those trained there.

The idea that aesthetic surgery was a sign of the modern was double edged, for the "modern" was also seen as the source of "unhappiness." Thus the anxiety about the increased pace of modern life was seen as affecting the body: "Good appearance is endangered by the ever-increasing tempo of our times." Similar arguments were made by the Jewish Hungarian physician Max Nordau (1849–1923) in his widely read *Degeneration* (1892–93) about the effects of the speed of modern life, such as the impact of train travel, on the moral constitution of modern "man." Aesthetic surgery promised to answer Nordau's complaint by reconstituting the mental health of patients, especially professional women, whose "psychological" pain stemmed from their unhappily formed faces. "The specific ethical value of aesthetic surgery lay in its treatment of the most difficult psychological load." For the Weimar public, aesthetic surgery was acceptable as a form of mental hygiene.

The erotic remained at the center of the sexologists' interest in aesthetic surgery. "How Does One Remain Young and Beautiful?" is a chapter heading in Lévy-Lenz's *Enlightened Woman* (1928).[41] Again the author created an archaeology of beauty, reminding his audience that even the Jews used cosmetics in the wilderness (p. 43). Cosmetics are a sign of all high cultures, as female beauty is a biological necessity (following Darwin) for reproduction of the fittest. The beautiful is not only a part of the biology of the female, it is "part of the woman's psyche" (p. 46). Once the modern began to undermine the erotic through the tempo of everyday life and the demands on the modern woman, aesthetic surgery became the only means to preserve or restore mental health: "Thus I recommend to women who have a wrinkle or a dimple to have them operated upon; thus I also recommend nose and breast operations even when they have nothing to do with actual health. [Such blemishes] are a burden on the soul of the woman, even if they are only imagined. Finally we suffer even from that which we imagine: feelings are and remain real to us" (p. 49). We suffer from what we only imagine—here Lévy-Lenz's words echo the rhetoric of the mistrust that young Jews came to have of their own bodies.

In the 1920s, the famed German Jewish author Jakob Wassermann (1873–1934) also chronicled the ambivalence of the German Jews toward their own bodies, their own difference. Wassermann articulated this difference within the terms of the biology of race. He wrote, "I have known many Jews who have languished with longing for the fair-haired and blue-eyed individual. They knelt before him, burned incense before him, believed his every word; every blink of his eye was heroic; and when he spoke of his native soil, when he beat his Aryan breast, they broke into a hysterical shriek of triumph."[42] Their response, Wassermann argues, was to feel disgust for their own bodies. Even when they were identical in *all* respects to the bodies of Aryans, they remained different: "I was once greatly diverted by a young Viennese Jew, elegant, full of suppressed ambition, rather melancholy, something of an artist, and something of a charlatan. Providence itself had given him fair hair and blue eyes; but lo, he had no confidence in his fair hair and blue eyes: in his heart of hearts he felt that they were spurious."[43] The belief in being able to "pass" was essential—and surgeons such as Lévy-Lenz needed to persuade their clients that they could "pass."

"Mundus vult decipi—the world wants to be deceived," begins Lévy-Lenz's introduction to aesthetic surgery in 1933.[44] By then, deceiving the world was no longer as simple as undergoing an aesthetic surgical procedure. In the 1920s, the climate was ripe for the development of a quick and relatively simple procedure to alter the external form of the body, whether breasts or nose. The procedures prior to the 1890s were not only more complicated (as well as dangerous) but they also did not come at a time when the need to "cure" the disease of the visibility of the Other was as powerful. Central to Joseph's process of nasal reduction as well as breast reduction, which will be discussed later, was the fact that there was "no visible scar."[45] Joseph's procedure began the craze for nose jobs and breast reductions in fin de siècle Germany and Austria. In the history of medicine, Joseph was the "father of aesthetic rhinoplasty." He came to be nicknamed "Nasen-Josef = Nosef" (Nose-Joseph) in the German-Jewish community.[46]

NAZI NOSES

The clinic for *Entstellungsfürsorge* (for the care of the mutilated) was reopened in 1938, again as part of the department of dermatology at the Charité. The complexity of aesthetic surgery in Nazi Germany can be sensed in one anecdote told about a visit by Harold Delf Gillies to the thoracic surgeon Ferdinand Sauerbruch (1875–1951). Gillies lectured at the Berlin Medical Society after the reinstatement of the public clinic at the Charité. He had made a double reputation for himself in the years following World War I.[47] Not only was he the best known "British" reconstructive surgeon but also, as we have seen, he had broken new ground in the reconstruction of the "syphilitic 'squashed' nose." He presented grand rounds to the clinic in which he described augmenting syphilitic noses by relining them with transplanted tissue and by fitting a strut in them. " 'It is perfectly possible,' he told his dispassionate and credulous audience, 'for a patient to pocket several different-shaped bridges and change his racial and facial characteristics by a simple sleight of hand.' "[48] In a nutshell, this captured the ambiguous position of aesthetic surgery in the Third Reich. Surgery could, it might be claimed by the Jewish patients of Jacques Joseph, enable them to "pass" as non-Jews; but it also could "cure" German patients of the problem of possessing a "too-Jewish" or "too-degenerate" physiognomy.

In *Mein Kampf* (1925–27), Hitler's anxiety about Jews and his anxiety about syphilis took the same form—he saw both as threats to the body politic.[49] One of the central themes of Hitler's

Was kann der Sigismund dafür, daß er so schön ist? ...

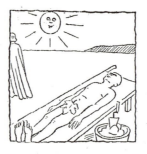

Als der liebe Gott den Juden schuf, formte er ihn, gleich Adam, aus feuchtem Lehm. Dann hieß er ihn in der Sonne liegen zu bleiben, damit er trockne.

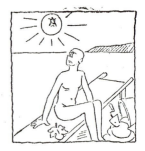

Weil aber der Jude von Anfang an das Licht scheute und das Dunkel vorzog, pfiff er auf das Gebot des wahren Gottes und verduftete lieber vorzeitig.

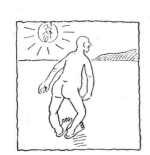

Da der Lehm noch feucht und weich war, bekam der Fürwitzige gleich nach den ersten Schritten nicht nur abnorme O-Beine, sondern auch Plattfüße.

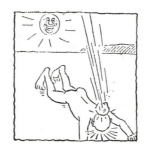

Als der Schöpfer dieses Zerrbild seines „Ebenbildes" sah, ergrimmte er und schleuderte dem Flüchtenden so heftig einen Meteor nach, daß dieser aufs Gesicht fiel.

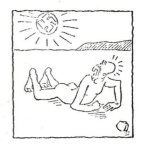

Der Jude erhob sich wieder. Nun war er auch im Gesichte gezeichnet. Was Wunder, wenn er da noch heute flucht und sich durch „Gottlosenverbände" zu rächen sucht.

The Nazi caricaturist Walter Hofmann, who drew under the name "Waldl," presented a series of images of the construction of the Jewish body in a cartoon strip ironically entitled "What can Sigismund do about the fact that he is so pretty?" The body of Sigismund, the archetypal Jew, was literally constructed, like that of Adam or the golem, from wet clay, but the Jew disobeyed the divine order and arose before his body was truly formed: "Since the clay was still damp and soft, the smarty developed after the first few steps extraordinarily bandy legs, but also flat feet."

anti-Semitism was that he learned to "see" Jews when he came to Vienna. They were no longer invisible to him as they had been during his childhood.[50] In seeing them, he claimed, he could now combat them. Could aesthetic surgery mask Jewish visibility? And what about those who only "looked Jewish"? Could they be made invisible, able to "pass" as what they really desired to be—

racially "pure"? Gillies commented ironically in 1934 that "already the dictatorship governments of the world are insisting on a perfection of form and uniformity of physique, and it may well be that at some future date they will insist on a uniformity of facial outlook. Believe me, there will then be some work for the plastic surgeon!"[51] The aesthetic surgeons' role under the Nazis should be to create the perfect racial body, but would it then be a real racial body?

In 1938 the annual meeting of the German Society for Surgery was opened by a session on congenital abnormality (such as that caused by inherited syphilis). The infamous eugenist, Otmar, Freiherr von Verschuer (1896–1969), began the conference with a talk on the inheritance of deformities, at the same moment when those bearing such deformities were being euthanized as "unwanted life."[52] For him, the line between aesthetic and reconstructive surgery was the line between life and death.

In Nazi Germany certain forms of reconstructive surgery were actually mandated. In 1936 the new law mandating military service authorized the State to reconstruct (*umgestalten*) the potential soldier's body "against his will if necessary, as to extract from it its maximum fitness."[53] Among the potential but unstated alterations of the body that would make the soldier more fit were changes to his physiognomy. Certainly the use of aesthetic surgery would enable the "too ugly" soldier, barred from military service, to become a "real" soldier, but it would also enable certain alterations of the body that would make the new soldier's body even more efficient. In the 1930s Benito Mussolini's (1883–1945) Italy also used aesthetic surgery to increase the performance of military officers. Mussolini ordered all officers over forty to report to have their eyelids examined because it was believed that drooping upper lids impaired vision. "Therefore, the Italians are removing excess skin from the upper lids of their officers since a tightened lid is an added aid to accommodative vision."[54] Aesthetic procedures that have a military significance were made mandatory under fascism.

There was one further addition to the image of aesthetic surgery in the Third Reich. Hitler felt that a contented female electorate depended on his maintaining those aspects of society that he thought women desired. He enabled beauty parlors and hairdressers to remain open during the entire course of the war because of his fear that women would revolt if these sources of their aesthetic pleasure were closed. Josef Goebbels (1897–1945) noted in his diary that Hitler observed on May 10, 1943 (well after Stalingrad and the beginning of German reverses) that "women after all constitute a tremendous power and as soon as you dare to touch their beauty parlors they are your enemies."[55] This also had eugenic significance. In 1940 Robert Ley (1890–1945), the head of the Nazi Labor Front who had a pronounced lisp, dedicated the "House of Beauty" in Berlin. In his opening remarks, Ley defined the beautiful as follows: "What benefits me and my people is beautiful; whatever makes me weak or ill is ugly." He noted that "party affiliation and the army are the institutes of beauty for men. In the case of women, many things are still lacking to secure charm and gracious living to them. We do not want the athletic type woman, neither do we want the Gretchen type."[56] Neither the liberal "New Woman" nor the passive, melancholic naive was the ideal for Nazi Germany. Beauty and aesthetic surgery thus both had roles in achieving the end of creating better soldiers and better mothers.

Under the domination of the Third Reich, Jews again turned to aesthetic surgery as a means of remaining (in)visible. We have one very late case description of one of Jacques Joseph's rhinoplasties, dating from January 1933, soon after Hitler's election and before Jewish physicians were forbidden to operate on non-Jewish patients except with special permission. Sixteen-year-old Adolphine Schwarz followed the lead of her older brother and had "her nose bobbed." She commented that her brother had written to Joseph and informed him that he had very limited means. "Joseph was very charitable," she later said, "and when he felt that someone suffered from a 'Jewish nose,' he would operate for nothing."[57] The image of "suffering from a 'Jewish nose'" is a powerful one.

Joseph's own view in 1931 was that "among patients of Semitic as well as of Aryan origin, a common desire is to be rid of their

Semitic nasal shapes, especially when these are of the unattractive exaggerated kind, in order to blend in appearance-wise with the remainder of the population. . . . [T]he crucial fact is that these patients undoubtedly suffer emotionally; this realization leads inescapably to the conclusion that their emotional balance should be restored by means of surgery whenever possible" (p. 85). It is, therefore, both Jews who look "too Jewish" and non-Jews who look "Jewish" in any way who "suffer" from being seen as Jewish. Being seen as a member of the wrong group has dire social consequences. The aim of both types of patients was thus "to go their ways inconspicuously and unnoticed . . . to achieve average looks, and therefore, to become inconspicuous" (p. 85). Young "Germans" who looked too Jewish were labeled as "Mischlinge," of mixed race, whether they had Jewish ancestry or not. The psychoanalyst Wilhelm Stekel (1868–1940), for example, reported a case of a twenty-five-year-old man who fixated "about the extraordinary size and ugliness of his nose." He "related his suspicion that he might be of Jewish extraction, an idea which was most unpleasant for him because he was a Nazi. . . . He did not suspect his mother of marital infidelity, but thought that there must have been a Jew among his ancestors."[58] Stekel most certainly saw this young Nazi in Vienna before the Nazi seizure of power in 1938 (when Stekel fled the country), but the situation would have become even more pressing after the Nazis' seizure of power.

Young Jewish men and women needed to become (in)visible, needed to alter their bodies, as their visibility became even more marked, but surgery provided only a momentary respite for them in Nazi Germany and Austria. For the virtual invisibility of any Jews in the German Reich vanished with the introduction of the yellow "Jewish star" and eventually the tattooing of Jews' bodies in the concentration camps. (Tattooing violates one of the basic Jewish religious taboos against "wounding the body," a taboo as powerful as that against cremation. In tattooing, killing, and burning Jews, the Nazis violated their bodies in every way central to Jewish religion.) Tattoos would be a permanent marker of their difference, which neither a nose job nor decircumcision would disguise.

"Nosef" died in February 1934 from a heart attack, before he was forbidden to practice medicine completely. His scarred face, at the last, did not make him (in)visible as a Jew, nor did his surgical interventions make those Jews whose noses he "bobbed" any less visible. But, as a Hungarian Jewish physician Alfred Berndorfer commented well after the fact, it is possible that

> the great number of persons persecuted by Nazism . . . were qualified as a 'foreign race' on the basis of the Laws of Nuremberg. Their looks caused them psychic troubles that were increased by the fear of racial persecution. This feeling was projected upon their faces, and the psychic problem aggravated their facial expressions. They objectively judged that the change of form would solve their psychic conflicts and relieve them of inhibitions. . . . [After surgery] they were sure that . . . they blended and therefore their behavior also became positive.[59]

Berndorfer illustrates how the Nazi belief in Jewish visibility formed the self-image of Jews remaining in Germany after the promulgation of anti-Jewish legislation in 1935. Aesthetic surgery liberated them. They came to believe that they no longer looked Jewish and, relieved of this dangerous visibility, were no longer terrified of being seen in public.

Such alterations of the psyche had, however, only transient value. Heightened anti-Semitic attitudes assumed that the permanence of the Jew's face marked the inherent difference between the Jew and the Aryan. The German Jewish poet George Mannheimer, writing in exile in Prague in 1937, could evoke the "strange face" of the Jew:

> I know, you don't love us.
> We are not like the others.
> People who rest and people who wander
> Have a totally different face.
>
> I know: you don't love us.
> We have swum through too many streams.
> But: let us come to rest,
> Then we shall have the same face.[60]

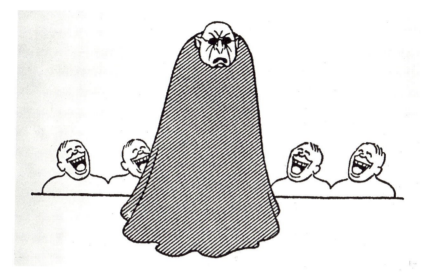

The claimed visibility of the Jewish body in the first half of the twentieth century was absolute. It was the Jew's difference that was to set the Jew apart from the society in which he or she dwelt. Here, the difference of the body is the cause of laughter.

Mannheimer's text evokes the potential elimination of any "ugliness" associated with the "nomadic" nature ascribed to the Jew. Here it is not surgical intervention, but rather acculturation that will alter the internalized sense of alienation that marks the face of the Jew. Given the Nazi belief that the physical characteristic that is "permanently common to all Jews from the ghetto of Warsaw to the bazaars of Morocco: [is] the offensive nose, the cruel, vicious nostrils," the fear of the Other's response to one's own face was not without grounding.[61] This image of the unalterability of the Jew's nose is internalized as a sign of the unalterability of the Jewish character. The dilemma is that of the body that is changed and cannot yet trust its changed self, or of the body that is unchanged and doubts its ability to be transformed.

Following the war, aesthetic surgery became associated in complex ways with the Nazis. Thus there is a recurring theme in postwar novels and films that Nazi leaders vanished by having their faces and hands rebuilt so that they could "pass," often as victims.

In the survivor-author Edgar Hilsenrath's (1926–   ) great novel on the Shoah, *The Nazi and the Barber* (1971), a Nazi takes over the role of his childhood Jewish friend after he murders him.[62] He has himself circumcised, his SS tattoo removed from his armpit, and a tattooed camp number added. Thus he can hide—in Israel! In the mid 1990s, it was believed that at least one leading Nazi war criminal, Alois Brunner, who was responsible for deporting 128,000 Jews from Slovakia, Greece, Austria, and France to Nazi death camps re-entered Europe in 1993 "with a new identity and a new look from cosmetic surgery."[63] "The old Nazi, believed sheltered by the Syrians since 1960, was reported to have undergone cosmetic surgery as part of the identity change, the sources said. They displayed a grainy photograph said to be of the 'new' Brunner, the face of a man looking distinctly younger than the fugitive would in his advanced years."[64] The model of the putative criminal, such as Vincent Parry in *Dark Passage,* who escapes identification by disguising himself becomes part of the legends associated with the disappearance of the Nazi leadership after World War II. Such transformations are not means of changing the psyche of the individual, only of masking his identity.

Even today, fascist groups understand the potential of aesthetic surgery. American neo-Nazi groups both use and hate aesthetic surgery. They use it for the purposes of self-transformation, so that they can become "like everyone else." David Duke, the former Grand Wizard of the Ku Klux Klan, had extensive surgery prior to 1987, including a nose job and a chin implant. According to one commentator, "Duke was transformed from a mustached nebbish with a dark, greasy forelock (disturbingly reminiscent of you-know-who) to a blond, blow-dried replica of a young Robert Redford."[65] In 1991, when he briefly held national attention, a columnist observed, sarcastically, that "David Duke, the former Nazi and Ku Klux Klan leader . . . , with some cosmetic surgery and barely moderated views, pronounces himself to be just another Republican. He sure looks like one to me."[66] The assumption was that the "true" Duke never changed and that the "cosmetic" changes were a sign of his hypocrisy.

Also in 1993 Jonathan Haynes, a young neo-Nazi and a former

chemist with the Federal Bureau of Alcohol, Tobacco, and Firearms, shot the aesthetic surgeon Martin Sullivan in his Wilmette, Illinois, office. Haynes later condemned aesthetic surgery because it "dilutes Aryan beauty." One could no longer recognize the true Aryan because of "plastic surgery, hair coloring and tinted contact lenses."[67] Haynes was sentenced to death in 1994. The claims of contemporary Nazis of all stripes are about the authenticity of the "real" Aryan body as opposed to those who merely try to "pass." Among people whose worldviews demand a consistency of body type as the marker of difference, aesthetic surgery plays a complex role in enabling them to change while also enabling their opponents to change. For them the consistent relationship between external, perceived reality and internal reality must be maintained, but only for the Other. Nazi ideology, in all of its manifestations, needs this consistency, even if it is only the consistency of the illusion of difference.

In the aftermath of World War II, the center of the Jewish world shifted from Central Europe to two Promised Lands, the United States of America and the new state of Israel. In these countries, it could be hoped, a Jew would never again need to "pass" as anyone but a Jew. Yet although safe havens in America and Israel meant that the survival of the Jews as a people was no longer in doubt, the definition of a good Jew's appearance could, ironically, be almost as problematic in New York City and Jerusalem as it had been in Berlin.

CHAPTER SIX

Assimilation in the Promised Lands

HELPING JEWS BECOME AMERICANS

$\mathcal{A}$s AESTHETIC SURGERY was
being developed in Berlin and Vienna, Western European Jews
seemed to have become indistinguishable from other Western Europeans in matters of language, dress, occupation, location of
their dwellings, and the cut of their hair. Indeed, if Jacques Joseph
was himself a model, his dueling scars matched the physiognomy
of masculinity that dominated German culture of his time. According to Rudolf Virchow's (1821–1902) extensive study of more
than ten thousand German school children (1886), Jewish children had also become indistinguishable in terms of skin, hair, and
eye color from the greater masses of those who lived in Germany.[1]
Virchow's study sought to show that wherever a greater percentage of the overall population had lighter skin or bluer eyes or
blonder hair, a greater percentage of Jews also had lighter skin or
bluer eyes or blonder hair. Although Virchow attempted to provide a rationale for Jewish acculturation, he still assumed that
Jews were a separate and distinct racial category. George Mosse
has commented that Virchow saw Jewish children as a separate
category, which must have made "Jewish schoolchildren conscious of their minority status and their supposedly different origins," especially because many of them were the product of
mixed marriages or no longer identified themselves as practitioners of the Jewish faith.[2] Nonetheless, even though they were
labeled as different, Jews came to parallel the scale of types found

elsewhere in European society, and the remaining difference could be effaced, many thought, through aesthetic surgery.

A parallel shift in the perception of the Jewish body can be found during the early twentieth century in the United States. In 1910 the famed German Jewish anthropologist (and the founder of modern American anthropology) Franz Boas (1858–1942) authored a detailed report for Congress on the "Changes in Bodily Form of Descendants of Immigrants."[3] This report documented the change in body size, cephalic index, and even hair color of the offspring of Jewish, Sicilian, and Neapolitan immigrants born in the United States. Unlike their siblings born abroad, first-generation immigrants were bigger and had greater brain capacity and lighter hair color. Boas argued that racial qualities, even hair color, changed when the environment shifted, and that racial markers were at least to some degree mutable. Bodies changed from generation to generation in America, which gave the lie to the claims of fixed racial types advocated by both the scientists and the politicians of the time who wanted to limit immigration of "bad" stock. Needless to say, Boas's view was contested in the science of his time. Arguments against his view postulated alternative causes for the changes he observed, ranging from the shift from rural to urban life to the true elimination of the "degenerate" types that had developed in Europe. According to the latter view, the "pure," and therefore healthier, original European types reemerged in the United States. The notion that there could be a "new human race" evolving under American conditions startled European scientists, who observed not only that these Eastern European Jewish immigrants were physically becoming more and more like other Americans, but also that they were growing into American culture.[4] As their body type altered, observers noted, their culture also changed, just as had happened with the Irish in the United States a few decades earlier. And yet even in the United States, there was the sense that no matter how much the Jewish body changed, certain markers, such as the Jewish nose, remained constant. These were the final racial markers, which could not be effaced—except through surgery.

In 1944 the American Jewish poet Karl Shapiro (1913–   ) stressed the malleability of the Jew's body. He was aware that the final reconstitution, not of the Jew but of the Jewish nose, would be the domain of the aesthetic surgeon:

> The name is immortal but only the name, for the rest
> Is a nose that can change in the weathers of time or persist
> Or die out in confusion or model itself on the best . . . [5]

Shapiro argues for the mutability of nose and character of the Jew as the new American, like all Americans, different but the same. Not acculturation or assimilation but the wizards of aesthetic surgery will make the new American nose. When the "objectivist" Jewish American poet Carl Rakosi, born in Hungary in 1903, looks down at "Jennifer Ebin, my eighteen-month-old granddaughter," and asks:

> Whose face is so fair
> that her eyes look blue
> though they are brown
>
> and bubbles fresh
> and sits in men
> like a nut in a shell?[6]

The transformation of the American Jewish body is thus almost complete—at least when seen through the eyes of those American Jews whose very desire for transformation enables them to metamorphose from generation to generation. How very different for the German-language Jewish poet. Under the Nazis the notion of the mutability of the Jewish nose was a topic for surgeons and poets alike. After the Shoah, when the greatest of the Jewish poets in German, Paul Celan (1920–70), imagined the fate of the Jew, he thought of it as having twisted the Jewish nose:

> Where is my beard, wind, where
> Is my Jew's badge, where
> my beard, blown by you?
>
> Twisted is the path, which I went,
> twisted it was, yes,

for, yes,
it was straight

Heia.
Twisted, so too my nose.
Nose.[7]

For Celan, the experience of being Jewish shapes the face so that it is marked as being that of the Jew. It is not acculturation but history that alters the physiognomy. The visible face, changed either by surgery or by history, defines what is seen as Jewish. The nose job (as in Berlin) comes to signify the erasure of visible difference and the permanent alteration of the perception of difference, disease and "bad" character.

The too-long nose came to be the final divide that separated the Jew from the society in which the Jew lived, and that marked the future by a nose. John Hunter, the British aesthetic surgeon, recounted the following anecdote concerning "a rich Jewish business man [who] came to have his nose straightened and, while he was waiting for the anesthetic, began to quiz Archibald McIndoe [the New Zealand–born surgeon and cousin of Harold Delf Gillies] about the operation. Patiently the surgeon explained how the operation would be handled. Then the patient said quite seriously: 'If my nose is straightened and my son has his done, do you think we shall begin to pass on the straight nose to our children?'"[8] The belief that aesthetic surgery changes not only the present but also the future is a reflection of the desire for permanent invisibility through individual transformation. It is also part of the oblique promise of aesthetic surgery. In 1990, a Canadian aesthetic surgeon wrote that "patients sometimes misunderstand the nature of cosmetic surgery. It's not a shortcut for diet or exercise. It's a way to override the genetic code."[9] If so, it "overrides" the genetic code only in the individuals operated upon, not in their offspring. But such hopes persist among patients.

Robert Goldwyn recounts the story of a rhinoplasty patient who, after the surgery, sent him a picture of her newborn: "I wondered whether Joan and Mel had secretly expected Lamarckian inheritance to work for them, so that the new baby would have

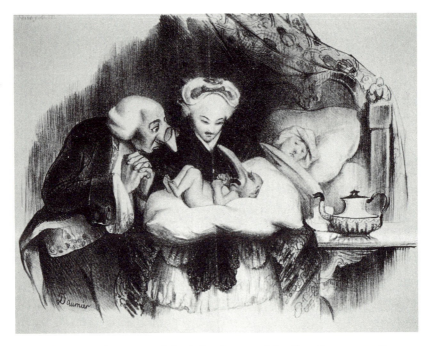

Henri Daumier's image of the inheritance of the "too-long nose."

an adequate chin and a good-looking nose. Would sexual selection be different, and natural selection also, if other forms of life, not just human beings, could have their own plastic surgeons?"[10] The mistaken belief that acquired characteristics, individual changes to the body such as a smaller nose, will be passed down through one's lineage, remains a powerful part of modern consciousness. Goldwyn's fantasy (of frog aesthetic surgeons operating on the frog-prince to make him "normatively" beautiful) aptly matches that of his patient. But until there is a union between aesthetic surgery and medical genetics, one can only mask the body, never reform it. The aesthetic surgeon's scalpel cannot sculpt a patient's genetic code. The genetics of "race" encouraged the fantasy of operating on the psyche through the alteration of the body to remove the fabled "Jewishness" of the spirit. Goldwyn's notion is quite similar—improve the patient's psyche through aesthetic surgery so that one falls in love not only with the physical aspects of one's beloved, but with his or her newly happy soul. Goldwyn's acknowledgment of this ability to transform the psyche is very much in line with Jewish Americans' expectations for their own transformation.

Philip Roth, in his *American Pastoral* (1997), reflected on the meaning attached to "looking American" in the 1940s and 1950s.[11] The protagonist of this novel is "Swede" Levov, whose "steep-jawed, insentient Viking mask of this blue-eyed blond born to our tribe" marks him culturally as the first generation of Jews to be truly American and therefore "happy" (p. 3). A third-generation American Jew who played varsity football, basketball, and baseball, he appears to the somewhat younger narrator Nathan Zuckerman as the personification of the happiness of Jewish acculturation. He is a real American and seemingly the antithesis of his model, Ernest Hemingway's Robert Cohn in *The Sun Also Rises* (1926), who came "out of Princeton with painful self-consciousness and [a] flattened nose," the result of boxing to prove that even a Jew could do sports.[12] For Roth, the mask of acculturation hides the decay of the Levov family. It obscures the "Swede's" desperation concerning his daughter, who is lost in and to America after perpetrating a bombing during the Vietnam War demonstrations: "I remember when Jewish kids were home doing their homework. What happened? What the hell happened to our smart Jewish kids? If, God forbid, their parents are no longer oppressed for a while, they run where they think they can find oppression. Can't live without it. Once Jews ran away from oppression; now they run away from non-oppression" (p. 255). This tension between the struggle to free oneself from stigma and the heavy identification with the stigmatized becomes a leitmotif of the transformation of the Jewish body in the 1980s. Physical transformation is shown to be a form of false acculturation. Whether accomplished through intermarriage, the identification with American goals, or aesthetic surgery, the ideology of progress and improvement is shown to be unobtainable. This is Roth's careful response, in the late 1990s, to the desire to change Jewish difference present among some American Jews in the 1940s and 1950s.

This awareness was projected not merely onto but also into the

Jew. In a startling series of studies undertaken during the 1940s and 1950s in the United States concerning the visibility of the Jew, the question was raised as to how and why the Jew could be seen. Raphael Isaacs in 1940 had discussed the "so-called Jewish type" in a Jewish medical journal, and his focus was on the "so-called 'hooked' nose." For him the "hooked nose, curling nasal folds (ali nasal)" were the salient markers in the representation of the Jew. He cited a University of Michigan study in which "only 51% showed a definite convex nasal outline," that is, "nostrility." Isaacs's work, like the earlier work by Joseph Jacobs (1854–1916), argued against the importance of "nostrility" as a marker of the Jew while illustrating the central importance of this sign for the culture in which he lived.[13] Jacobs's work, written in England in the 1870s, had tried to question the "nostrility" of the Jews.[14] The assumption that "nostrility" marked the Jew continued well after the Shoah. Jacobs's sketches of supposed Jewish "nostrility" were reproduced, counter to his intent, as "evidence" of Jewish physical difference in a respected textbook of physical anthropology in 1974.[15]

But did Jews actually look different from everyone else? The more analytic work of the Harvard psychologist Gordon Allport (1897–1967) in 1946, followed by a series of papers in the late 1950s, attempted to understand what was being measured when Jewish and non-Jewish judges were asked to sort images into the category "Jewish" and "non-Jewish."[16] Jews had a greater ability to identify "Jewish" photographs, as did those non-Jewish judges who showed a higher index for anti-Semitism. Was it that these two groups were more closely attuned to what the subliminal signs of Jewishness were, or was it that they simply judged more of the images to be Jewish? The former seemed to be the case.[17] Jewish judges "tended to give more false positives and were more accurate than non-Jews." They began to believe that hidden under the seeming non-Jewish images were Jews who were "passing." The conclusion was that they "were particularly sensitive to possible cues in others which would enable them to ascribe group membership to these others and that this disposition was directly related to the degree of acceptance of the majority stereotype."[18] One could add—even if the subjects were believed to be hiding their Jewishness. What was being measured was the anxious perception of a "Jewish" physiognomy. Non-Jewish as well as Jewish participants identified Jewish subjects as Jewish more than 30 percent of the time. This exceeded their identification of Jewish subjects as Jewish when the experimenters supplied speech, gesture, and name. In other words, Jews (and non-Jews) were attuned to the meaning of the image of the Jew because of the culture in which they lived.

The desire for invisibility, to "look like everyone else," still shaped the Jew's desire to alter his/her body. The greatest increase in the growth in rhinoplasties in the United States was in the 1940s, at a time when awareness of the dangers of being seen as a Jew was at its peak.[19] Through the 1960s more than half of the patients seeking rhinoplasty were first- or second-generation American Jews.[20] In 1960, a Johns Hopkins survey of predominantly Jewish female adolescents saw their desire for rhinoplasty as rooted in their ethnic origin. Indeed, the assumption of this study was that these young women were articulating their negative identification with their parents, specifically their desire to alter the appearance of their noses, which they said resembled their fathers'. They wished to mask the image of their fathers as Jews and its associations. These young women gave no sign of wishing to abandon their Jewish identity, only their Jewish visibility: "We were interested to know whether the quest for rhinoplasty was perceived as a disavowal or disassociation from a Jewish identity. Whereas this would seem to be true at a superficial level, the patients came from practicing religious homes and there was no hint they wished to marry or have male friends outside of their religion or that they contemplated any deviation from the patterns of religious beliefs of the family. In the attitudes and response of parents also, there was no evidence of their being perceived as a desertion of religious or racial identifications."[21] The internalization of the negative image of the Jew is one model of response to the sense of being seen as "too Jewish," or, indeed, being seen as Jewish at all. One desires not to be seen as a Jew, yet retain one's identity as a Jew.

Such fantasies can be read in the American context of a revised meaning ascribed to the Jewish nose. Herbert Lindenberger, professor of comparative literature at Stanford University, writes about his uncle, an aesthetic surgeon, offering him a nose job in the 1950s. Uncle Fred stated that his nephew's nose would be "bad for your career the way it is." Lindenberger replied that "in my particular field people usually took you for bright if they also took you for Jewish."[22] Jewish noses mark smart Jews.[23] But is it necessarily good to be seen as a smart Jew? And can observant Jews actually have aesthetic surgery?

Among religious Jews the prohibition against *chavalah* (wounding) has not been uniformly applied to aesthetic surgery. One respected authority dismisses the psychological rationale for aesthetic operations: "I very much doubt if, as a rule, the psychological stress, in merely pathological terms, resulting from the facial malformation to be corrected will outweigh and thus neutralize the health and other risks involved in such an operation. In other words, the chief indication for such surgery, I suspect, is cosmetic pure and simple and not medical."[24] Aesthetic surgery, from this point of view, is permitted only for social reasons: if the feature to be improved (1) prevents a woman from finding a marriage partner, (2) prevents a happy relationship with her husband, or (3) prevents a person from fulfilling a constructive function in society—"this applies especially to men who without such improvement could not earn enough to support their families." This would perhaps have covered Lindenberger's case. Some rabbinic authorities have even cited *Deuteronomy* 22:5: "A man shall not put on a woman's garment," seeing aesthetic surgery as gendered and thus prohibited for men.[25] The other view, slightly less limiting, sees that social isolation (citing *Tosafot, Shabbat 50b*) constitutes psychic "pain."[26] This authority finds the "psychological anguish normally attendant upon not being able to find gainful employment or a suitable marriage partner is, for him, a form of 'pain.'" The expansion of the permission is tied to the culture in which the opinion is given. The more limited view was held by a British rabbi trained in the 1950s, the broader view by a contemporary teacher of medical ethics in New York City. Culture (*min-hag*) determines how aesthetic surgery is understood within Jewish religious practice.

Although in Israel the orthodox religious prohibition against wounding is still in effect, Israel is becoming an aesthetic surgery society. The rise of tattooing, a prohibited act among traditional Jews (with even further negative overtones of the Shoah), has been defended based on the spread of aesthetic surgery. Tattooed Jews are supposed to be refused burial in consecrated ground. "What about all the Jewish women who get nose jobs and face-lifts?" asks one young Israeli. "The whole thing is about changing your body, but where do you draw the line? Do you draw it at tummy tucks?"[27] Certainly this debate centers on aesthetic surgery as psychosocial therapy (rather than "merely" ornament).

In the mid twentieth century in the United States, the "nose job" came to represent a gender distinction, although it also continued to be rooted in fears of looking "too Jewish," just as in pre–World War II Germany. But the form of the desired nose had become Americanized. The ideal nose was the "upturned nose," the Irish "pug nose" that John Orlando Roe and others had sought to correct in the century before. "By the mid-sixties, an upturned nose had practically become a middle class status symbol, and hundreds of teenage girls in New York [read: Jewish girls] seemed to be wearing the same design. The bone was narrowed, the tip pinched into a triangle, and there were two distinct bumps above the nostril."[28] Such noses were consciously understood as "Irish." "I want to look typically American. You see a typical American and she turns out to be Irish so I guess that's what I want," said one candidate for rhinoplasty in the 1960s, and another stated that to "look like an American" would mean having "a turned-up Irish nose."[29] In Britain, the introduction of the "too-small" Irish nose seems to have a specific history. Evidently the reconstructive surgeon Archibald McIndoe operated on the British comedienne Kay Kendall's nose in the late 1940s and gave her a retroussé nose. McIndoe's response was that "he hated it and said: 'I really must take you back and do it again.' She, however, adored the little thing, so McIndoe allowed her to hang on to it, so long as she didn't reveal who had done the deed." At least that is what the London aesthetic surgeon Eric Gustavson claims.[30] Who wants to take credit for having given a young Englishwoman an Irish nose?

With the rise of a heightened feminist and Jewish consciousness during the late 1980s, this association became the focus of some concern. This is nowhere better illustrated than in the feminist *Wimmen's Comix* entitled *Little Girls* (1989), subtitled *Case Histories in Child Psychology.* One of the most striking of these case histories is Aline Kominsky-Crumb's "Nose Job." Aline Kominsky-Crumb was one of the founders of the feminist comic book movement in the late 1970s with her creation of *Twisted Sisters,* and she is presently the editor of *Weirdo* magazine. "Nose Job" is a cautionary tale about a young woman "growing up with cosmetic surgery all around [her]," who avoids cosmetic surgery in her forties by recalling her earlier temptation as a teenager on Long Island in 1962. There "prominent noses, oily skin & frizzy hair were the norm. . . . (No, we Jews are not a cute race!)" This self-conscious admission of the internalization of the norms of her society even in 1989 underlies the dangers lurking even for those who can articulate the meaning ascribed to the Jew's body. As all about her teenagers were having their noses restructured, she held out.

Her "sensitive folks kicked this already beaten dog" by pushing their daughter to have a nose job. She eventually fled to Greenwich Village, where she "felt hideously repulsive." After she ran away, her parents agreed to postpone the procedure. And she "manages to make it thru High School with [her] nose." The story, at least in the "comix" has a happy end: "6 months later styles had changed and she looked like the folk singers Joan Baez or Buffy St. Marie." In other words, one could look as "beat" as one wanted, as long as one did not look "Jewish." The "Jewish" nose came to signify the outsider, but that outsider was never identified as Jewish. The moral of Aline Kominsky-Crumb's tale is that fashions in appearance change and that women should not

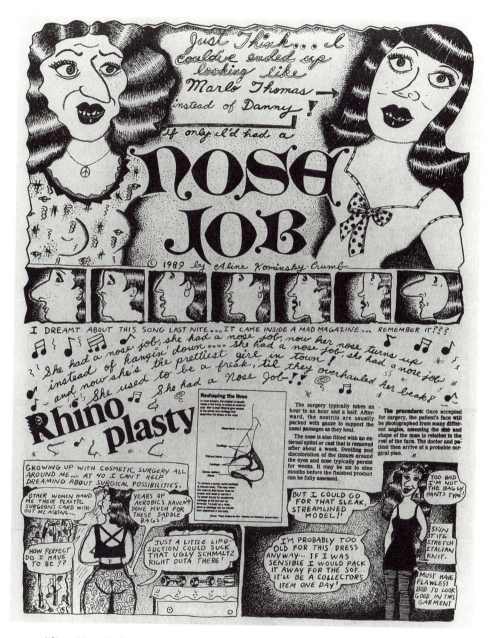

Aline Kominsky-Crumb's "Nose Job," 1989.

succumb to the pressures of fashion to homogenize their bodies, but the hidden meaning is that it is all right to look Jewish as long as you can be taken for someone other than a Jew.

What is still left within the memory of Aline Kominsky-Crumb is the sense that looking Jewish is looking different, looking marginal, not "looking cute." Even the heightened awareness of feminism does not diminish the internalized culture's power to judge one's appearance. Looking like a beatnik folksinger may be a step up from looking like a Jew, but in no way can it be understood as looking "cute." This consciousness of the negative aspects of the body leads to the sense that some type of alteration of the body is a potential need, even if it is rejected.

The racial nose is, of course, not only a "Jewish" nose. The too-long nose is read in other cultures as racially marked and, therefore, the source of unhappiness. In Mexico, over the past few decades there has been an explosion in the number of rhinoplasties, as wealthier Mexicans seek to obscure their Indian ancestry.[31] Increasing affluence has made aesthetic surgery widely available, and the desire to efface the Indian within has now spread to small-town Mexico. Even in the small town of Nezahualcoyotl, procedures to alter the shape and meaning of the Indian nose can be found in the local clinic for "aesthetic surgery." The operation of choice in such clinics is rhinoplasty, even at $1,500.[32] With such effacement of racial identity, the patients are made "happy" with their bodies.

The plastic surgeon Mark Gorney noted, "Patients seeking rhinoplasty . . . frequently show a guilt-tinged, second-generation rejection of their ethnic background masked by excuses, such as not photographing well. Often it is not so much a desire to abandon the ethnic group as it is to be viewed as individuals and to rid themselves of specific physical attributes associated with their particular ethnic group."[33] It is in being visible, in "the body that betrays," that the Jew is most uncomfortable.[34] The shift in the third and forth generation (using Gorney's three-generational sociological model) is a return to "origins," to the "Jewish nose."

Indeed, by the 1990s too-small noses had become the stuff of mass cultural satire, as in Marissa Piesman's Nina Fischman mystery *Heading Uptown* (1993), in which one of the characters is described as

> having a nose job too early, before the plastic surgeons had
> grasped the concept of subtlety. So swimming in this sea of big-
> ness was a too-small nose. Nina . . . had gotten used to those odd
> little cartilage vestiges set at such awkward angles on the faces of
> the city's ethnic women. . . . You had gone to some guy on Park Av-
> enue back in the early sixties, when he was practically the only
> game in town. And he had done, with the limited technology avail-
> able to him at the time, the best he knew how. And now you had
> to walk around with this porcine look and there was nothing you
> could do about it.[35]

Even more aesthetic surgery could not correct such a nose, for the
nose was a sign of the failed attempt at acculturation. Here may
be one answer to Bichat's question of what would happen if *everyone* were beautiful: when everyone looks like everyone else, a moment comes when there is a claim on the "more authentic," on the
original appearance—and at that moment there is a need for the
old nose made new again.

THE ISRAELI EXPERIENCE

The tradition of rhinoplasty as the dominant mode of altering the
Jewish body continues in Israel today.[36] Most procedures are undertaken in the most secular area of Israel, in greater Tel Aviv,
with Haifa second, and the religious center of Jerusalem a distant
third. Rhinoplasty remains the most frequently performed procedure on both men and women, with one Tel Aviv–area medical
center performing hundreds of rhinoplasties each year, compared
to several dozen procedures for all other aesthetic surgeries combined. These procedures are performed at a much younger age on
women, who come in as young as fourteen, whereas their male
counterparts have rhinoplasty performed somewhat later, usually before the age of twenty-five or thirty. In Israel, aesthetic
surgery is not covered by the state health system. Such surgery is

relatively expensive, with a rhinoplasty costing at least a month's salary.

The ideal of the "Israeli" face seems not to be completely identified with the image of the "Jewish" face, thus it is notable that both men and women have nose jobs in today's Israel. Only 5–10 percent of all other aesthetic surgeries performed in Israel is done on men. The goal of aesthetic surgery in Israel, as elsewhere, is "happiness." Israel is inherently an "Enlightenment" state, with its central ideal of the transformation of Diaspora Jewry into "modern" Israelis: "I make people happy. They leave my office with a smile on their faces," states Daniel Yachia, head of urology at the Hillel Yaffe Medical Center in Hadera about his aesthetic surgery patients. "If the surgery doesn't make them sexier, happier and wealthier, they blame the doctor," according to Professor D. J. Hauben, head of plastic and reconstructive surgery at Rabin Medical Center–Beilinson Campus in Petach Tikvah. "Happiness" is the goal of physical transformation, and the inability to achieve happiness can only be the fault of the physician.

A large proportion of the men who have aesthetic procedures are teenagers who have surgery on their noses, ears, breasts, or penises just before they begin their compulsory military service. Moris Topaz, an aesthetic surgeon in Ráanana, notes that they want to "pass." "They want to look like everyone else when they go into the army. These may be boys who were able to conceal protruding ears under long hair that will now be tightly shorn. Or boys who wore shirts at the beach to conceal feminine breasts, and now will have to shower naked with dozens of other young men." Rhinoplasties do not figure into this rush for surgery before military service.[37] "These patients have lived with large noses all their lives, whereas large breasts, for example, typically appear at puberty because of excess weight or hormonal changes. It's a new problem they're facing as teenagers, and they're quite ashamed. It makes them look female, and they want to get rid of it immediately." As a young man, one must look hypermasculine to be seen as a soldier. And that visual definition of masculinity is rigorously defined. The army experience, created to shape all Israelis into a single national identity, also shapes them to imagine their male bodies as identical.[38] Despite universal military service in Israel, young women recruits seem not to have this rush for surgery, perhaps because they have already had procedures (such as rhinoplasty) done well before the age of military service.

The military experience reifies the construction of the "new" Israeli (not: "Jewish") male body that defines the Israeli male. Not only are breasts unacceptable on men, as we shall see in our later discussion of gynecomastia, but the wrong shape or form of the penis comes to be read as a major sign of difference in a world where the two defining groups, Jews and Moslems, are both circumcised. Daniel Yachia, himself a pioneer in penile aesthetic surgery in Israel, notes that most of his patients for aesthetic surgery of the penis are between the ages of sixteen and eighteen. Either they imagine that their penises are oddly shaped or they are indeed differently shaped because of congenital or surgical changes, such as botched circumcisions, which left behind scars or extra skin. "These boys are ashamed of the shape of their penises, and dread taking showers with the other boys," he explains. "They want to have 'normal-looking' penises." The increase in aesthetic surgery of the penis has become noticeable in contemporary Israel. Amitzur Farkas, head of Shaarei Tsedek's urology department, noted that "in Israel, [in the past] if a child does not have the 'perfect penis' it's not a big deal, so we haven't done many operations in which there is merely an esthetic problem. But now, parents are more aware and ready to allow cosmetic surgery to correct problems that don't interfere with functioning."[39] Here the notion of an idealized penis is the obverse of the cry for the return of the foreskin; it is the perfectly shaped, circumcised penis. All "real" men need to look "normal," and that is defined culturally. "Passing" here is not having one's foreskin reconstructed, but making sure that one looks like "everyone else" within one's cohort.

Israel today has become the aesthetic surgery capital of the Middle East. Well known as the culture with the most modern system of medical care in the area, Israel has served unofficially as the host for patients from throughout the Middle East since the peace accord with Egypt in 1979 and Jordan in 1994. Now women from the Arab lands are coming to Israel in ever-increasing numbers for surgical procedures that they feel they cannot have in their homelands. Women from Jordan, Egypt, the Gulf states, and other Arab countries have their noses, mouths, or breasts altered in Israeli clinics each year. "They come from conservative societies. I guess it's a little more comfortable for them to go away and come back with a new nose than to do it at home," according to Yaakov Golan, head of the Israeli aesthetic surgery association and a surgeon at Jerusalem's Shaarei Tsedek hospital.[40] Given the meaning associated with the changes of the shape of the nose in the Middle East and the anxiety about having one's nose "misread," such crossing of borders to undertake aesthetic surgery provides a commentary on the globalization of both the field and the models for acceptable and unacceptable appearance.

THE IMPORTANCE OF BEING BARBRA

In the United States, the new "ethnic-specific" aesthetic surgery aims at alleviating the fear not of looking Jewish, but of looking "too Jewish."[41] Leslie Fiedler commented in the 1970s: "As the case of [Barbra] Streisand makes clear, we have begun to deliver ourselves from the tyranny of such ethnocentric norms in the last decades of the twentieth century; so that looking Niggerish or Kike-ish no longer seems as freakish as it once did, and the children of 'lesser breeds' no longer eat their hearts out because they do not look like Dick and Jane in their Primers."[42] The image of Barbra Streisand (1942–   ) has come to represent, for the general public as well as for young artists in the 1996 "Too Jewish" show at the Jewish Museum in New York (and elsewhere), the acceptable level of looking Jewish.[43] By 1997 Streisand attained the role of an icon of beauty—exotic beauty, "Jewish" beauty, but beauty nevertheless: "The word 'ugly' is defined as 'displeasing to the eye.' Is Barbra Streisand uncomfortable to look at? With her hideously large and misshapen nose, she is recognized as one of the most beautiful people in the world. Her ugly nose only makes her beauty more distinguished. This is only one example of how a bit of ugliness can achieve an uncommon magnificence."[44] This is a far cry from the early reception of Streisand's appearance, which is now transvalued as aesthetically pleasing or at least interesting.

John Simon wrote, upon the release of Frank Pierson's *A Star Is Born* (1976), with Streisand playing the role originated by snub-nosed Janet Gaynor in 1937: "O for the gift of Rostand's Cyrano to invoke the vastness of that nose alone as it cleaves the giant screen from east to west, bisects it from north to south. It zigzags across our horizon like a bolt of fleshy lightning; it towers like a ziggurat made of meat. But the nose is only a symbol, or symptom, of what is wrong with Barbra Streisand. She could easily have had it fixed; she had no problem, after all, shaving the middle 'a' out of her given name."[45] By the opening of the "Too Jewish" show in 1996, Streisand had come to represent the problem of "Jewish identity in American culture, and the struggles Jewish Americans face in balancing assimilative urges with the need to preserve a distinct identity and a heritage." She is central to the artists' vision of the Jew's physiognomy: "But first and foremost, there is Barbra. There are no fewer than three pieces featuring the charming and enigmatic Ms. Streisand and all that she and her defiant nose symbolize. Two works are Warhol knockoffs, with Barbra's image supplanting that of Elvis or Jackie O. Nice, but the funniest example is Rhonda Lieberman's little white Christmas tree, decorated with Star of David–shaped ornaments bearing Barbra's likeness. The piece is called Barbra Bush."[46] Another review of the show stresses the representations of the nose as an icon of difference that, now that the Jews are acculturated, can be seen and represented: "In a more serious vein, Adam Rolston offers a series of painful, dramatic drawings depicting the surgical procedure of the 'nose job.' "[47] According to Rolston, the inspiration for his six-plate series on the nose job was my book *The Jew's Body.* Thus art comes from criticism and returns to art.

Deborah Kass pays tribute to Barbra Streisand's nose in a Warholesque silk screen of repeated images of Streisand's profile, which she subtitles "the Jewish Jackie Series." Here the ethnic nose has become the emblem of non-acculturation in the work of

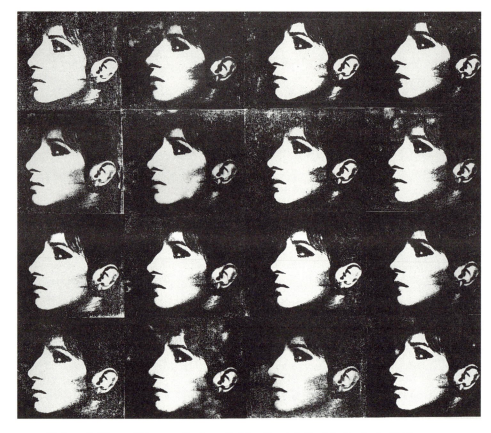

Deborah Kass, "Sixteen Barbras" (The Jewish Jackie Series), 1992.

artists who are clearly mainstream within the new claims of the multicultural ethnic identity that is America of the 1990s. How very different from the (Ruthenian) Czechoslovakian American artist Andy Warhol's (1928–1987) *Before and After*, a portrait of an aesthetic surgery nose job: there are no possible "before and after" images for Streisand—even though at the very beginning of her career she for a fleeting moment thought about it.[48]

Barbra Streisand's image in 1996 is a far cry from that of the Jewish vaudeville star Fanny Brice (1891–1951) in 1923. Brice, whom Streisand played in her first starring role, in William Wyler's *Funny Girl* (1968), had a rhinoplasty performed in her apartment at the Ritz during August 1923 by Henry Junius Schireson. Her employer, Flo Ziegfeld, was opposed: "I can get all the classic beauties I want. There are a hundred pretty girls with nice noses for every place in the chorus—and they're all alike. They cost fifty dollars a week. This nose cannot be replaced or imitated. It's a million-dollar nose."[49] Dorothy Parker, in one of her most telling observations, claimed that Brice "had cut off her nose to spite her race." (This moment is, of course, completely missing from Streisand's film.) Brice defended her actions, saying that "no woman on the stage of today can afford to have a nose that is likely to keep on growing until she can swallow it." Brice's role as a comic figure was certainly tied to her facial image; the Italian-American comic Jimmy Durante, whose nickname was "Schnozzola," paralleled her on the vaudeville stage. In altering her appearance, she altered her limiting role as an ethnic comic, but her audience knew full well what the nose job meant. The *New York Times* (with its powerful assimilationist leanings) stated that Brice could "change her style by changing her nose."[50] Ethnic identity—whether Jewish American or Asian American or African American—is validated as long as the general aesthetic norms of the society are not transgressed. Being too visible means being seen not as an individual but as an Other, one of the "ugly" race. The realm where these distinctions matter most, of course, is in the sphere of sexual relationships and the erotic.

CHAPTER SEVEN

After the Nose

Erotic Bodies

𝒪ne of the major themes in our history of aesthetic surgery has been the association of the recontouring of the body with the erotic. The wish to be erotic is the desire to "pass," not to "pass" as unnoticed, but to "pass" as desired, to "pass" into the group that silently acknowledges itself as erotic. It is to identify so intensely with the idealized image of that group that you will yourself to become one with them. Indeed, "passing" is never vanishing, but rather merging with a very visible group. The boundaries between the beautiful and the ugly, between the happy and the unhappy, are also those between the erotic and the unerotic. "Black" and "Jewish" and "Irish" noses are unerotic; the missing foreskin is a turn-off. The missing nose may well be the greatest antierotic sign of them all—at the midpoint in the nineteenth century, Eduard Zeis claimed that "the eye is so used to seeing a nose on a human face, that even an ugly one is preferable to one that is partly or completely missing."[1] That missing nose marks the person as sexually contagious. Horror, not sexual excitement, results from seeing this face.

The history of aesthetic surgery on the racialized face is the first installment of a history of modern procedures for the aesthetic alteration of the body. Once the "visible" body is seen to be mutable, and the patient is seen to be able to "pass" "in public," then the "hidden" aspects of the body become the materials of the surgeon. Although early nineteenth-century operations for decircumcision may provide the roots for the distinction between reconstructive ("real") and "beauty" surgery and thus serve as the model for "beauty" surgery of the racial face, they were preceded by aesthetic procedures that repaired the face understood as damaged by syphilitic infection. Analogous to the fear that sexual misadventure or sin could be read into the damaged face of the syphilitic is the anxiety that the "damaged," that is, circumcised body will be read as dangerous. After the mid nineteenth century, the popularization of facial procedures without risk of pain, infection, or residual scarring was followed by the development of new approaches to the invisible, sexualized body.

The boundary between the erotic and the unerotic body is imagined as permanent. Actually, like the boundary between "reconstructive" and "aesthetic" surgery, it is always being changed. The claim is that one is attracted to or envious of another body because of that body's appearance. If one could only acquire such a body and be able to "pass" as sexy! The ideal erotic body changes from time to time, place to place, and cohort to cohort. One powerful presupposition of aesthetic surgery, as we have shown, is the transformability of the body. By extension, it is believed that aesthetic surgery can change the unerotic into the erotic. This belief is present whether one alters the shape of the nose or of the buttocks.

The erotic is a quality that seems to be rooted in the body, but, as the long discussion of the origins of sexual arousal have shown, it is also perceived as a quality of the mind or the psyche.[2] Bodies are what we make them to be, and when we change the rules as to what body parts can be altered and how they should appear, when we alter what orifices of the body should be entered, we change the erotic nature of the bodies themselves. Judith Butler has observed that the very construction of gender relies on a fixed understanding of the body.[3] When aesthetic surgery acquired the technical ability to transgress the boundary that arbitrarily defines the body as either erotic or unerotic, it disrupted the notion of the fixed gendering of the body. Yet, ironically, transgressing this dichotomy constantly reestablishes it.

The body that is erotic in one decade may not even be attractive in the next. The erotic body is always a healthy body, even though the meaning of "health" will also change. Eroticism as a quality, however, ascribed to both sexes (in all combinations and contexts) means a healthy body and a healthy psyche—this linkage is seen as absolute and desirable. It is to be acquired by crossing the boundary from the unerotic, and the unerotic, as we have seen, is clearly defined in the history of aesthetic surgery by racial models. Becoming "erotic" also has its downside. The anxiety about the erotic body in the West is omnipresent. The erotic body may cause terrible diseases such as syphilis and AIDS, which are then written on the body for all to see (thus the attraction of seeing this played out in *The Phantom of the Opera*). This secular transformation of St. Paul's disgust at the erotic as diseased and corrupting is also part of the "Protestant ethic" of Western culture.[4] How can the erotic body make you "happy" when you know that the body is corruptible and will eventually die?

At the last fin de siècle, the female body was imagined to be infinitely malleable. Women could become anything and everything. This was Frank Wedekind's (1864–1918) fantasy of Lulu in his *Earth Spirit* (1895) and *Pandora's Box* (1904), which reappeared as G. W. Pabst's (1885–1967) *Pandora's Box* (1929) on the screen and as Alban Berg's (1885–1935) *Lulu* (1935) on the operatic stage. The protagonist Lulu was all women to every man. Female bodies were universally transmutable, but always retained their feminine essence. This was perceived as the source of female erotic attraction, for good or for evil, as Christina von Braun has argued.[5] Racial bodies, too, are both immutable and infinitely malleable, as we have seen. They shift and change; their malleability becomes one of the hallmarks of their identity. They are everyone, and everyone has the potential of being they; thus anxiety about aesthetic surgery becomes anxiety about the potential of infinite transformation and the inability to judge who is "passing." Is my erotic feeling real or is it merely a simulacrum?

What happens when you operate on the "unerotic" body in order to make it erotic and the psyche "happy"? In 1934 Harold Delf Gillies (1882–1960) saw breast reduction as "the borderline of what is justifiable" for the aesthetic surgeon. He argued before a medical school audience that the condition of virginal hypertrophy of the breast . . . is a quite common condition and in its very worst form constitutes one of the great tragedies of life. . . . They are enormously heavy, affecting the patient's physical attitude, for they frequently occur in young girls with otherwise slim figures and thus cannot adequately be hidden. Almost invariably the patients give the history that they shun the opposite sex and refuse the pleasures of the ballroom or swimming-pool. . . . Even in the milder conditions many of the patients are unduly sensitive and the happiness given to them by reconstruction is a delight to the surgeon.[6]

At the end of the twentieth century the situation has changed little. As the Pittsburgh plastic surgeon H. W. Losken claimed in 1990: "In the final analysis, breast surgery, whether it be augmentation, reduction, lift, or reconstruction, is associated with a very high percentage of happiness. So many women say that it is the best thing they ever did or that it has made such a difference to their lives. The objective for which we strive is the happiness of the patient. That is the criterion of success of any cosmetic operation."[7] While desiring it, popular Western culture also distrusts this happiness with the body as strongly as St. Paul would have. The formerly underendowed and now aging dancer in Michael Bennett's *A Chorus Line* (1975), turns to her colleagues and sings:

Tits and ass can change your life,
They sure changed mine.
Have it all done. Honey, take my word.
Grab a cab, c'mon, see the wizard on Park and Seventy-third
For Tits and Ass. Orchestra and balcony.[8]

"T&A," to use the formula from *A Chorus Line*, may make you successful as a dancer (it is claimed) but, as the musical shows, they may not make you happy as a human being. This is the Pauline struggle that accompanies the construction of the erotic through aesthetic surgery. In this age of aesthetic surgery, you can only mask the corrupt nature of the body, you can never change it. Have you become sufficiently "real" to allow you to cross the boundary into the erotic? Or do you remain a mere simulacrum, a virtual reality now possible in our age of technical reproduction?

Buttocks Have Meaning

The erotic is located in the sexualized body, and that body is juxtaposed in our imagination with the ill, the different, and the unerotic body. Often such juxtapositions focus on the meaning ascribed to what a culture labels as secondary characteristics; thus, in the West when we publicly imagine the erotic, we fantasize about the buttocks and breasts, but only the buttocks and the breasts of the *female* are accepted as secondary sexual characteristics within this play of the erotic. Even gay eroticism, in its more public forms, plays on the "fem" aspects of the female and male alike. The question is what the female (or perhaps better: feminine) buttocks and breasts come to mean as a sign of the line between the erotic and the unerotic—and whether one can ask such a question in a manner that highlights the complex meaning of the breasts and the buttocks for a history of aesthetic surgery.

The buttocks (also called the nates, ass, clunes, breech) were represented in equally complex ways during the late nineteenth century and the rise of aesthetic surgery. The breasts (which both men and women don't have and want, or do have and don't want, or any combination of the above) are culturally defined as female or feminizing in the light of the reading of the mammae as the sign of female reproductive functions. The buttocks are also read in the light of the meaning ascribed to the breasts.

The buttocks are the prominence formed by the gluteal muscles of the upper legs and hips. As the hip bones are less mobile than the leg, the huge muscles at the hip are mostly concerned with moving and stabilizing the hip joint. This joint also has a complete complement of muscles, the largest of which is the *gluteus maximus* (Latin for "biggest in the buttock"), which is important for locomotion. Although hip shape and pelvic form have been read as secondary sexual characteristics, structured by the

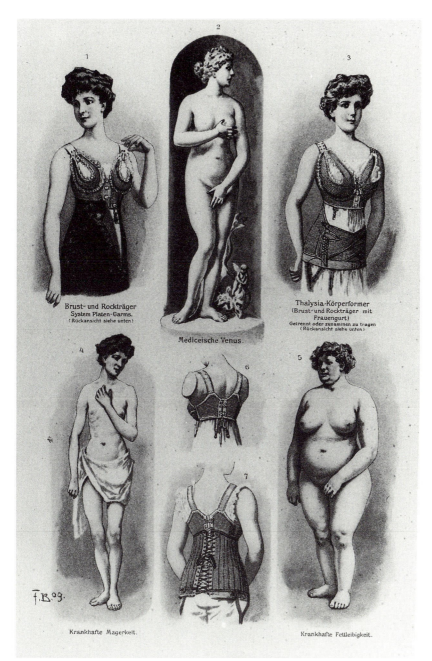

Image of the healthy and therefore beautiful female form, contrasted with the too fat and too thin, 1901. Classical sculpture remains the model for the "normal."

birthing process, the complexity of reading the buttock points to the cultural construction of the erotic body. Both men and women have breasts and buttocks—and yet these are defined as feminine, making the male breast and buttocks virtually invisible.

Charles Darwin's *Descent of Man and Selection in Relation to Sex* (1871) assumed a relationship between the "natural" form of the buttocks and the reproductive meaning associated with the human female pelvis.[9] (Darwin built upon the work of earlier anatomists such as Georges Cuvier [1769–1832].) The pelvis was seen as the most prominent secondary sexual characteristic, and the buttocks were read as the visible sign of the pelvis. The buttocks thus became eroticized as the visual sign of the reproductive system. The human breasts came to be understood as a sign of the anomalous nature of the human female body, as other female mammals do not have prominent mammae. Only human females do. The prominent (primitive) breasts came to be perceived as mimicking in their form the protruding (primitive) buttocks, the "real sign" of the sexual.[10]

Beginning with the expansion of European colonial exploration, describing the form and size of the buttocks became a means of describing and classifying the races. The more prominent, the more primitive. Thus Darwin's view is a further elaboration on the adaptation of the human form for reproductive purposes. This is a continuation of the cultural presupposition that "primitive" races have a "primitive" sexuality, which is represented in their bodies by physical signs of their "true" nature. Thus Khoikhoi (called Hottentot by the first Dutch explorers) and San (named Bushman by early Anglophone explorers) women of southwestern Africa were represented from the sixteenth century on by their exaggerated buttocks (steatopygia) and labia (Hottentot apron). Although these images suggested a greater size for the buttocks, they also claimed that these women (once anatomized) had a smaller pelvic size. The steatopygia was seen as a pronounced, localized accumulation of fat or fatty-fibrous tissue on the upper part of the buttocks. It was understood as rarely manifested prior to puberty, and as an accumulation that enlarged gradually and was a *normal* physical characteristic in

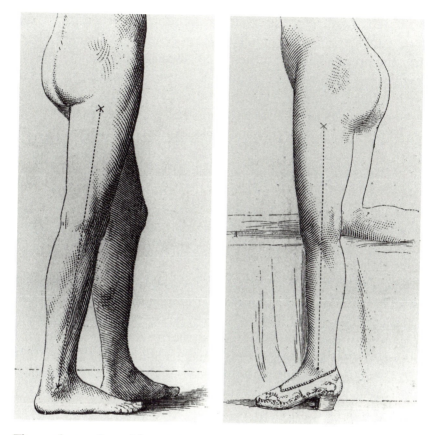

The perfect male and female leg, foot, (and buttocks).

women who otherwise might not be obese. The fascination with the body of the black woman was evidenced by white scientists from the nineteenth-century French anatomist Cuvier to Weimar Germany's Magnus Hirschfeld, who analyzed the black woman's body in relation to the range of "normal" body shapes.[11]

As greater pelvic size was understood as analogous to increased cranial capacity as a sign of "progress," the small pelvic size of the "primitive" was understood as proof of her actual place in the great chain of being. The exaggerated buttocks were understood as an attempt to "mimic" the higher stages of evolutionary development. Similar representations can be found in the images of the native peoples of South America in the earliest illustrated accounts of European exploration published by the de Bry publishing house in seventeenth-century Holland.[12] Here too, the breasts and the buttocks are seen as natural signs of the barbarism of the native. Although they were initially represented as idealized "Roman" types, these native inhabitants came to be seen as in need of domestication and conversion. Thus their body form, including their buttocks, come to be represented as grotesque.

Works such as Havelock Ellis's (1859–1939) multivolume *Studies in the Psychology of Sex,* following Darwin, stressed the buttocks as a female secondary sexual characteristic highly fetishized in European culture. Ellis associated the erotic practice of whipping with the overemphasis on the buttocks in British culture. Ellis related this symbolic reading of the buttocks to the primary sexual characteristics (the genitalia) and other secondary sexual characteristics (such as the female breasts). In his case study of "Florrie," he showed how "Florrie" came to displace the meaning of the buttocks onto other body sites.[13] It is "the pronounced development of the gluteal region and thighs" that makes them "specially fitting to become the seat of the symbolism" (p. 197). For Ellis this was a sign of the restructuring of the meaning of the buttocks, "especially in girls" (p. 196). Buttocks came to replace the breasts in a system of representing their own sexuality, because the young girl's emphasis on her buttocks as the site of fat deposits was to the exclusion of the breasts, which, according to Ellis, showed little development.

Ellis's work on the meaning and the history of the buttocks was paralleled in Austria by Sigmund Freud's discussion of the meaning of the anal phase, worked out in detail first in his *Three Essays on the Theory of Sexuality* (1905). Freud understood the anal phase as the second of three stages of bodily fixation—beginning with the mouth, then the anus, and then the genitals. "Normal" development proceeded along this path, but development could be fixated at the earlier stages. Freud sees anal fixation as the origin of homosexuality. The buttocks become the place where a "primitive" fixation takes place, thwarting the movement of the erotic interest of the individual to the genitalia. It is not the anus per se that comes to function as the symbolic reference in Freud's system, but rather the buttocks. It is not the proximity of the buttocks to the genitalia that is of interest, but rather their position adjacent to the anus. Thus the buttocks become the sign of the female as "primitive" or of the male as "fixated" at an earlier stage of development.

The buttocks have ever-changing symbolic value. They are associated with the organs of reproduction, with the aperture of excretion, as well as with the mechanism of locomotion through discussions of gait. They never represent themselves. Indeed, the very problem of whether they are singular or plural is a sign of their nature as a floating signifier.[14] When aesthetic surgery is performed upon the buttocks, it is to enhance their sexual attraction.

Buttock lifts, like the reduction and lift of the breasts, come to be gendered female.[15] The Brazilian aesthetic surgeon Ivo Pitanguy (1926–   ) in the 1970s developed a buttock lift that was widely copied.[16] Pitanguy was trained at the faculty of Medicine in Rio de Janeiro and served on the staff of the Pronto Socorro Hospital, where he did reconstructive surgery.[17] At age twenty-one he left Rio and traveled to the United States to study at Bethesda Hospital in Cincinnati. Later he worked with surgeons in France and the United Kingdom, including Archibald MacIndoe, who taught him rhinoplasty and prepared the way for his encounter with Harold Delf Gillies. Thus the line from Pitanguy's development of aesthetic surgery in Brazil, where he opened his first clinic in 1963, led in a straight line back to the beginning of aesthetic surgery at the turn of the century.

It is not surprising that the buttock lift came out of Brazilian aesthetic surgery. Brazilian aesthetic surgery can justifiably claim a history of more than one hundred and fifty years, and it came to dominate certain areas during the 1980s.[18] Just as the Brazilians deemphasized the breasts, they reemphasized the buttocks, creating an image of the female body strikingly similar to that of Ellis's English "girl." According to one of its leading practitioners, Ricardo Baroudi, the emphasis on the "culture, genetics, and race" of the patient in Brazil also shaped the Brazilian's attitude toward "the concept of beauty, body fat distribution, and body weight." In this context, according to Baroudi, women, seen primarily in terms of their reproductive abilities, became conflicted with the cultural norms of physical beauty: "Maternity takes its toll on a woman's body. It is difficult to maintain body contour, skin tautness and turgor, and breast shape after one or more pregnancies. This fact explains why mammaplasties and abdominoplasties are the most frequently requested procedures, second only to requests for facial surgery" (p. 396). The claim is that the woman, having fulfilled her maternal duty to country and race, now wishes to return to the role of the erotic female, but to do so she must maintain her image as someone able to excite the male with the constant promise of reproduction; otherwise, she is of no sexual interest. Such views combined with the racial reading of the body have made Brazil one of the centers of aesthetic surgery.

The overcapacity generated in the limited homegrown market, however, has meant that aesthetic surgeons have turned Brazil into a center for international aesthetic surgery. In an age of ever expanding globalization of medical markets, Brazil is now firmly on the map (along with Israel in the Middle East and South Korea in Asia) as one of the places to go to have aesthetic surgery. With sixteen hundred trained aesthetic surgeons, the Brazilian market relies on attracting clients from throughout the world.[19] When you check into a hotel in Rio de Janeiro, you find pamphlets for the local aesthetic surgery clinics on your bedside table along with a Gideon Bible. Procedures such as those developed by Pitanguy aided in this quest for the perfect Brazilian bottom.

A series of procedures to "firm" and "tighten" the buttocks to restore youthful contours, including the use of liposuction to remove localized fatty deposits (from other parts of the body as well as the buttocks), has become a relatively common procedure.[20] Until the 1970s the classic method of removing fatty deposits from the buttocks, stomach, and thighs was by "block lipectomy with skin resection," surgery that removed fat tissue as well as excess skin.[21] The result was a slimmer body, but one marked by scars, which often became the locus for new fat deposits. These procedures grew directly out of the reduction operations beginning in 1886 with Howard Kelly's removal of fat and skin from the abdomen and thighs. Through the 1970s various procedures, including those by Pitanguy, were developed to hide the scars.[22] Some of these combined surgery with the use of a sharp curette to remove fat from below the skin.

Various methods of subcutaneous surgery were tried to replace these procedures. The use of the uterine curette often led to catastrophic results, as one was never quite sure what was being removed from under the skin. Thus the first malpractice suit for aesthetic surgery in France was brought against a surgeon who used a curette to reduce the calf of a dancer. He damaged a blood vessel and she had to have her leg amputated.

Modern liposuction, using blunt instruments to create tunnels and pass between major blood vessels, was developed by Yves-Gerard Illouz in France in 1977 and introduced into the United States in 1981.[23] It quickly became the most popular means of shaping the body, especially the buttocks and thighs. Illouz noted that he wanted to develop a procedure for "removing riding breeches," without scars.[24] His first patient was a young woman who wanted a lipoma removed from her back and did not want to have a scar. He undertook this procedure, and there was little scarring but also no excess skin to signal that fat had been removed. It was essentially "invisible" surgery, replacing earlier procedures in which "the resulting scars did not compensate for the prior deformities."[25] It is the increased invisibility of such procedures to shape the body that makes each generation of procedures acceptable. It also turns the now-visible results of the prior generation into signs that aesthetic surgery had taken place. "Passing" is always tied to the expectations of visibility in one's own moment of history.

With the anxiety over silicone implants, silicone buttock implants for the augmentation of the buttocks are no longer as sought after as they once were. New surgical techniques in addition to liposuction hide scars at the superior bikini line rather than at the inferior gluteal fold.[26] Yet all of the procedures on the buttocks have as their purpose the "happiness" of the patient. As Baroudi and Moraes note: "Patients who are candidates for body contouring surgery are not happy with their image" (p. 16). The truly unhappy, according to Baroudi and Moraes, are those who "go from office to office, searching for solutions to their problems but do not try to improve their body contour, depending totally on the surgeon to solve the problem." They present as patients who will never be "happy" (p. 17). These patients use their autonomy not to exercise but to seek the Holy Grail of thinness in the surgeon's office.

How does one deal with a fat body, with heavy buttocks? Is it sufficient to have fat removed, or must one change one's life? Is aesthetic surgery an answer, or must one alter diet and exercise? Most important, what do you change when you have your bottom lifted? Do you change your soul? Do you now "pass" as someone who is not "primitive" but rather erotic? The buttocks become both the site of the "primitive" but also (and often simultaneously) replace the breasts as the site of the fetishization of the erotic—in men and women.

Big Breasts and Bellies

In the world of the fat, the obese abdomen and pendulous breast have evident if complicated (and often contradictory) meanings. A recent history of the breast in Western culture has provided the baseline for any contemporary discussion of the breast. Marilyn Yalom's *History of the Breast* provides a rich, illustrated vocabulary of images concerning the meanings associated with the breast. Her history of the "medical breast" rests on the assumption that any discussion of the breast is defined by its role as a sign of femininity (as opposed to masculinity).[27] This binary opposition (women have breasts, men don't) immediately presents a set of further questions concerning the medicalization of the breast, much as the binary opposition between "happiness" and "unhappiness" evokes problems in defining the outcome of aesthetic surgery.

The modern history of the aesthetic surgery of the breast begins with breast reduction. Parallel to their development of procedures to reduce the size of the nose in the 1880s and 1890s, aesthetic and reconstructive surgeons devoted much effort to developing techniques to reduce the overly large breast. The distinction between reconstructive surgery and aesthetic surgery is nowhere drawn more clearly than in the history of the breast. One can examine the literature on aesthetic breast reduction (reduction mammaplasty or mastoplasty, alterations undertaken not as a result of cancer or other invasive tumors) from the perspective of the notion of the perfect breast at the turn of the century, a breast that is smaller rather than larger, and rounded rather than pendulous. On the surface, aesthetic surgery to reduce a woman's breast size relieves stress on her back muscles, but it is also supposed to boost her self-esteem.

By the 1930s breast reduction crossed out of the realm of reconstructive surgery and entered that of aesthetic surgery. The American surgeon Hans May described breast reduction as "not merely a cosmetic operation due to vanity of the fair sex. . . . Pendulous breasts are apt to be a psychical and psychic handicap, resulting in inferiority complexes. When it is possible to correct a breast deformity safely and satisfactorily and thus restore the happiness of the patient, plastic reconstruction of the breast is a justifiable operation."[28] Maxwell Maltz (1899–1975) seconded this opinion, noting that such a problem "causes psychological disturbance in the growing girl who feels physically abnormal."[29] The abnormality is being seen as different within the model of the racialized (or primitive) body. Women with large, pendulous breasts are not yet "New Women" with small, firm breasts.

Even a hundred years later, in an age that emphasizes the erotic nature of the large breast, the question of how breast reduction is to be read is ambiguous. The public image of Roseanne (then Barr) in 1994 can serve as an example. She had a breast reduction because she suffered "from backaches and pains because, like other big-breasted women, she finds it hard to hold them up."[30] But at the same time she acquired a "whole new body after spending more than $60,000 on new eyelids, cheek implants, liposuction, a face-lift, nose job, chin implant and breast reduction."[31] In late twentieth-century America we have all become victims of biology. Stardom is incomplete without a grounding in victimhood. Constructing the beautiful body may alleviate discomfort and pain, but it is pain of the psyche as much as of the body.

To examine the origins of aesthetic breast reduction, one must understand that, like many of the other aesthetic procedures, the reduction of the pendulous breast came to have meaning within another system of representation, that of race. In the 1890s Ernst Brücke wrote about the specifically racial nature of the breast. For him, the "German" breast was a youthful, underdeveloped breast, smaller and more juvenile than the "Italian" breast[32] Thus breast form, as one can see in the almost fetishized popular and semipopular cultural histories of the breast published by Brücke's contemporaries, came to represent images of idealized racial body types. Smaller breasts represented "Germanness," as opposed to large, pendulous breasts, which were read as a sign of the primitive.

The history of the racial breast is the history of the aesthetics of the breast. In his *Beauty of the Woman's Body* (1904), the Viennese ethnologist Friedrich S. Krauss (1859–1938), a friend and colleague of Freud's, presented a descriptive study of the woman's body. The images he presented, however, focused on the representation of the breast.[33] Even with chapters on eyes and cheek

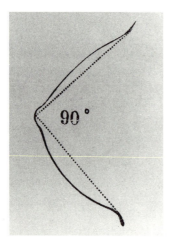

The perfect female breast.

and neck, the book visually represents in the breast the racial divisions that underlay Krauss's study. Yet he did not devote a separate chapter to the breast because it was understood as a ubiquitous sign. Krauss's work is typical of the popular sexological cultural histories of women's bodies, which used racial categories as their basic model for categorization.

The most comprehensive study of this type is Hermann Heinrich Ploss's (1819–85) ethnographic study of "woman," which first appeared in 1885 in two illustrated volumes and grew under other hands until the eleventh edition of 1927, when it featured more than a thousand images in four volumes.[34] It was a middle-class cultural phenomenon rather than a merely scholarly publishing venture. Ploss distinguished among racial classifications on the basis of the form of the breast. Thus he quotes another authority that the breasts of the "white" and "yellow" races are virginally compact, while those of the "black" race are like a goat's udder (1:314). Likewise, the form and size of the areola has specific racial implications, and size is the determining factor. The farther south one goes from Germany, the more pendulous the breasts and the larger the areolas seem to get. Jewish women, according to the work of Sarah Teumin, also present racially determined forms of both breast and nipples (1:334). The forms of the breast reflect specifically the characters of the races. Ploss's images of the ideal female body as found in the various races followed the contemporary sense of "what is beautiful." For one of his plates he compared the physical form of various races using images extrapolated from ethnographic photography. The two exceptions are images of the ideal and perfect Western woman represented by a Greek sculpture and a Viennese analogue.

As with the nose, the discussion of the racialized breast is always a discussion about character. The anthropologist Hans Friedenthal (1878–?) saw in the physiognomy of the breast the origin of language.[35] In an essay published in 1927 he postulated that the form of the nose and lips was determined by the racial form of the mother's breast, and the structure of the language was formed by these noses and lips. The suckling of the child at the breast formed the shape of the child's mouth and nose through

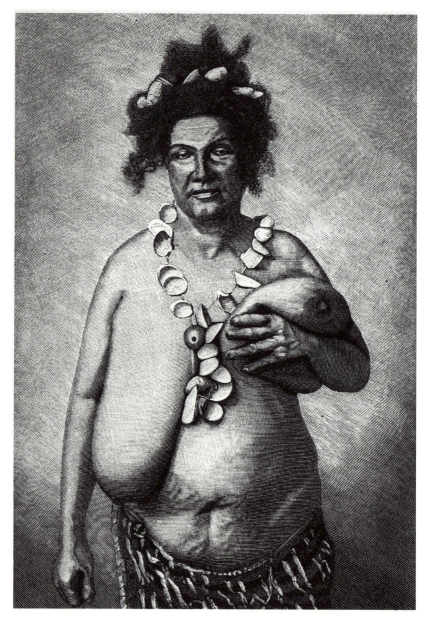

The Ethiopian woman.

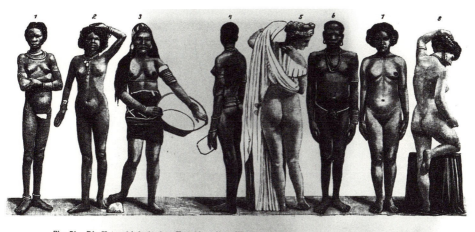

Fig. 71. Die Unterschiede in dem Körperbau (dem Wuchs) verschiedener Rassen. (Nach Photographien.)
No. 1. Makraka-Mädchen (Central-Afrika). — No. 2. Australier-Mädchen (Nord-Queensland). — No. 3. Dajak-Mädchen (Borneo). — No. 4. Madi-Weib (Central-Afrika). — No. 5. Griechische Idealfigur (Venus Kallipygos). — No. 6. Mondú-Weib (Central-Afrika.) — No. 7. Mädchen aus Samoa (Polynesien). — No. 8. Mädchen aus Wien.

The scale of the female body.

the pressure of the shape of the racial breast. (This sounds like an early twentieth-century scientific parody of the analogous argument in Sterne's *Tristram Shandy*.) Thus the breasts of black women (in Friedenthal's words, the "Hottentots and Bushmen") form the "strange sounds of their languages which is in harmony with the club-shaped breasts of the mothers which shaped the lips of the nursing child." Character (the nose), race, and even culture are shaped by and shape the form of the breast.

The breast functions as a racial sign even in the basic aesthetic surgical guides to breast reduction, such as that of Jacques Joseph.[36] He described the "anthropology" of the breast as basic to any discussion of aesthetic surgery of the breast: "Certain racial differences exist with regard to the shape and growth pattern of the breast. Whereas among Caucasians the hemispherical breast shape is the most common, the pointed breast shape seems to predominate among Black women" (p. 743). Race for Joseph was inscribed in the difference between the "white" and the "black" breast, whereas most other discussions emphasized the difference between the breasts of Europeans and other racial types, including the pendulous breasts of Jewish women.[37] In all cases, the

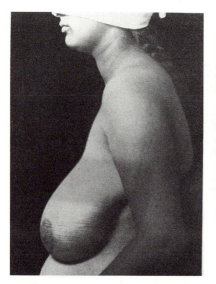

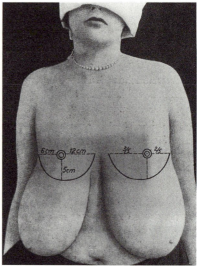

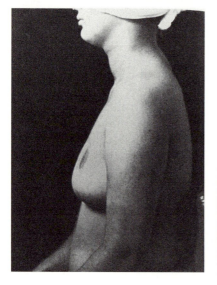

Jacques Joseph's case of large,
pendulous breasts before and
after surgery, first published in
1925.

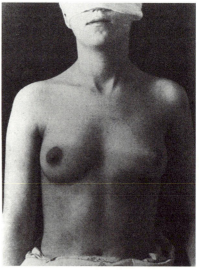

By contrast, "normal breasts in
an eighteen-year-old girl."

writers of the turn of the century figured the breast as a marker of the female as opposed to the male. Having breasts, as we have seen, defines the individual as "female." All other associations seemingly result from the form of the breasts.

At the end of the twentieth century the meaning of the breast remains associated with race. In Brazil today breast reduction has become commonplace among upper-middle-class families, so as to distinguish their daughters from the lower classes, who are imagined as black. Farid Hakme, the president of the Brazilian Plastic Surgery Society, attributes Brazil's fascination with aesthetic surgery to "the country's mix and match of different races, which can create physical disharmonies. 'What happens is the nose sometimes doesn't match the mouth or the buttocks don't match with the legs,' he said."[38] Fantasies about symmetry and balance reflect a Brazilian anxiety about looking "too black."[39] And this is represented by the "pendulous breast." "The women who want to reduce their breasts here [in Brazil] would probably want to increase them in the United States," Oswaldo Saldanha, the vice president of the Brazilian Plastic Surgery Society, noted. His explanation for this avoids the specificity of race; rather, for him, "beauty ideals and cultures are different in every country." The healthy and erotic body in Brazil is not the black body. As with rhinoplasties among Jews in the United States during the 1950s and 1960s, Brazilian breast reductions are often "sweet sixteen" birthday presents. By means of such gifts, parents enable their daughters silently to "pass" as members of an erotic cohort and find appropriate mates.[40]

The noted Brazilian anthropologist Roberto da Mattas stated the cultural context for the desire to reshape the female breast in terms of Brazil's racial culture. He believed that Brazil's body cult has its roots in the institution of black slavery, which was not abolished in Brazil until 1888. According to Da Matta, in the relationship between slave and master, the slave's body was the key element, the main instrument of economic and social survival for both.[41] It represented both "labor" and the "erotic." But in modern Brazil, such colonial dependency came to be a mark of opprobrium.

Racial identity is keyed to the desire for (in)visibility and the ability to "pass." One of Robert Goldwyn's patients from South America came to him with a "very personal" problem: "I looked up my family history and I found that way back we have black blood in it. . . . My question is, can you change my skin? Can you give me the skin from a completely white man?"[42] Becoming "completely white" means effacing all of one's own difference from the idealized ("white") cohort so that one can blend into it without comment. Achieving such "whiteness" becomes the domain of aesthetic surgery, at least in the fantasy of the patient. The desire is not merely to change but to vanish and to have all markers of difference, such as the pendulous breast, eradicated from the present and the future. It is necessary to become "completely white," for the negative image of the male Brazilian is that of the ugly, deformed and very *black* trickster Macunaím. Macunaím has a deformed body that defines the anxiety of masculinity; the supposedly pendulous breasts of the black woman define the anxiety of the feminine.

If Brazilian women wish to reduce the size of their breasts, young Argentinean women often opt for extensive breast enlargements, fulfilling the "Spanish" fantasy of the large-breasted woman as the icon of the erotic.[43] In Argentina, a million operations have been performed since 1970, one for every thirty Argentines. Argentina has the world's highest ratio of silicone implants per person. Jorge Weinstein of the Organization of Argentine Plastic Surgeons has commented that aesthetic surgery is popular among the working classes as well as the middle class.[44] Public hospitals offer nose jobs, breast implants, and liposuction. Their goal is happiness. "It's complete madness," Dr. Weinstein says. "People come in here describing how they want to look as if it were as natural and simple as going to the hairdresser. And I seem to spend more time listening to people's fantasies about what surgery will do for their sex life or marriage—and advising against treatment—than actually practicing." The search for happiness in Argentina is keyed to the erotic, but an erotic of imagined European beauty. It is a means of curing the "unhappiness" of the psyche. Luis Majul, the author of a popular book on the rise of aesthetic surgery in Argentina, notes that the increase in aesthetic surgery is the latest manifestation of a neurotic society, which often looks to psychotherapy as its path to happiness.[45] In aesthetic surgery it has simply found a form of external psychotherapy.

Concern for the health and proper size and shape of the breast has focused on different aspects of the breast at different times and places. Initially the major question confronting the surgeon was the reduction of the size of the breast.[46] Concern with the excessively large breast is documented as early as the time of Paulus of Aegina (635–90).[47] The seventeenth century worried about the repositioning of the nipple (and the areola) in case of breast reduction. William Durston described the drooping breast (ptotic or diffuse hypertrophy of the breast) as a medical problem as early as 1669. His description virtually vanished from the medical literature soon after it was published. Such mammoth breasts were understood as a pathology (or even a sign of the monstrous) and fell into the same category as tumors of the breast within the purview of the physician, but the surgical procedures for the reduction of the mammoth breast left ghastly scars, marking the body as having been ill.

The first nineteenth-century approaches, such as those suggested by Theodor Billroth (1829–94), did not concern themselves with "aesthetic" questions.[48] Removal of the breast, not its reduction, was the procedure of choice, even though Johann Friedrich Dieffenbach a generation before had already recognized the need for a procedure short of complete removal. According to contemporary comments, the first "modern" reduction mammaplasty took place in 1897. Alfred Pousson (1853–?) undertook the excision of the upper half of such breasts from the armpit (axilla) to the sternum by making two half-moon flaps.[49] The patient was a "still young woman" whose "breasts hung down to the inner aspect of the thighs" when she was seated. The result of the surgery was recognized to be "aesthetically mediocre [moyen]," but it did relieve the patient's somatic complaint, her back pain. The aesthetics of the procedure became more and more vital to its successful completion, which was to result not only in the reduction of physical pain, but in the constitution of psychic happiness. Pousson's awareness of the poor aesthetic result of his procedures marked a major step in the transformation of such breast reductions into aesthetic surgery. "Happiness" is an unscarred body with an erotic breast.

Such early procedures simply removed the excess breast tissue (whether tumorous or not) and did not make much of an attempt to reconstitute a breast that appeared and functioned like a natural breast. The definition of the "natural breast" evolved in the surgical discussion of the late nineteenth century. In 1882 Theodore Gaillard-Thomas suggested submammary incision to rescue at least part of the glandular disc. Scarring of the breast was evident in this procedure to rescue the breast's nursing function. This was virtually the same moment that surgeons began to be concerned with the scarring of the face following rhinoplasties. The "natural" breast was overtly unscarred and had a functioning nipple. Function, in this context, meant a nipple and breast that could lactate; there was no discussion of the role of the nipple in the erotic stimulation of the woman's body. By this definition of the "natural" body, the preservation of the areola was first successfully undertaken by the Heidelberg surgeon Vincenz Czerny (1842–1916), who transplanted the nipple following a simple mastectomy.

It was only in the first decade of the twentieth century that Hippolyte Morestin and Eugen Holländer specifically undertook aesthetic breast reduction.[50] In cases of "gigantomastia," it was necessary to rescue the nipple to make the breast both aesthetically pleasing and functional. But in no discussion of "function" is there any mention of the erotic. In 1922 Max Thorek in Chicago introduced wedge incisions, which made the preservation of the nipple an intrinsic part of the procedure.[51] But this nipple only looked real. It was Jacques Joseph who first proposed a two-stage surgical procedure for breast reduction with preservation of the areola's vascularization.[52] Thus the reduced breast came to be a functional and erotic breast as well as an aesthetic breast. Scarring was minimal and the breast with its aesthetic shape and form looked "natural." The operated woman could now "pass" as a

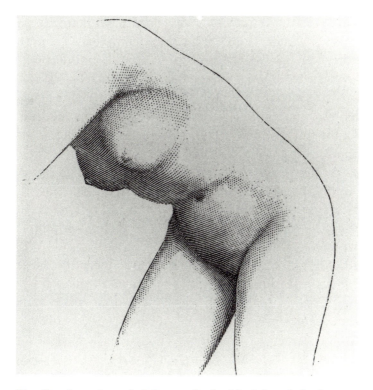

The firm breasts and abdomen in the ideal female body.

new woman with a complete breast, including a nipple. It was a truly erotic breast—it appeared erotic and was able to be erotically stimulated. As one of Robert Goldwyn's patients commented: "After all, a breast is not a breast until it has a nipple."[53] But it has to be a nipple as defined by the woman's experience of the function, feel, and response of her breast, not by the aesthetic visualization of the surgeon.

The cultural reading of breast reduction stressed the modernization (read: deracialization) of the woman's body. Big breasts are signs of the primitive. The advocates of surgical breast reduction in Weimar Germany stressed that pendulous breasts are unaesthetic and encumbering.[54] "Sporty women" do not want to have pendulous, lopsided breasts. Women who are "full of life, undertake sport, swim, and dance" want breast reductions so that they can "pass" as "modern." Truly elegant women with pendulous breasts suffer from "inferiority complexes." Sport and the sporty female body become an icon of the modern woman. This modern woman is not seen as "reproductive." This "New Woman" was also not a member of any race; her new body transcended racial categories. Indeed, according to the medical literature of the time, women who are in a happy marriage with children, and who have a husband happy with the form of their breasts do not need breast reduction. Their breasts signify the more traditional role of mother. The boundary is evident. Such breasts are the sign of the primitive, of racial difference, and of maternity. All of these categories are contrasted with the "modern" woman.

"Pathological" breast size and the reduction of breasts to acceptable *aesthetic* dimensions were connected from the very beginning. Hypertrophy of the breasts was understood as both a physical and an aesthetic problem. Aesthetic surgery of the breast increasingly aimed to remedy psychological as well as somatic complaints. Yet the central surgical problems to be overcome were the problems of scarring and those of the repositioning of a totally functional nipple. Once these problems were overcome (by the 1930s), breast reduction became commonplace. In the age of the flapper, the large breast was a sign of the proletarian, the common, the racially different. Nursing was part of the meaning ascribed to the large breast, and this was understood as antithetical to the erotic meaning inscribed on the "modern" breast. All of these qualities were racialized in the 1920s. Large breasts were seen as "primitive," not "modern." As standards of beauty shifted from the nineteenth to the twentieth century in Europe, the smaller breast came to provide an image of the erotic. The smaller breast enabled the woman to "pass" as a "New Woman," rather than a racialized woman. The latter was not free, she was encumbered by her role as mother, reproducing the race. The smaller breast enabled a woman to "pass" as free and erotic. In providing a breast that looked and responded as the woman expected, the surgeon enabled her to "pass" into the world of the "New Woman."

The primitive is understood as an anachronism, a sign of a past that refuses to go away, or as a degenerate throwback to the world that existed before the modern age. In conceptions of the racialized woman, huge breasts became identified with obesity, represented by the enormous belly, another sign of the racial body. Thus extremely large bellies and breasts were linked as signs of difference. Recently, Richard Klein has noted the oddity of a culture that has so much food stressing the thin body as an ideal.[55] By the close of the nineteenth century, the meaning of fat in American society was negative. Obesity had become a diagnostic category in medicine, and the "fat" body was no longer seen as a sign of social success, as it had been in the world of Franz Kafka's father. Kafka's (1883–1924) inordinate, self-conscious thinness was a sign of the modern. The stoutness that marked the "primitive" bodies of his parents was a sign of an age past.[56]

Late nineteenth-century aesthetic surgery dealt with the obese stomach of the racialized woman by removing her "apron" of fat.[57] The "apron," with its reference to cooking, another female role in addition to reproduction, marked the racialized body. Abdominal apronectomy or dermolipectomy for abdominal panniculus (in order to reduce obesity) was developed by Howard A. Kelly in Baltimore. On May 15, 1899, he removed the "pendulous abdomen" weighing 14.9 pounds from a 285-pound woman.[58] The piece removed was 90 cm long, 31 cm wide, and 7 cm thick, and was, according to the surgeon, "larger than the ordinary woman's whole belly." The rebuilding of this obese female body had begun with a breast reduction. In 1896 J. W. Chambers of Baltimore removed twenty-five pounds of this woman's "large, flabby and . . . very pendulous breasts."

Kelly saw the removal of the abdominal fat as a reconstructive procedure analogous to the removal of the pendulous breasts. It is no surprise, given the discourse on the racial breast and the racial body, that "the woman was a Jewess, Mrs. M., thirty-two years of age . . . with the complaint of 'excessive fat over the lower part of the abdomen.'" She also suffered from a "'neuralgic headache'" (p. 300).

The body that began the history of the aesthetic surgery of the

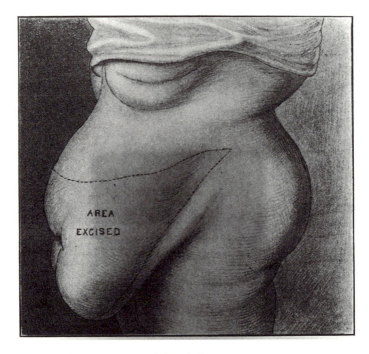

H. A. Kelly's resection of the abdomen.

abdomen was a Jewish woman's body. One of the most evident visual stereotypes of the Jewish woman was that of the heavy-set female. Thus Hans Günther, in representing the Jewish woman, chose the intensely anti-Semitic image of "Susannah in the Bath" by Arnold Böcklin (1827–1901), with the naked, very large figure of Susannah representing the female Jewish body in a "scientific" context.[59] Günther stands in a long German tradition of the ethnological understanding of the Jewish female body. The expansive image of the Jewish woman's body had become a commonplace at the turn of the century. Hugo Obermaier (1877–1946), the Viennese archaeologist who in 1908 discovered the "primitive" statue he labeled the "Venus of Willendorf," entered the following note into his diary about it: "a schematically degenerate figure, which represents a higher, exemplary school [of art], such as the Tanagra. No face, only fat and feminine, prosperity, fertility, compare today's lazy/rotten [faule] Jewesses."[60] This image

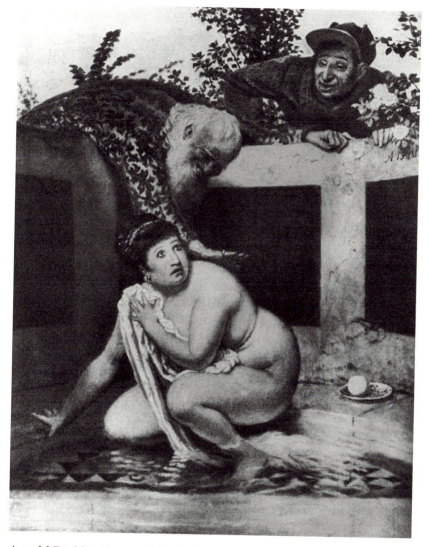

Arnold Böcklin, *Susannah in the Bath.*

served as the basis for the anxiety about the "primitive" Jewish woman's body.

Such images had particular salience in the "melting pot" ideology of the United States. The American eugenist Albert Wiggam (1871–1957) complained that the United States was being invaded by "ugly women" who are "broad-hipped, short, stout-legged with big feet [and] faces expressionless and devoid of beauty."[61] Wiggam also stressed that "good looking people are better morally, on average, than ugly people." Can aesthetic surgery make "good-looking people" out of ugly people? Can aesthetic surgery also change one of the ugly body's most salient "universal" characteristics, the "natural" (read: primitive) form of the body?

From the history of breast reduction, it is evident that J. W. Chambers would have removed Mrs. M.'s nipples when he reduced the size of her breasts. In his operation to remove the fat, Kelly was unable to retain the umbilicus, which "was situated about at the center of the mass."[62] To be lacking a belly button is to be marked in a very specific way. It sets your body apart as much as do missing nipples or a scarred face. Its importance can be noted if we turn to Clarence Darrow's question of William Jennings Bryan during the Scopes trial as to whether or not Adam had a belly button. If he did, what function did it have? and if he didn't, how are we made in the image of God? Does God have a belly button?

Twenty months after the surgery, Kelly contacted his patient, sans breasts, sans nipples, sans belly, sans belly button. She was alive but suffering from "extreme nervousness." This was the "normal" mental state attributed to the Jews and indicated to Kelly that the surgery had had a limited impact on her "happiness." Perhaps you can change the ugly body but not the unhappy psyche. She was not a "happy" patient, though clearly a smaller one, and "racially" her essence did not change.

Fat removal by surgery, the reduction of belly and buttocks, enabled overweight patients to turn to the aesthetic surgeon for their "cure." The cure of obesity was inevitably also an attempt to cure their psyches and their characters. Following Kelly's report of his successful procedure, no more than a dozen cases were reported between 1886 and World War I. Historians of the procedure commented that the absence of reports may be attributable to the "stigma that existed in the past toward 'cosmetic surgical improvement.'"[63] Yet it is evident that Kelly's procedure was the surgical and conceptual extension of breast reduction. Reductions, whether of the nose, the breast, or the abdomen, formed the "boundary cases" for the contemporary differentiation between "reconstructive" and "aesthetic" surgery. Reduce the racial signs and the person can "pass."

It was only in the 1920s that the "fundamental principles" of contemporary dermolipectomy were developed. By 1922 Max Thorek pioneered the first procedure to remove the fat on the belly as well as on the thigh simultaneously. He removed only the fat and skin below the umbilicus. He saw that the removal of fat could make patients happier.[64] The patient became a work of art formed by the surgeon. Thorek stressed that "localized fat deposits are the ones which most often call for surgical removal. . . . This work is, in truth, a very high type of sculpture—surgical sculpture—and the surgeon who undertakes it must possess the artistic sense of a sculptor besides being a thoroughly trained surgeon."[65] Joseph's model of the surgeon and the patient rooted in neoclassical aesthetics is part of the mind-set of the aesthetic surgeon. The body becomes a work of art and thus sheds its primitiveness. When the surgeon imagines himself as a sculptor, the patient becomes a classical statue.

In 1957 S. Vernon described the transposition of the umbilicus, which modified Thorek's procedure and made the results even more aesthetically pleasing.[66] Ivo Pitanguy's 1969 abdominal reduction procedures made the scars even less noticeable by having a horizontal excision located a bit above the pubic hair and thus made the psyche even happier.[67] But surgeons did not make a distinction between reconstructive removal of fat and aesthetic removal. Everything seemed to be defined as reconstructive following Kelly's first procedure. In 1971 at a meeting of surgeons in Rio de Janeiro it was decided that removing *excessive* fat (dermochalasis) could be distinguished from aesthetic surgery of the body for the removal of less evident amounts of fat tissue.[68] Now one could distinguish between reconstructive and aesthetic surgery. The reconstructive procedures reshaped the truly obese body; the aesthetic surgeons concentrated on the nuances among the various types of the aesthetic sculpting of the body.

The extensive tummy tuck now retains the belly button, limits

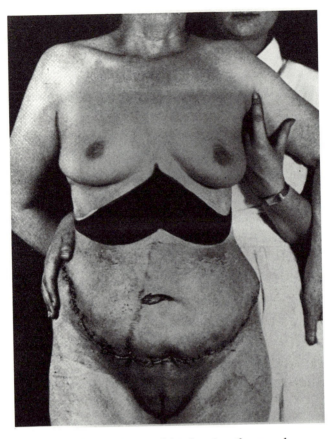

The removal of abdominal fat, leaving the navel.

scarring, and has become aesthetic surgery. But is the new belly with its intact belly button a "real" belly or is it merely a disguise for an obese body and thus pathological character? When Roseanne had her extensive aesthetic surgery in 1994, she also had a "tummy tuck." "A tummy tuck sounds almost gentle until you think about what it is. Incisions are made in the lower abdomen and fat sucked away; the navel is 'freed' from the abdominal wall; skin and fat are removed, and the wound sutured; the navel is 'relocated.' This is not embroidery we're talking about here. Does having your navel relocated make you any less real than before, though?" asks Suzanne Moore about the new "reality" of Roseanne Barr's body.[69] Moore's question raises the specter that Roseanne's body is not quite a real body because of its new shape, and certainly, the surgery seems to have had little impact on Roseanne's public character.

During the 1980s, a new procedure for removing the fat from the body was developed. Known as lipoplasty or liposuction, it will be discussed in more detail below. The reason liposuction was developed by Yves-Gerard Illouz was to replace another Pitanguy procedure for the reduction of "riding breeches" deformities which left "a long depressed scar."[70] Liposuction claimed to remove fat without scarring. Liposuction is clearly aesthetic surgery. The shift from the removal of the obese belly to the shaping of the body took place over the past century. Fat remains the mark of a pathological state of the psyche and its removal makes the patient-statue and the surgeon-sculptor happy.

SMALL BREASTS = NO BREASTS?

When does an aesthetic procedure on the breast count as "medical" and when is it merely "vanity"? There was a loud, public debate about the problems believed to be attendant to female breast augmentation in the 1990s. It was sparked by the claim that the use of silicone gel breast implants for breast augmentation, which had been seen as a cure for the unhappiness of the unerotic female body, actually caused physical illnesses.[71] Breast augmentation suddenly was split into two distinct categories: the "voluntary" patients, who underwent breast augmentation out of personal vanity (and paid for it themselves), as opposed to the reconstructive breast patients, who had cancerous breasts removed and then reconstituted through augmentation (and often had the cost reimbursed by third-party payers). In 1994, 20 percent of breast implants were employed in reconstructive procedures after cancer surgery.[72] Each group of patients received breast implants, but different qualities were ascribed to the resultant happiness of each group.

All of the early attempts at breast augmentation in Europe focused on breast replacement, as we shall discuss later. Certainly there was some early attention to the small breast as a surgical problem, as in the work of Fanny Brice's surgeon, Henry Junius Schireson, but this was evidently tangential to the greater focus on breast reduction.[73] Too-small breasts, as opposed to missing breasts, which had been surgically removed, were not seen as a significant medical problem that affected the psyche of the patient until after World War II. As late as 1948, Marguerite Clark noted in the American women's magazine *McCall's* that surgeons did not deal with small breasts "because women with small, infantile breasts do not suffer so much physical and psychological discomfort. These conscientious surgeons have neither time nor sympathy for vanity and vague longing for a beautiful body."[74] Clark's statement dates the switch from reduction to augmentation as the central concern of aesthetic surgery of the breast, for during the 1930s and 1940s the "primitive" racialized breast came to be seen as the erotic breast.

One might imagine this as part of a dialectic of the breast. The small breasts of the "New Woman," which were defined by her function as a sportswoman, were replaced by the very breasts the absence of which defined the "New Woman" as new—large breasts. Beginning in the United States in the 1950s, there was a concerted effort to search for cures for this new disease of "too-small breasts." This became medicalized in the 1950s. H. O. Bames observed that "hypomastia causes psychological rather than physical distress. Its correction has been receiving increased interest only since our 'cult of the body beautiful' has revealed its existence in rather large numbers."[75] Here the shift is complete and the "too-small" breast has been medicalized. Today many more women are persuaded that their breasts are too small than are persuaded that their breasts are too large. Breast augmentation is now a cure for a psychological problem, the lack of happiness. The new "body beautiful" is the old racialized body—in the country that spawned Rock and Roll out of the Jazz Age.

The charge that the implants that made them happy were the cause of illness made these newly "erotic" women with implants anxious about their potentially "unhealthy" (and therefore "un-

erotic") bodies. What was it in their bodies that was causing illness? Silicone had first been used in 1953 in the form of subcutaneous injections for body augmentation. Thus injected into the
body, it was soon shown to have the risks of migration and infection.[76] Other problems such as hematoma, visible lines of implantation, and, most frequently, capsule contracture (abnormal
firmness of the breast to the touch) also were experienced by
women who had had silicone injections. Alternative substances
were experimented with: Ivalon, a derivative of polyvinylic alcohol, in 1949; Polistan, a derivative of polyethelene, in 1950;
Etheron, a derivative of polymethane, in 1960; and Hydron, a derivative of polyglycomethacrylate, in 1960. Each had a spongy
texture and was advocated for short periods as the "ideal" sub-
stance for breast augmentation. And each had extremely negative
outcomes for the health of the patient.

In 1963 the Houston surgeons Thomas Cronin and Frank
Gerow developed a "silastic gel" prosthesis, which contained
saline and provided a preshaped form and size.[77] Gerow came to
the idea of a silicone sack filled with liquid by observing a plastic bag filled with blood used for transfusion. He saw in its form
the shape of a breast. Thus "aesthetic" augmentation had its conceptual origin in the context of "real" surgery. Gerow implanted
the first such prosthesis in March 1962. It broke and released the
saline. A week later he implanted a prosthesis filled with silicone
gel, and this was successful. The result was a patient who "was
healed and happy," according to one account. Thus the surgeons
neglected to pay much attention to actual negative outcomes such
as the hardening of some of the breasts with the prosthesis (contracted capsules). The surgeons relied on initial success, ignoring
long-term problems until confronted with them. With insertion of
the implant under the muscles of the chest wall (submuscular
augmentation mammaplasty) and the introduction of Franklyn
L. Ashley's silicone-gel implant covered with polyurethane foam
in the 1970s, which reduced the risk of contracture, many of the
initial problems associated with breast augmentation seemed to
have been overcome. Although improved saline-filled implants
reappeared in the 1970s, they remained less attractive until the at-

tack on the silicone implants two decades later. They were "felt" to be less "natural" and did not give the illusion of the breast form and texture that physicians and women wanted. Silicone held its own for augmentation of the breast for all purposes.

In 1990 a House committee chaired by Representative Ted Weiss held its first hearings on the safety of silicone implants, and this quickly became a major media event. The claim was that the improved procedures still masked long-term major medical problems. By 1991 the first court case was resolved with findings that the silicone implants had caused immune system illnesses in patients. A $7.3 million-dollar damage claim was lodged against Dow Corning, the developer of the gel implant. A number of recipients of silicone breast implants then claimed to have developed a wide and divergent set of symptoms ranging from chronic fatigue to rheumatoid arthritis (and other inflammatory illness of the joints), lupus, damage to the immune system, and scleroderma (a hardening of the skin and internal organs).

The unhappiness of a minority of breast augmentation patients became manifest. There had been 237 legal cases concerning breast implants from 1973 to 1991. Following the publicity concerning breast implants, more than thirty thousand lawsuits were filed against the primary manufacturer of silicone breast implants, Dow Corning. As of September 1994, half a million "unhappy" patients with breast implants intended to participate in the proposed global settlement with Dow Corning when the corporation declared bankruptcy. Equally important was the fact that at least 37,853 women had their breast implants surgically removed in 1994, virtually the same number (39,247) as had their breasts augmented that year.[78] (In 1996 the number of augmentations increased to 87,704 and the number of removals dropped to 3,013.)[79] These women's marked unhappiness with their bodies was now a matter of public record. The courts came to be the arbiters of the happiness of the patients and set a price on their unhappiness. What had happened too is that this cadre refused to be silent. Their silent validation as "happy," erotic women with large breasts had vanished as the implants were shown to them to be the source of a new unhappiness. The seemingly uniform cohort of erotic women with large breasts had fractured into two groups. The first comprised women with breast implants who began loudly to articulate their unhappiness. This defined them in public. The other group, the still silent cadre of "naturally" large-breasted women, happily had their own authenticity validated by the fact that women with implants now spoke about their unhappiness with the "artificial" breasts.

The findings of the court centered on the "unhappiness" of the patients. The implants, which were intended to cure their psychological unhappiness with their bodies, could now be seen as causing somatic illness and therefore psychological dis-ease. "But there certainly is a group of women who are unhappy and believe that their symptoms may be in some way related to their breast implants," wrote Diana Sugg in the *Sacramento Bee*.[80] R. Merrel Olesen, an aesthetic surgeon who directed the La Jolla Cosmetic Surgery Center, which provided a large number of breast implants over the decade of the 1980s, observed that if "breast implants were harmful, we would demand new products. We understand that all surgical procedures carry risks, and if the risks are too high, our patients are unhappy, and so are we. Breast implants are important because they are used to reconstruct cancer victims as well as to boost self-esteem and address psychological issues."[81] Darcy Sixt, a mastectomy patient and soon-to-be patient advocate, reported to the *New York Times* that the silicone implant "allowed her to throw away a prosthesis that chafed her skin and floated out of her bathing suit. And once she felt 'normal,' she felt less cheated by her illness."[82] The restoration of symmetry is the restoration of health and beauty. The psychological issues addressed in the late 1990s are those associated with the meaning ascribed to the breast in Western culture, such as the definition of femininity. These meanings, however, have come to have complex significance in the ability to shape and / or remove the breast as a means of defining the "happy" and the "unhappy" psyche.

One aside should be made here. We began by noting that the erotic when it is associated with the breast becomes gendered female—it is the female breast that Marilyn Yalom writes about with such passion. The discussion of breast implants in the media assumed that breast implants were the only silicone gel implants actually used in aesthetic surgery. Clearly they were the most numerous. But, as with the American discussion of breast cancer as *purely* a feminist issue in the 1990s, the assumption is that only women were concerned by the question of the health risk posed by silicone implants.[83] In the breast cancer discussion, male breast cancer rates were ignored; questions of the reconstruction of the male breast, while a subject of the clinical and surgical literature, seemed to carry no psychological baggage. Breast cancer in men does exist and is treated with therapies and interventions analogous to those used on women. According to the National Cancer Institute, male breast cancer accounts for less than 1 percent of all breast cancers, but that still means that some fourteen hundred new cases will be diagnosed this year, with a mortality rate of about 30 percent.[84]

A closer analogy to the anxiety generated by breast implants may be the use of male genital implants. They, too, seemed to have little room in the popular consciousness even though a case that dealt with silicone penile implants was brought before the courts in 1994.[85] In 1961, Harvey Lash had developed the silicone penile implant as a treatment for sexual impotence. Even the inflatable penile implant, introduced in 1972, is a silicon elastomer-based device. There had been a dramatic increase in the use of such implants in the 1980s. In the late 1980s there had been a 31 percent annual growth rate, and the devices reached sales figures of $110 million by 1989 from a 1984 base of $24 million.[86] In addition, shunts, chin implants, hiatal hernia implants, and most tellingly, testicular implants (cancerous testicles are replaced by a plasticor gel-filled implant designed to look and feel like an actual testicle) are commonly constructed out of silicone gel.[87] Little if any attention was paid to the potential risk in these cases, since they could not be clearly and publicly coded as violating the promise of (re)constructing the "erotic" and therefore "happy" psyche. *Male* impotence, castration, and breasts seemed to be taboo subjects in modern Western society.

With seemingly great speed, the U.S. Food and Drug Administration accepted claims that the use of silicone *breast* implants created the wide range of complications listed above either by rupture of the elastomer bag or by "bleeding" of the gel over time even through an apparently intact prosthetic envelope. In April 1992, David Kessler, then the commissioner of the FDA, banned the use of silicone gel implants for aesthetic reasons, but stated that they could be used for post-mastectomy reconstruction.[88] Kessler believed that the implants were dangerous to women's health and stood in opposition to the medical establishment such as the American Medical Association. He stated, however, that the danger of the post-mastectomy patient's unhappiness with her now scarred body was greater than the physical risk from the implant. (Indeed, a Swedish study seemed to imply that women who have augmentation after mastectomy are substantially happier than a control group of women who elect to have rhinoplasty.)[89] Kessler's formulation was oblique: "Breast reconstruction with implants is a recognized, widely used component of breast cancer treatment; for some patients, breast reconstruction with an implant is a vital part of their recovery process" (p. 2607). This implied the psychological (rather than physical) well-being of the mastectomy patient.

Because one out of ten women has had or will develop breast cancer, the question of reconstructive breast augmentation remained a major political question in the early 1990s. It seemed to people in authority, such as David Kessler, that it was worthwhile risking long-term health dangers from silicone gel implants only if there was a compelling advantage. According to his statement, there was a risk "including implant rupture, gel bleed and migration, and contractures" in as many as 75,000 of the "estimated 1 million to 2 million women with implants." This risk was, for him, still worth taking if it improved the mental health of mastectomy patients.

The mental health ("happiness") of women who underwent breast augmentation without first having cancer was evidently too trivial to warrant their being permitted to take such a risk themselves. Here the assumption of the autonomy of aesthetic surgery is drawn into question. Only a greater good could permit such a procedure. The individual's right of choice was canceled by the risk entailed. Kessler dismissed the American Medical Association's demand that the women "be fully informed about the risks and benefits associated with breast implants and that once fully informed the patients should have the right to choose" (p. 2602). That a woman be allowed to make the choice after having heard the public debate as well as her physician's counsel was not acceptable to Kessler. His sense of the space for appropriate risk mirrors the dichotomy between the reconstructive breast replacement and the act of breast augmentation. In each case the woman desires to "pass"—in both cases to be understood as a "normal" woman within the cadre with which she is identifying.

The debate came to be about the degree to which the government would permit a woman to "pass" as whole and, therefore, as healthy. If she was missing a breast, went the argument, she would be "unhappy" about her body and would need augmentation surgery to make her happy. This was worth the risk. If she only wanted to be "happy" without having first suffered cancer, that was not worth the risk. The reconstruction of the erotic, female body in the first case was seen as a goal of reconstructive surgery; the construction of the erotic body in the latter case was "merely" aesthetic surgery and a sign of false vanity.

This view was very much against the model set by some feminist writers and thinkers, such as Audre Lorde (1934–92), who themselves suffered from breast cancer and underwent mastectomies.[90] Lorde even advocated creating new clothing to emphasize the missing breast as a sign of survival. The visual artist Matuschka represented her own mastectomy scar in a wide range of self-portraits, which include the widely discussed *New York Times Magazine* cover image in 1993 (titled *Beauty Out of Damage*).[91] In an interview she said, "I'm very unhappy that I had to have a breast and 24 lymph nodes removed, I believe, unnecessarily, but I am happy about the extent that my work has helped to publicize the breast cancer epidemic."[92] Other visual artists who have represented the amputated breast include Helke Sander, who produced the series *So Help Me Hannah: Portrait of the Artist with Her Mother* (1978–81) documenting her mother's breast cancer,

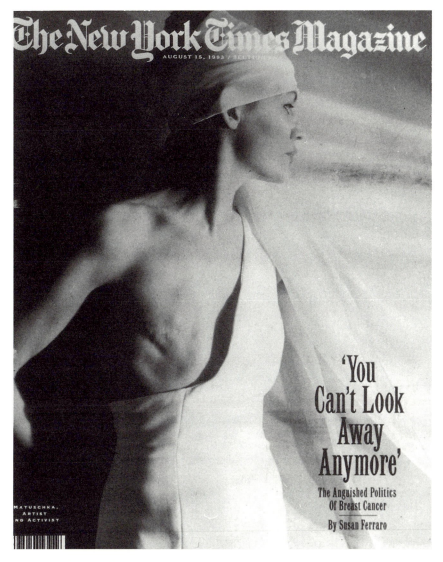

Matuschka, self-portrait.

Intra-Venous (with her early 1990s series documenting her own treatment for lymphoma), and Hella Hammid, whose photo of Deena Metzger (a one-breasted woman with a vine tattoo) has been widely shown. In Chicago, Hollis Sigler has taken breast cancer as one of the major themes in her work. All have argued

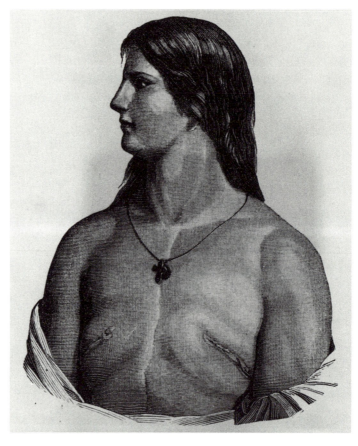

The ritual removal of the breasts.

that the "damaged" body of the woman after a mastectomy should be seen and understood as an acceptable body, even as an erotic body. This is quite the opposite of Kessler's argument. The artists stress that the female body without a breast can represent a "happy" psyche.

The response to such public representations has been positive even though it has not become a dominant representation of breast cancer. Seeing such art representing mastectomies enabled some women to imagine a "connection and creativity."[93] One woman commented on her response to seeing artwork that represented the woman's body after a mastectomy: "art is a very creative process for me, and through art I have come to know the courage, joy, and fortitude of women in this group." Matuschka has carried on the gospel of the beautiful, damaged body after Lorde's death. Her view is that the damaged body is a sign of the potential in all women for suffering and it creates a bond among women who have suffered cancer as well as those who have not. "Hearing other women's poems and admiring others' photos and paintings drew out a flood of conversation amongst us," commented one of the women at a workshop with Matuschka. Such responses must be placed within the overall debate about the reconstitution of the psyche through augmentation or through the acceptance of the scarred body. These feminists argued that the missing breast should be seen as a source of feminist strength and solidarity, following the model of the mythical Amazons, who removed a breast to enable themselves to better draw a bow.

Eventually David Kessler capitulated, and silicone breast implants (as well as saline-filled implants) were permitted for all women who desired to have them. But the firms manufacturing silicone implants have ceased to produce them because of lawsuits, and saline-filled implants are not the choice of patients and surgeons. The erotic body was no longer divided into the acceptable and the unacceptable, the real and the false, the healthy and the corrupt. The drawing of such boundaries was the cause of this debate and was a permanent part of the social construction of the erotic.

Some recent court decisions have rejected the claims of a high incidence of somatic illness as "not scientifically valid."[94] Studies such as one at the Mayo Clinic have determined that patients with silicone breast implants tend to have no greater risk of illnesses such as lupus or rheumatoid arthritis than a control group.[95] Given the accepted idea that any surgery will have a potential for failure in a relatively small percentage of patients, the unhappiness of breast implant patients has some basis in experience. In the case of silicone breast implants, the problems of leakage or of capsule contracture have been shown to be an ongoing problem in a relatively small number of cases.

But the general claim that such implants *necessarily* lead to illness and unhappiness is a striking reversal of the claim for aesthetic surgery. Now aesthetic surgery makes the patient unhappy. As one patient stated who had had bilateral implants eighteen years before the interview: "I get sick. I usually always get sick when I go out into traffic, even, almost immediately, even getting into my car. . . . I'm so sick . . . for fifteen years I've been sick, constantly sick all the time."[96] In many cases, the very thought of having the implant now makes the individual "ill." Such feelings are real. But their etiology may well be a psychological state experienced as a physical illness (conversion disorder), which in this case is labeled "chronic fatigue syndrome."[97] The somatic experiences of a minority of patients who spoke out in public fractured the uniform assumptions of health and happiness held by women with breast implants. They could no longer "pass" as erotic, and the antithesis of the erotic is the ill. The result of the breast implant debate is the conviction that breast augmentation can make you sick and therefore "unhappy" so that you need further surgery to remove the implants and cure your psyche. Indeed, in a few cases, self-mutilation occurred as women desperately tried to remove their implants themselves.

The 1990s debate about breast augmentation continued the obsessions of late nineteenth-century surgery. Whereas breast reduction demanded the evolution of specific surgical techniques that were closely related to "reconstructive" procedures for mastectomies, augmentation demanded the introduction of some form of supplemental material. The discussion about what materials could be used for implants in the body traditionally had been undertaken in regard to the correction of the problem of the sunken nose.

As breast size and form became the field of the "aesthetic" surgeon, the question of the use of materials for augmentation became important. As early as 1887, the Viennese surgeon Robert Gersuny (1844–1924), following attempts at breast reduction, gave serious thought to the problem of breast augmentation. Initially, his concern was to restore the breast following amputation (mastectomy) because of tumor or localized infection.[98] Yet it was clear that there was also a limited interest in correcting what in the mid twentieth century came to be called micromastia or hypomastia, the "pathology" of too-small breasts. In addition, surgeons began to consider the sagging of the aging female breast as an aesthetic problem. Large breasts are read as signs of race and the happiness about being identified with (or the unhappiness about being seen as belonging to) a specific race. Small breasts come to be seen as infantilizing, and the sagging breast as a sign of the ravages of age. All these signs can be read as "natural," in which case any changes are seen as nonmedical, or they can be turned into pathologies of the body, in which case all interventions are medical.

Gersuny condemned the aesthetic reshaping of the breast as vanity surgery, giving into the "hunger for beauty of old coquettes who . . . wish me to give their sagging breasts a youthful vigor."[99] His breast augmentations and treatment for sagging breasts were medical, and he reserved them for those who had suffered cancer or other serious diseases. They provided a means of altering the unhappiness of the patient, not simply pandering to her vanity. Vanity here is defined as going against the perceived force of nature. Such vanity demeans the surgeon, who is put in the place of the cosmetologist. With the emphasis on the alteration of the psyche, a new medical rationale is provided for precisely these procedures. The question remained as to what could be used as the means for the augmentation of the breast as well as other body parts in those procedures understood as "medical" rather than as "vanity" surgery.

The first modern breast augmentation took place on November 24, 1893, in Heidelberg, and thus followed the initial procedures for reductive rhinoplasty and breast reduction. Vincenz Czerny's patient, a forty-one-year-old singer, had a growth in her breast removed.[100] Given her profession, Czerny decided that the asymmetry of her breasts resulting from the procedure had to be modified. Luckily, the patient also had a growth (lipoma) on her back. The fat for the augmentation was harvested from the lipoma on her back and was transplanted into her breast. When she was discharged on December 20, 1893, "the left breast was well shaped and was similar to the right." Her augmentation was therefore

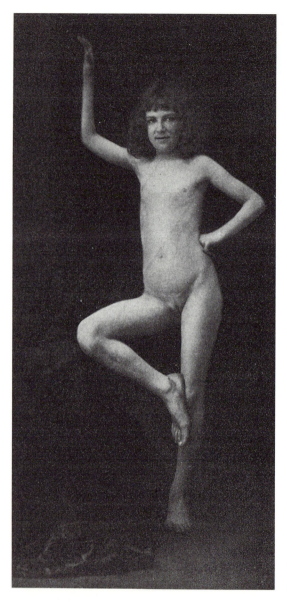

The breastless
child-woman.

understood as "reconstructive" even though it was guided by
aesthetic considerations.[101] One might note here that although
Czerny (like Gersuny) was best known as a student of Theodor
Billroth, among his other teachers in Vienna was Ernst Brücke.
Aesthetics had motivated Czerny in the first breast reconstruc-

tion, and in his imagination there was a classical body—that represented in the work of his teacher, Brücke.

Vincenz Czerny's symmetrical breast reconstruction in 1893 rested on the earlier work of Gustav Neuber (1850–1932), who had first used fat transplantation for the repair of a tubercular eye socket and the "saddle nose" of the syphilitic.[102] Later, Martin Bartels in Strasbourg in 1908 and the Anglo-Swiss "beauty surgeon" Charles Willi in London used body fat transplants for other forms of facial and body augmentation. Such procedures eventually failed in their goal because the fat was relatively quickly reabsorbed into the body.

Charles Willi falsely claimed that he too had studied with Jacques Joseph in 1908 or 1909 while Joseph was working on breast reductions. Actually self-taught and without any formal medical training, he became the most widely sought after aesthetic surgeon in London during the first half of the twentieth century. Willi's procedures were effective and popular (at least until the fat he injected was reabsorbed into the body). He evidently also knew of Neuber and Czerny's work on augmentation. By the time Willi began to experiment with "aesthetic" breast augmentation after World War I, the shift in the meaning of breast size among specific groups was beginning to take place.[103] Even though the complete shift occurred after World War II, there was interest in both breast reduction and breast augmentation from the beginning of the modern aesthetic surgery of the breast in the 1880s. What shifted was the perceived relative importance of these procedures. Willi's patients who wanted breast augmentation in the 1930s were clearly "aesthetic" patients, whose desire was to have larger (read: more erotic) breasts. Fat transplantation soon showed itself to give but temporary relief for the unhappiness of his female patients with their too-small breasts. These autogenous procedures using body fat reappeared after World War II and in the 1980s with the same poor results.[104]

Aesthetic surgeons also tried paraffin. In Vienna the craze for paraffin injections began with Robert Gersuny, who had been appointed by Theodor Billroth to head the surgical department of his hospital, the Rudolfinerhaus, in 1888.[105] He had developed the first "island flap" in 1887, in repairing with subcutaneous tissues the floor of the mouth of a young woman suffering from cancer. He had initially and unsuccessfully injected his patients with a mixture of paraffin and Vaseline for the remedy of "saddle nose."[106] Here he followed the earlier suggestions of the Berlin dermatologist Hugo Eckstein.[107] Such procedures had the advantage of using what was perceived as a relatively inert material that could be easily shaped.

Gersuny proposed the injection of paraffin to shape and augment the breast and, indeed, all other areas, including replacement of missing testicles.[108] Gersuny had most probably developed this procedure by observing Billroth's use of paraffin as a means of replacing resected joints. Earlier experiments by the New York City neurologist J. Leonard Corning (1855–1923) in 1887 using paraffin injections to treat muscular spasms seem to have been unknown to him. It is also quite possible that he knew of the first use of paraffin injections in the 1880s by dermatologists who used them to deliver mercury compounds for the treatment of syphilis. Paraffin augmentation was attractive because it was easily done and because it seemed not to leave overt initial lesions.[109]

When Martin Gumpert's Berlin institute was created in the early 1930s, a great number of individuals came for treatment, many of them disfigured because of earlier "cosmetic quackery," especially paraffin injections.[110] Paraffin injections were used, as Stephen Paget (1855–1926) noted in 1902, to repair sunken noses. He endorsed only reparative uses of paraffin and condemned the use of such injections "to try to conceal the advance of years by padding out sunken cheeks, or leveling up wrinkles, or by filling up the hollows of thin necks" as counterproductive to the invisibility desired by the patient. "Even if one could be sure of doing the thing right at the time, the unhappy patient could be left for the rest of her life with a lump or a plaque of stuff as hard as cartilage under her skin, which would steadily become more obviously false, till in her old age it would look and feel like a disease."[111] Such therapies were known to be risky, and surgeons such as Paget advocated them only for "reconstructive" patients,

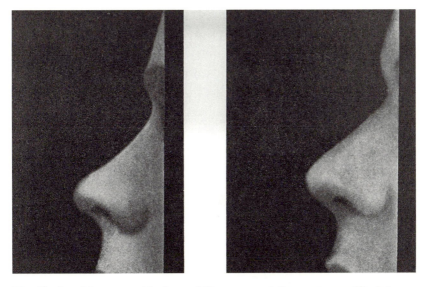

The "before" image, with the saddle nose and the post-paraffin injection.

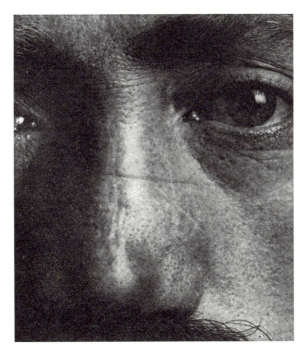

The scarring caused by paraffin.

not aesthetic ones. The acquisition of perpetual youth through the use of paraffin injections placed the patient in the category of the young who would come to naught as the inevitable aging process revealed the means by which this pseudo-youthfulness was created. This was similar to the belief that Jewishness revealed itself in the aging process. As Roland Barthes noted in his *Camera Lucida:* "Proust . . . said of Charles Haas (the model for Swann), according to George Painter, that he had a short, straight nose, but that old age had turned his skin to parchment, revealing the Jewish nose beneath"[112] The Jewish nose always reveals itself, even if once it went masked and unrecognized.

Paraffin therapy itself becomes a disease because it turns the "happy" patient into an unhappy individual. Indeed, in the case of the repair of the "saddle nose" of the syphilitic, the marks of paraffin branded the sufferer as much as the symptoms of mercury treatment had in the eighteenth century:

> A young man had had paraffin injected along the bridge of his nose. Years later an attempt had been made to remove it by an incision from the glabella to the tip. He had a wide grayish ugly scar, extending the whole length of the nose with wide areas of red on both sides. The man was an artist and felt his disfigurement very keenly. The scar was excised, the paraffin removed, and the wound resutured. At a second operation, a piece of rib cartilage was inserted along the bridge. The psychologic condition improved greatly.[113]

Being marked by the failed operation not only made him "ugly," but made people "turn to take a second look at him . . . as he walks down the street." It is this inability to "pass" as healthy that is corrected by the aesthetic surgeon.

The intent of paraffin injections was to assure a "happy outcome."[114] The actual result was catastrophic. Shortly after injection, the paraffin wandered and clumped, resulting in disfiguring lumps and permanent draining fistulas in virtually all patients. Among the other complications were blindness, pulmonary embolism, inflammation, and necrosis. Disfiguration or death resulted all too often. The best-known victim was Consuelo, the duchess of Marlborough, called the "most beautiful woman in the world." Her extraordinary portrait as a young mother by Giovanni Boldini (1906) hangs in the Metropolitan Museum of Art in New York as testimony to her contemporary reputation as a beauty. In 1935, her beauty fading, she had paraffin injections to remove wrinkles. The paraffin wandered over her face and formed bumps and grooves. She felt herself so disfigured that she withdrew from society, remaining a recluse until her death in 1977.[115] Such patients showed up at Martin Gumpert's clinic in the early 1930s demanding treatment for their now too visible disfigurements, disfigurements that were seen as resulting from their "vanity."

Paraffin was used for a wide range of aesthetic alterations of the body. Among women it was used for breast augmentation, and thus the procedure presented problems for aesthetic surgeons well into the late twentieth century.[116] It was used in transsexual surgery to augment the male breast and led to unexpected lesions.[117] It was also used as recently as thirty to forty years ago in Asia for penile implants.[118] In the former Soviet Union paraffin was injected under the skin of the penile shaft to thicken the penis, leading to infection and complications. Israeli surgeons are now dealing with the rather catastrophic results of such procedures among recent Russian immigrants to Israel.[119]

The "unhappiness" with the results of the paraffin augmentation seems to parallel the discussion about the dangers of silicon breast implants in the 1990s. The physical problems caused by paraffin injections destroyed any "happiness" created by the initial operation. But *everyone* who had paraffin injections had massive physical problems. The difference with silicone gel implants was that the relatively *small* number of patients who had purely physical symptoms such as scarring structured the response of many of the women who had had implants. Such physical symptoms gave raise to the anxiety that even worse illness, such as cancer and lupus, would result from the implants. Women became convinced that they too were ill and unhappy. The psychological experience of seeing oneself as at risk shaped the physical experience. The end result was that both cohorts, those with physical complaints and those without, were "unhappy." "Passing" was no longer a possibility, as patients claimed their ill bodies now marked them as mere simulacra. The response of the patients treated with paraffin was analogous.

Writing in 1911, before the dangers of paraffinoma were fully known, one of its greatest advocates, the American surgeon Frederick Strange Kolle, wrote: "Let the author warn the operator against the 'beauty cranks,' especially those who are just about to engage in great theatrical ventures, circus performances, or 'acts,' and very desirable marriages. These are patients who are not only difficult to deal with, but the first to harm the hard-earned, well-deserved reputation of the surgeon and to drag him into courts for reimbursement for all kinds of damages, especially backed up by events, losses, and sufferings largely imaginary and untrue, and oftentimes entirely impossible."[120] The response of the patient to the painful growths caused by injecting paraffin and silicone (paraffinomas and siliconomas) is quite correctly "unhappiness," and this is articulated in a different professional sphere, that of the courts. It also then becomes a response to the altered body in general.

When patients articulate their unhappiness with their new bodies in public, this makes them visible as "false" and therefore "unhealthy" bodies. The "unhappiness" of the specific illness becomes a quality associated with the "new" body part, and the unhappiness of the patient, whether suffering from specific illnesses or not, results. The failure of paraffin caused aesthetic surgeons to experiment with substitutes, with much the same result. Similar psychological and physical problems arose when the American aesthetic surgeon Charles Conrad Miller (1880–1950) suggested substituting rubber and gutta percha for paraffin in the 1920s. His goal, too, was to raise the "depressed nasal bridge."[121] This suggestion was accepted by a number of surgeons such as the American Vilray Papin Blair (1871–1955), who used rubber, gutta percha, celluloid, ivory, and metal as well as autogenous bone grafts.[122] The search for a means to augment the body that did not cause the body further harm was ongoing in the history of aesthetic surgery. Various substances had different responses in different patient cohorts, some positive, some not. The mass response to the silicone implant in the 1980s is a form of conversion disorder after the model evoked by Elaine Showalter in other, related contexts from this period.[123] Triggered by physical illnesses in a small number of individuals, it manifested itself in the psyches of many more as that which was to be cured by aesthetic surgery. No longer able to "pass" as "happy" and "erotic," the patient with a silicone implant becomes "unhappy" and "ill."

As we have seen, nearly all the late twentieth-century arguments about large or small breasts and buttocks presuppose that it is appropriate for women to have aesthetic surgery, but not for men to do so. In this context, if women have the right body for aesthetic surgeons to sculpt, men emphatically have the wrong body.

Such assumptions ignore the extent to which anxiety about appearance, especially the appearance of the sexual self, is not at all gendered. Judging by the increasing rates at which they are having aesthetic procedures, men, too, are susceptible to the fear that without the help of aesthetic surgery they will be condemned to live in the wrong body. Let's now take a closer look at what that means for men—and for the women who wish to become men.

CHAPTER EIGHT

The Wrong Body

MEN WITH BREASTS

𝒯HE REDUCTION or augmentation of the breasts is central to aesthetic surgery in our day. As we have seen, it is defined at almost every point as the alteration of the *female* breast. Yet beginning with Aristotle in the *Parts of Animals* (688b1), one of the ironic questions posed about human anatomy is why women have "functional" breasts (which "scientifically" define us as mammals, that is, as animals who have mammae [breasts] and nurse), but men have only rudimentary breasts with "nonfunctional" nipples.[1] (The erotic plays no role in this discussion.) Much ink has been spilled over this question by writers from medieval theologians to contemporary biologists, but for the aesthetic surgeon the question was one of correction rather than speculation. If the replacement/augmentation of a female breast removed for pathological reasons is one of the most contested places for asking the question of what aesthetic surgery really does and really means, then the most unquestioned, unexamined problem is that of the male breast. The topic of men with breasts would seem to test "passing" as a means of understanding aesthetic surgery. What can having breasts "mean" for "men"?

In his standard handbook on aesthetic surgery, Jacques Joseph dealt with the male under a discussion of malformation (teratology) of the breast, summarizing that "I should also like to mention at this point the male breast. . . . The male breast is quite rare."[2] Excluding questions of breast augmentation in transsex-

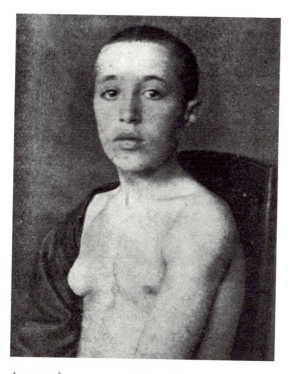

A case of gynecomastia in a fourteen-year-old boy.

ual surgery, males are not supposed to have breasts.[3] Yet in the United States in 1992, 39,639 breast reductions were performed, of which 4,997 were done on men.[4] Thus, at least at the end of the twentieth century, male breasts are not as rare as was imagined at the beginning of the modern procedures for breast reduction.[5]

The male body, too, has its specifications, which define its masculinity. For male bodybuilders in contemporary American culture, "pecs" are fine; breasts ("bitch tits") are not. Having breasts is the cause of the "embarrassment [that] these men suffer in locker rooms, barracks, or on the beach."[6] Men with breasts are "unhappy." This seems to be equally true in Asia. Japanese commentators note that having breasts makes a man's "psychologic pain ... great. If he has to bare his chest frequently, he suffers tremendous embarrassment, especially in the Orient, where the daily custom of public bathing still remains."[7] Having breasts precludes a man from "passing" as truly male among his peers; it is seen as androgynous in a world that divides the sexes into clear antitheses—those with breasts (female) and those without (male).

Male breasts are caused by the body's estrogen reaction to testosterone onslaught. As part of his advertising on the Web (phudson.com), the aesthetic surgeon Patrick Hudson provided the following narrative:

> "Doctor, I have bitch tits. Am I f***ed?" These are the words that a young body builder used to introduce himself. He went on to describe how he followed a cycle of anabolic steroids and then afterward noticed a swelling of his chest that he thought was the muscle growing. It soon became tender and progressed to a sizable mass of tissue, to the point where he was embarrassed to take off his shirt and show the physique he'd worked so hard to build. Dieting and building up his pecs only made the problem worse. He couldn't even hug his girlfriend without discomfort.[8]

The discomfort is psychic unhappiness, not physical pain, and the strong suggestion is that the only appropriate response is aesthetic surgery.

The Alexandrian physician, Paulus of Aegina, defined this discomfort in the seventh century as a *medical* problem to be cured through surgery. Its technical name is gynecomastia (woman-breast), the presence of breasts on the male. Gynecomastia is also ascribed not only to bodybuilding but also to primary testicular failure such as that found in genetic errors of development like Klinefelter's and Reifenstein's syndromes. Klinefelter's syndrome occurs when individuals are genetically "male" but exhibit a characteristic phenotype including tall stature, infertility, gynecomastia, and hypogonadism; Reifenstein's syndrome is marked by gynecomastia, and is a form of androgen resistance caused by a faulty receptor protein. Some of the young "men" who develop breasts turn out to be true or pseudo-hermaphrodites, and thus not "men" (according to medical diagnosis) at all. This comes, as we shall see, to present quite a different reading of male breasts. Another culturally linked cause of gynecomastia at the end of the twentieth century is the use of "forbidden substances," such as bodybuilding steroids and marijuana.[9] The treatment for nondevelopment gynecomastia is usually the use of testosterone (to turn the boy into a real man); but in cases of chromosomal deficiency, only the use of testosterone and surgery ensure that the masculine body is restored to its "authentic" masculine self in spite of its ambiguous chromosomal definition.[10]

Men with breasts are either born or made. If the body is born with the potential for gynecomastia, it is a pathological body. But if it is a result of bodybuilding, it is also pathological. The cult of bodybuilding began in the 1890s at exactly the same moment that aesthetic surgery took on its modern form. Its goal was the building of a beautiful, healthy body to provide for a beautiful, healthy race, which would in turn ensure individual and collective happiness.[11] Yet such "happiness" quickly became "unhappiness" caused by the development in supposedly heterosexual male bodybuilders of protuberant breasts, with or without steroids. Among male bodybuilders today anabolic steroids are seen as a leading cause of gynecomastia. These synthetic derivatives of testosterone trigger a variety of other deleterious side effects as well in their role of transforming "mere" men into "real" men.

Problems with breasts haunt bodybuilders. In contemporary Israel, bodybuilders turn to the aesthetic surgeon for the relief of such problems. Amit, a twenty-seven-year-old Tel Aviv bodybuilder who developed excessively large nipples and breasts, felt that they marred a beautiful physique he had worked long and hard to create.[12] They were, he says, "not aesthetic." He had surgery in secret. "No one knows I had plastic surgery, and no one will know," he vows. "I did it strictly for myself, not for anyone else. And I feel much better now." Aesthetic surgery is "just not accepted" in contemporary Israel in his bodybuilding cohort. He is afraid that his surgery will become known and that people will think of his body as merely a simulacrum created by a surgeon: "I don't want people to stare at my body and think, 'a doctor created that.'" The anxiety about the "authenticity" of the bodybuilder's body seems to transcend all national conventions. Authenticity has to do with the absence of surgical intervention.

The feminizing side effect of "bitch tits" (indeed the very name) draws the constructed masculinity of the steroid user into question. His "hypermasculinity," to use Theodor Adorno's term, is really a form of "pseudo-masculinity" that is represented by character traits such as "determination, energy, industry, independence, decisiveness, and will power." This is undermined by the very body that the steroid user wishes to construct.[13] The "feminized" body, seen in the "maternal" breasts, comes to represent the stereotypical antithesis of this hypermasculinity. Men with breasts are an oxymoron.

The breasts of female bodybuilders are read as a positive sign of the female body. As one woman bodybuilder remembered: "people used to laugh at my chest" before she began to pump herself up.[14] Another woman stressed that "one of the things I enjoyed most about body building was going from flat-chested and being razzed about it to people all of a sudden noticing my body. I had this nondescript body. Now men say, 'Wow, check out the bod!'" (p. 180). Breasts on the "male" body in this context create unhappiness; breasts on the "female" body in women bodybuilders create "happiness," even if they are the result of steroid use.

Paulus of Aegina recognized gynecomastia as a medical problem because of the resulting psychological damage. He advised the surgical removal of the breasts because they "bear the reproach of effeminacy."[15] He saw the reduction of these small breasts as analogous to the reduction of the size of women's monstrous breasts. The "reproach of effeminacy" is still implicit in present-day psychological explanations. Peter Hall could write in 1959 that the treatment for gynecomastia depends "[on] the extent to which the patient complains of the gynecomastia."[16] Hall's question was one of self-perception. How much do you see your body as having breasts? If you feel yourself in a cohort of those with breasts, you will want to become (in)visible in the cohort of men without breasts, but can the result of the surgery be just as stigmatizing as the "affliction"? Paulus of Aegina's procedure, a semicircular incision (or mastectomy), is no longer used as it leaves "a large scar, which constitutes as great a source of embarrassment as the gynecomastia itself."[17] Scarring marks the body as altered and inauthentic, as the Tel Aviv bodybuilder commented.

This was already evident in the surgical procedures of the 1920s. With the work of Louis Dartigues (1869–1940) in 1927, the male nipple was preserved and the scar minimized.[18] The procedure used a truism of aesthetic surgery, that scars placed at the junction of pigmented and nonpigmented skin were virtually invisible. Later procedures in the 1940s introduced surgical interventions through the areola, which left minimal scars and in which the excess skin more or less retracted itself.[19] Recently, the improvement of the techniques of liposuction for gynecomastia has meant that even less scarring can be expected if such procedures are generally introduced.[20] In 1994 the members of the American Society of Plastic and Reconstructive Surgeons undertook 4,416 procedures to reduce male breasts; this was 0.6 percent of all of the plastic and aesthetic procedures done in the United States that year.

The unhappiness associated with gynecomastia became material for psychologists. Alfred Adler (1870–1937) provided a long case study of a young Jewish man who suffered from his sense of sexual inferiority in relation to his older brother, whose maturity seemed better and more complete than his own.[21] Suffering from an undescended testicle, the younger brother feared that "he is perhaps a girl after all. . . . The marked development of his breasts lent considerable weight to his uncertainty" (p. 198). The occurrence of gynecomastia in this case came to be proof for Adler of the sexual confusion of the child. The patient narrated a dream: "I felt as if I were witnessing an ape nursing a child" (p. 199). The patient was called an ape by his brother "because of his excessive hairy growth, which he nevertheless exhibited with pride." Adler continued: "The ape, which is nursing the child, a female ape, is he himself—that is, he sees himself, he feels himself in a feminine role, along with the nursing is to be considered a gynecomastia which came up during the dream analysis. . . . Thus the patient enters upon the treatment with the disclosure that he feels himself belittled—and permits us to divine from the choice of his figure of speech, that he evaluates this inferiority as feminine" (p. 200). The desire to be a man and the sense of being a woman were signs of "psychic hermaphrodism" for Adler. Thus the patient's original thought, "I have imperfect genitalia, I will not be a complete man," became transformed into the Oedipal desire to be a complete man like the father (p. 206).

Adler's therapy for this pre–World War I patient was clearly the "talking" rather than the "cutting" cure. Psychoanalysis will eventually enable him to "pass" as a "real" man, a man who has come to terms with his body and his psyche. His breasts will become part of his body with which he has come to terms. By the 1920s, Adler's concept of the "inferiority complex" came to be the generalized shorthand for that which was "cured" through aesthetic surgery.[22] His original concept was crafted from his earlier theory of organ inferiority. He noticed that a biological weakness in an organ or organ system seemed either to strengthen the body through "compensation" or to weaken the body to such a degree that the patient needed medical intervention.[23] After his break with Freud in the fall of 1911, Adler began to rethink his purely somatic model of the "inferiority complex" and its relationship to aesthetic surgery. In his study of the neurotic constitution, written in 1912 under the influence of Hans Vaihinger's (1852–1933) philosophy, he claimed that one lived as if one could attain the idealized goals set for oneself in childhood. Inferiority is a problem of the internal, fictive life, rather than the organ. This view is worked out in greatest detail in his foreword to Maxwell Maltz's book *New Faces, New Futures* (1936). In this introduction Adler, now well entrenched in American psychological social work, emphasized the question of the acceptance of the individual by the peer group. What mattered was neither the weakness of the organ nor the question of the actual, physical nature of the individual but rather "the manner by which the people around him judge others. As we live in a group and are judged by the group, and as this group objects to any departure from normal appearance . . . a facial deformity can have a very deleterious effect on behavior."[24] Thus, according to Maltz, it is the surgeon who enables this individual to "pass": "the surgeon . . . seeks to ease the mind by remolding the . . . features to a conformity with the normal. Once normality is attained, the mind throws off its burden of inferiority, of fear of ridicule and of economic insecurity . . . behavior responds to normal social contacts, the personality relaxes into naturalness and character is transformed" (p. 303). At this point Adler's patient would have had his breasts removed surgically, rather than undergoing the talking cure.

No literary text represents with more force the dilemma of men with breasts than Philip Roth's extraordinary novella *The Breast* (1972).[25] The story is about the transformation of a man into a breast—a female breast. The tale, like Adler's idea of inferiority, moves between notions of gender and race in complex and often surprising ways.

One morning after a restless night, David Kepesh, professor of comparative literature at the State University of New York at Stony Brook, awakens to find himself transformed into "a mammary gland such as could only appear, one would have thought, in a dream or a Dali painting" (p. 13). His doctors are puzzled at this transformation and have multiple explanations. It is "a phenomenon that has been variously described as . . . 'a massive hormonal influx,' 'an endocrinopathic catastrophe,' and/or 'a hermaphroditic explosion of chromosomes'" (p. 13). All of these explanations, we shall see in the rest of this chapter, come to be models for the rationale of why men have (not necessarily are) breasts. Kepesh is transformed into a *man* as a female breast, not into a male breast.

According to his physicians, Kepesh's new form is at least attractive: "my flesh is smooth and 'youthful,' and I am still a 'Caucasian'" (p. 14). These notes read as if they are from his medical chart, phrased by his endocrinologist. The breast is beautiful and white (read: erotic), as this image follows the construction of racial as well as sexual identity in Roth's account of Kepesh's life. Kepesh is well known to the reader of Roth's oeuvre from *The Professor of Desire* (1977), in which his hypersexual, unfocused existence is charted from his Jewish childhood to the sexual adventures of a student life in London to a sad and isolated adulthood in New York City. Kepesh is the Jewish intellectual as represented in Roth's world—hypersexual, and extraordinarily isolated and lonely in his sexuality.

Pleasure and happiness seem to stand at the center of Kepesh's life as well as at the center of this novella. Kepesh's fetishization of the female breast as the source of his erotic pleasure becomes his nightmare of pleasure, for this giant, 155-pound breast is the site of erotic pleasure. His nipple, massaged and sucked, provides him with orgasm after orgasm. This fantasy of being transformed into one's own object of desire and experiencing the pleasure one imagines providing is a narcissistic form of identification with one's own sexuality. The pleasure that he imagines the breasts of his female sexual partners receiving is the pleasure that he himself receives.

His nipple, the source of his pleasure as a breast, is truly his own penis. The "wrinkled, roughened skin of the nipple . . . was formed out of the glans penis" (pp. 15–16)—needless to say, given the description of both breast and penis, a circumcised penis. The sexuality of the Jewish male stands at the very center of Kepesh's transformation. The Jewish male is traditionally feminized, and simultaneously the circumcised penis traditionally represents hypersexuality. But at least he is "white"! In racial terms, the blackness of the Jew was one of his hallmarks and was written on his body. Adler's patient, too, was a Jew. His sense of his feminizing body must also be read in the light of the cultural definition of all male Jews as feminine. Here, this is translated into the world of the breast. Kepesh is transformed into a giant breast, which is the concrete representation of his own hypersexuality.

Kepesh first notes the beginning of the transformation in his groin. He hysterically calls his doctor to complain that he has developed a "pale red" stain at the base of his penis (p. 5). This stain and the heightened sensitivity in his groin during his erotic activities signal the beginning of his transformation. He notes that he had initially taken his increased erotic sensitivity as a "sign of health rather than disease" (p. 7). But he understands his transformation into a breast with all the sensations of a penis as a "disease" (p. 11). This breast remains, evidently, a man. He loves being manipulated and sucked by women (including his wife) and cannot imagine having the same response from contact with men (p. 44). This man as a breast remains hypermasculine, at least in his fantasy.

Kepesh eventually comes up with his own explanation for this transformation. He has been teaching too much Franz Kafka (1883–1924) ("The Metamorphosis") and Nikolai Gogol (1809–52) ("The Nose") (pp. 60, 65–66). He has gone mad and imagined himself transformed as their characters were transformed. He is mad and thus his transformation is "merely" a delusion. "Did fiction do this to me?" he asks (p. 81). Is this dysmorphophobia, the contemporary psychiatric category that encompasses bodily illusions? If treated as a neurosis, will the giant breast vanish and the male body reappear?

His psychoanalyst tells him that such an explanation is avoiding the reality of his transformation and is certainly "the way into madness" (p. 61). "Hormones are hormones and art is art" (p. 81). The transformation is "real," not merely psychological. His unhappiness lies in his body, not in his soul. His choice is clear: "I am indeed a wholly authentic breast—or else . . . I am as mad as any man has ever been" (p. 75). But he understands his situation finally not in terms of Kafka or Gogol, but in the rejection of the "Age of Reason." Kepesh is Jonathan Swift's (1667–1745) Gulliver among the Brobdingnags: "How the maid-servants had him strolling out on their nipples for the fun of it" (p. 85). This sense of the necessary transformation of the hypersexual Jewish male into the female breast provides a double reading. It is a comment on the power of sexuality in the "Age of Reason" to shape our very sense of our selves; but it is also a commentary on the problems and potential of the transformation promised to everyone in the Enlightenment. Here it is brought to an evident and ludicrous conclusion, but not beyond the bounds of the promise of transformation in the age of aesthetic surgery. One can have a new body and a new spirit!

Indeed, the contemporary (as well as the nineteenth-century) debates about body dysmorphic disorder rest on the question of whether distortion in body images is a psychological problem.[26] The clinical category of "dysmorphophobia" was developed by

Enrico Morselli in the 1890s to explain the unhappiness of many aesthetic surgery patients.[27] It has been expanded in the various *Diagnostic and Statistical Manual of Mental Disorders* of the American Psychiatric Association to become a means of excluding patients from aesthetic surgery.[28] With DSM-IV, unhappiness with the body (in addition to eating disorders) has come to hold a major place in the psychiatric discussion of body distortion as mental illness (300.7; pp. 466–69). The favored treatment of body dysmorphic disorder is now psychopharmacological intervention rather than surgery.[29] The differential diagnosis to body dysmorphic disorder in DSM-IV is gender identity disorder (302.6; pp. 532–38). If a patient focuses on any part of his or her body *besides* his / her primary or secondary sexual characteristics, one can diagnose body dysmorphic disorder; if the focus is *on* the primary or secondary sexual characteristics, then one can diagnose gender identity disorder. Patients suffering from gender identity disorder are primary candidates for transgender surgery. The debate about transgender surgery as a treatment for gender identity disorder centers on whether the body is to be "restored" to an original (Platonic) self or whether it can only be transformed into a simulacrum of that self. By the end of the twentieth century, the outcome of that debate is still unclear. "I don't consider this a mutilation," said a male transsexual before his transformation under the knife of Stanley Biber, who turned the town of Trinidad, Colorado, into a center for transsexual surgery in the 1990s.[30] Yet it is a question whether the transformation of the body is a mutilation or a cure—or, indeed, both simultaneously.

Transsexual Surgery

There are men who desire to have breasts and women who desire to have none at all. For them, "unhappiness" is the result of their sexual assignment, the capricious lottery of birth producing males who desire to be females and females who desire to be males. In such dilemmas the absolute boundary between the genders is not only constructed but also reconstructed. Marjorie Garber, who has written the best account of the culture of transsexualism, has argued that the transsexual is utterly invested in the "age-old boundary between 'male' and 'female'" and thus stands for a kind of return to gender essentialism. "Transsexuals . . . are more concerned with maleness and femaleness than persons who are [not] transsexual. They are emphatically not interested in 'unisex' or 'androgyny' as erotic styles," for their central intent is to "pass" as a member of the "other" sex, to become essentially male or female.[31]

The history of transsexual surgery can be approached initially through questions about the transformation of identity and the body. Is this reconstructive surgery? Has there been a wrong sexual assignment? Is this a "man" (or a "woman") trapped in the body of the other sex? Does being so trapped mean unhappiness? "The physician is trained to alleviate suffering, and there can be no doubt about the genuine suffering transsexuals experience."[32] Or, as with Klinefelter's syndrome, if you know only the person's chromosomal identity, whether they are XX or XY, does this make sexual assignment or reassignment easier or more difficult? What of true or pseudo-hermaphroditic individuals born with what seem like or even are the primary sexual characteristics of both sexes?

It is of little consequence whether the transformation is on the level of morphological (the shape of the genitalia), hormonal, chromosomal, or social definitions of sexuality and gender. The discussions of sexual transformation center on the question of identity and the role aesthetic surgery plays in constructing or mimicking sexual identity. Gary T. Marx, in an insightful essay on "fraudulent identification," raises the specter of whether impersonation is a quality of modern culture.[33] In the age of the Internet and aesthetic surgery, can't we simply re-create ourselves as we desire? Aren't these new selves as valid as all other forms of identity? Marx sees "cosmetics and plastic surgery" as two of the "resources available that intentionally or unintentionally aid false presentation" (p. 151). Are transsexuals "merely" surgical cross-dressers? He contrasts two examples. The first is "the case of the New York model whose face was cut and who had undergone plastic surgery and wears cover-up makeup" (p. 151) She is not creating a fraudulent identity because "she can be viewed as trying to create what was once hers." In a sense she seeks a Platonic ideal, the authentic form of who she "really" is. He contrasts this with "a dark-skinned person who uses skin lightener or a person who undergoes plastic surgery to obtain a more Nordic look." As he notes, "there can be a tension in the cultural emphasis to be all you can be, make yourself over versus being yourself, accepting your identity" (p. 158). This is the dilemma of transsexual surgery as aesthetic surgery. Aesthetic surgery resolves ambiguities by allowing an individual to "pass" unspoken as a member of a definable class. The question remains whether the person truly belongs to that class.

The American psychologist John Money (1921–), the most outspoken advocate of transgender surgery during the latter half of the twentieth century, imagines a Platonic ideal of sexual and gender identity. "When you read about a grown man who has become a woman do you wonder if you yourself are a man or a woman? Of course not. You knew that you were a boy, or that you were a girl, long before you learned to read. And unless you are one of the very few exceptions to an all but universal rule, you've never seriously questioned it since."[34] Money advocates a restoration of the relationship between the inner and outer selves. An asymmetry between them causes unhappiness; the restoration of an ideal symmetry (dimorphism) results in happiness. There is never the possibility of ambiguity. One is either male or female—though sexual preference is not so defined. One can be a male in a woman's body (erotically attracted to either men or women) or a woman in a man's body (erotically attracted to either men or women).[35] Surgery is the path to happiness, and for Money transgender surgery is reconstructive along a spectrum running from the resolution of the ambiguous morphology present in fetal deformation to adult transsexual surgery. Surgery becomes the means of restoring order and making the psyche happy through the establishment of a unitary identity.[36]

The establishment of aesthetic surgery at the close of the nineteenth century made transgender surgery conceptually possible.

But it was as much the experience as the fantasies of mutilation in World War I that enabled surgeons to imagine how such surgery could be done. Sexologists, such as Magnus Hirschfeld (1868–1935), were concerned with the impact of castration as a war wound on the individual's sense of his own masculinity. Once it is claimed that the patient's autonomy defines the physician's approach as well as the "deformity," then transgender surgery becomes not only feasible but also inevitable.[37] It is the voluntary nature of the medical contract in aesthetic surgery that is central—patients come to the physician and request certain procedures to alleviate their unhappiness. In both aesthetic and transgender surgery, the link between mind and body is absolute and defines health and illness. Transgender surgery is aesthetic surgery if it is deemed to operate on the psyche.[38]

C. G. Jung (1875–1961) dismissed transgender surgery as "merely" aesthetic surgery in 1950 when he condemned transgender surgery as having nothing at all to do with medicine or psychology (as defined by him). "Any one, even the patient, could give advice that a surgeon be sought for the procedure."[39] If the patient initiates treatment, defines treatment, and defines the goals of treatment, according to Jung, this is not "real" medicine. Jung argued that it is as bad as if someone went to a surgeon and persuaded him to amputate a fully functional finger. The only difference is that the functional penis has a symbolic status in society. For Jung, any physician who undertakes such a procedure is to be roundly condemned: there is no possibility that such "cosmetic procedures" are medicine in any shape or form.

Of course, if you assumed that the transgendered individual is "simply" being restored to some type of Platonic ideal, Jung's position would be an anathema. Some American legal specialists have argued against this assumption that transgender surgery is aesthetic surgery. "There is a superficial resemblance between a transsexual's bodily gender projects and a cosmetic surgery such as breast augmentation. Perhaps if a woman who pursues breast augmentation is guilty of an abusive simulation, then a man or a woman who chooses to undergo the more radical procedures of sex-reassignment surgery is [also] guilty. . . . Instead of regarding sex-reassignment surgery as producing an imitation in the way that cosmetic surgery produces an imitation, one might say that the choice of such surgery stands in the same relation as masturbation to the appropriate use of one's gendered body: to participate in the 'conjugal good.'"[40] The contrast so advocated is parallel to that suggested by Gary T. Marx, but such distinctions always play one set of "real" experiences off against the illegitimate desires of those who are defined as merely vain. Other forms of aesthetic surgery produce only simulacra, while transgender surgery produces "real" bodies. Such arguments assume the parallel between the creation of bodies that are able to "pass" and "real" bodies.

The image of "gender identity disorder" as a psychiatric diagnostic category is rooted in the model of the restoration of a prelapsarian "happiness" with the body. In the 1920s, primarily through Magnus Hirschfeld's (1868–1935) Institute for Sexual Science in Berlin, a series of surgical interventions was developed by Ludwig Lévy-Lenz, as we discussed earlier, and Felix Abraham (1901–?). They surgically transformed male genitalia into simulacra of the external female genitalia (without, of course, the ability to reproduce).[41] The emphasis in such surgery was on the creation of the appearance of female genitals, which could be erotically stimulated. Reproduction was never even imagined as a goal, as the transplantation of ovaries for reproductive purposes never has been part of the conceptual strategy of "becoming female" in transsexual surgery.

In an earlier paper, Richard Mühsam (1872–?) of the City Hospital in Berlin recounted that as early as 1920 a male patient referred to him by Magnus Hirschfeld requested that he be castrated and that in 1921 he removed the ovaries of a female transvestite at her request.[42] One can add that in the 1920s and 1930s castration was understood as a medical practice that was a "form of therapy for neuroses, perversions, sexual crimes, sexual abnormalities, mental disease and even tuberculosis."[43] Mühsam's paper was read by his contemporaries in this broader context.

In all of the cases in which Mühsam undertook the removal of the gonads, there was no claim that the patient was either a

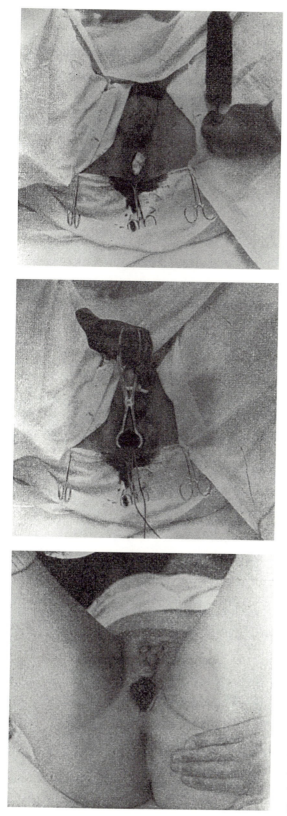

The construction of
the vagina in one of
the first transsexual
surgical procedures.

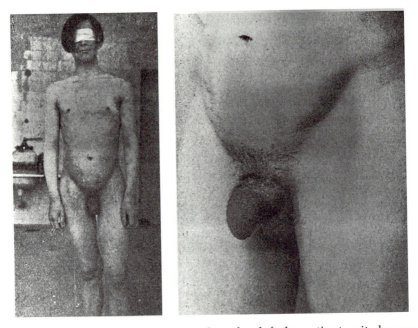

The incomplete transsexual procedure that left the patient quite happy with his lot.

pseudo- or an actual hermaphrodite. There had been a long history of the surgical reconstruction of "ambiguous" genitalia, usually as female genitalia.[44] Given that one out of a thousand births results in "ambiguous" genitalia, this surgical intervention was already an established part of reconstructive urology. Indeed the transgender patients all were represented as suffering from psychological difficulties rather than physical anomalies.

Mühsam's first patient, a twenty-three-year-old student, had been dismissed from a military school for "lack of guts." He served as an officer during World War I, testing his manhood, and came to Mühsam after the war when he no longer could function. "He gave up his medical studies . . . spent the day in bed and slept most of the day." When he was in public he wore a corset, women's stockings, and high heel shoes (1926: p. 452). Mühsam's text makes it evident that the patient desired to be castrated and transformed into a woman: "The fate of this man sounds like a novel," Mühsam wrote in 1926, "it shows that the most active fantasy cannot imagine what feelings, wishes, and imaginings one finds with sexual neurotics." On June 21, 1920, the young man was castrated, and on June 23, for the first time in a long while, he asked for a book and resumed his studies. He requested to have an ovary implanted to generate female hormones rather than for reproductive purposes, and this was done in March 1921. Following the surgical interventions, the patient developed breasts and wore women's clothing in private. He also began to sound "feminine." His larynx was examined and revealed a "laryngeal feminine type structure."

Mühsam could not bring himself to amputate the penis, so he created a mock vagina into which the penis was placed, so that it could be sexually stimulated. By August 1921 the young man returned to the surgeon and requested that he return his penis to a form more functional for intercourse, as he had a new woman friend. After this was done, he completed his medical studies and emigrated, informing his physician in a letter that: "My health is well. I am absolutely happy [zufrieden] with myself ... and my work pleases me greatly" (1926: p. 453). In this case, as with the other cases, he became both "happy" and, according to Mühsam, a productive member of society. Indeed, Mühsam stresses, the transformation of this young man from a suicidal, sexual neurotic to a productive member of society is one of the major results of the procedure (1921: p. 156).

None of the patients that Mühsam records was labeled a "hermaphrodite." All were "normal" in terms of their bodily structure and had been referred by Hirschfeld because of their psychological state. Magnus Hirschfeld's fascination with hermaphrodism was rooted in his own conviction that the homosexual was a "third sex" bearing psychic qualities of the other sexuality.[45] The hermaphrodite provided a biological model for people who were both sexes and yet neither. Since physical hermaphrodites were potentially the subject of "reconstructive" surgery, by analogy sexually troubled / transgendered individuals (psychological hermaphrodites) could also make this claim. But was it reconstructive or was it aesthetic surgery? Was it the restoration of a pre-existing body that would match the psyche within, or was it the manipulation of the external aspect of the body to make the individual happier?

Surgical procedures similar to those described in detail by Richard Mühsam and Felix Abraham were also undertaken by a Dr. Gohrbandt at the City Hospital in Berlin. They consisted of the removal of the penis and testicles and the creation of an artificial vagina. The cases reported by Abraham were not cases of hermaphrodism but of male transvestites who desired sex changes. The cases are exemplary. The first case, also reported by Richard Mühsam, was of Rudolph, a.k.a. Dora R., who at the age of six had attempted to amputate his penis because of his intense discomfort with his body. He had himself castrated in 1922, and in 1931 his penis was amputated and the procedure for the construction of the vagina was undertaken.

Arno, a.k.a. Toni E., was married, and after the death of his wife began to dress as a woman. He was "calm and intelligent" when dressed as a woman; "nervous and completely nonfunctional" when dressed as a man. Within two years he was surgically transformed into a woman. Abraham commented: "One could object that such operations are 'luxury' operations with only playful character, since those operated on after a certain time again and again return to the surgeon with greater demands. It was not easy to decide to undertake these procedures but the patients were not only not to be talked out of them, but they were also in a state of mind which led one to believe they would have mutilated themselves and would have had life-threatening complications."[46] Arno/Toni had procedure after procedure to alter the form of the body. Multiple surgery here is not a sign of neurosis or psychosis, as implied by many of the surgeons and psychoanalysts dealing with aesthetic surgery. Such requests are an indicator of the degree of transformation needed by the patient to turn him into as much of a woman as matches his sense of being able to "pass." Thus the initial transsexual operations, as with most of the earlier procedures, were modeled on the desires (and potential actions) of the client. They were also seen as cures, not of bodily anomalies, but of psychic unhappiness.

In his discussion of the central cases of aesthetic surgery during his own professional career, the Parisian aesthetic surgeon Jean Boivin (1907–   ) presented the best-known case of such sexual reassignment from the 1930s. It was the case of Einar Wegener (d. 1931), the first widely publicized case of a male (pseudo-hermaphrodite) to undergo surgical transformation into a female. Although Wegener did not leave an autobiography, s/he did turn a diary and letters over to a German journalist whose account reflected the temper of the time concerning this highly publicized case.[47]

Wegener's diary account is the first of a long series of autobiographies or ghosted autobiographies of transsexuals, which include (more recently) those of Christine Jorgensen, Caroline Cossey, and Jan Morris.[48] The popularity of such texts seems to speak against the silent acceptance of the individual "passing" into a new cohort. One can imagine that the new cohort is not at all the overt one represented in the autobiography; rather the new cohort is the world of the transsexual. Not surprisingly, transsexual surgery makes transsexuals rather than "men" or "women." This may well be why transsexuals need the boundary between the male and the female to be absolute. Acceptance into this cadre can indeed be signaled by public self-representation as a "man" or a "woman." The public's fascination with such books, as in the case of Jorgensen and Morris, may well express its anxiety about the fluid nature of sexual boundaries.

In many of the autobiographies of transsexuals, the theme of the restructuring of the body centers on the ability of the surgeon to alter the psyche. Certainly, traditional medicine in the 1920s was not seen as a source of solace by Einar Wegener. According to the fictionalized account, Wegener consulted three doctors: "the first had declared that he had never in all his life performed 'beautifying operations'; the second examined exclusively the blind-gut; the third declared [Einar] to be 'perfectly mad'" (p. 19). Here we have three of the most commonly held views of aesthetic surgery: it is "merely" cosmetic and can have no therapeutic value; unhappiness with the body is a sign of a diseased body; or unhappiness is a sign of insanity. One doctor "regarded the whole

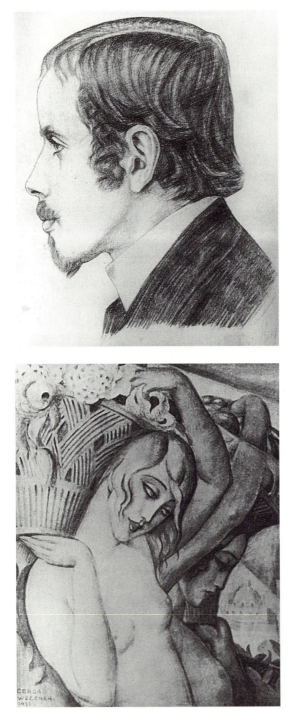

Einar Wegener with
beard in 1920, and
his alter ego "Lili
Elbe" with breasts
after her transforma-
tion. The latter
painted by We-
gener's wife.

thing as a fixed idea of mine, and exclusively as a 'diseased imagining without any physical foundation' . . . and one of them, the new specialist, even hinted I was really homosexual." The clinical psychiatrist sees the desire to change the body as a symptom of dysmorphophobia and the psychoanalytically oriented therapist reads it as a homosexual fixation at an earlier stage of development. These are two of the strategies to cut Wegener's "madness" in this world. Surgery offered another alternative (p. 110).

Wegener's body, however, began to change without any medical intervention: "His eyes looked hollow, his skin took on a pallor which was frightening to behold, and he was unable to sleep. His masculine organs atrophied and his breasts began to develop."[49] Examined by his physician, Werner Kreutz (a pseudonym), he is declared to be a true hermaphrodite—having ovaries as well as testicles, but only according to an external, physical examination, which could hardly establish the presence of ovaries (p. 25). Wegener needs to be seen as a person whose shift of gender is a "natural" one, resulting from the bisexual nature of his body (which mirrors his psyche). But the seemingly spontaneous transformation of the adult male body into that of a mature female hints at a psychological rather than a physical explanation.

According to Wegener, the physical and psychic pain arose out of the struggle for domination between the masculine and feminine principle. "I was both man and woman in one body, and . . . the woman in this body was in the process of gaining the upper hand. Upon this assumption I explained the disturbances, both physical and psychic, from which I was suffering to an increasing extent" (p. 100). The end result of this was extreme unhappiness even for his feminine alter ego: "Lili [Elbe] appeared; but she had lost all her gaiety. She wept every time" (p. 103). Unhappiness is the central marker of the illness.

Surgery enabled Wegener to begin to achieve some modicum of happiness. After the first operation in Dresden in 1930, he awakened castrated and asked: " 'Did I make much noise?' 'Well, just a little,' said one of the nurses with a smile, 'and the strange thing was that your voice had completely changed. It was a shrill woman's voice' " (p. 128). His transformation had begun; his "passing" as a woman was recognized by the women nurses, representing the group into which Wegener desired to enter. Wegener's (now called Lili Elbe's) diary for the time reads: "In the first months after my operation it was necessary above all to recuperate. When this had happened to some extent, the physical change in me began. My breasts formed, my hips changed and became softer and rounder. And at the same time other forces began to stir in my brain and to choke whatever remnants of [Einar] still remained there. A new emotional life was arising within me" (p. 243). Lili's new breasts represented the entire transformation, one of the soul as well as the body, as she wrote in a letter to her physician, "Werner Kreutz": "I feel so changed that it seems as if you had operated not upon my body, but upon my brain" (p. 244). Lili Elbe returned to Dresden for a third operation and died there, as Jean Boivin said in his account of her experiences, "obsessed by the idea that the professor whom she adored as if he were God had never regarded her as anything else but a guinea-pig on which to practice his skill."[50] This is missing in the "official" published account of the life and death of Lili Elbe, which concludes with happiness and love. Boivin's statement marks not the restoration of happiness but the anxiety of being the subject of an experiment. For the surgeon to treat the patient for his own ends undermines the patient's autonomy, even if the patient instigated the surgery. This ambiguity shadows Lili Elbe's death.

Sexual surgery is the realm of the gynecological surgeon undertaking procedures that are "aesthetic" in order to cure the unhappiness of the patient. Wegener makes the argument that he was a true hermaphrodite in order to argue that he truly was a woman trapped in a male's body and that body revealed its female essence by developing breasts. His/her body desired to "pass" and s/he was unhappy because her psyche could not understand the body's desires. The sexual identity of the psyche is embodied and/or contradicted by the apparent gender of the body. Correct the error of the physical and the unhappiness of the patient will vanish.

The culture of "passing" is thus closely related to the world of the transsexual. The extraordinary case of N. O. Body caught Magnus Hirschfeld's attention in 1907.[51] Karl M[artha] Baer (1885–1956) was a man who had been designated as a female at birth because of the ambiguity of his genitalia. Raised as a female, s/he found himself developing in ways that were at odds with her/his gender assignment. S/he recounts her/his growing confusion and intense unhappiness in her/his autobiography, published pseudonymously under the name N. O. Body and accompanied with an afterword by Hirschfeld. His/her confusion was exacerbated by the break of her/his voice (p. 58), which convinced the teenager that s/he was sick, indeed that s/he had developed tuberculosis. His/her schoolmates (in their all-girl school) were developing their "slim, virginal lines," while Baer remained flat-chested. The girls showed each other their breasts and reveled in the changes of their bodies (p. 70). This made the author question her/his own female identity: "What was I? Boy or girl? If I was a girl, why didn't my breasts develop?" (p. 79). Even more than the absence of menstruation, the lack of development of her/his breasts signaled not belonging to the cohort to which s/he had been assigned. Once s/he was sexually reassigned as a man (which was undertaken with a court order to alter her/his birth certificate), his body was allowed to develop as a man. S/he did gymnastics and became "stronger and broader" (p. 154). No trace of a woman's body remained except for the mark of the corset. Hirschfeld's lesson from N. O. Body's account was that "the sex of a human being rests much more in his/her soul than in his/her body, or to express myself in a more medical manner, more in the brain than in the genitals" (pp. 163–64). Happiness according to this model, is when the soul and the body are in alignment.

Baer's reassignment does not necessitate any surgical procedure. His ambiguous genitalia were actually male and, although his education as a "girl" later caused some difficulties in his life as a man, the absence of breasts was the "true" sign of his sexual identity. In Imperial Germany "real" men did not have breasts. However, Baer's narrative contained a double "passing." He published it pseudonymously and successfully disguised all aspects of his identity, including the fact that he was Jewish. In the narrative he represented this "exotic" background as "French." Indeed, this effacement of Baer's Jewish identity is noticeable only where he stresses the difference of his own body. He praises his body as having a "fine body shape, long, small feet, and a long, oval face" (p. 10), quite the antithesis of the anti-Semitic image of the Jew at the turn of the century, with his squat body form, misshapen feet, and face marked with the curse of "nos-trility." To "pass" in the autobiography, an account of an unin-tended, unconscious "passing" as a woman, meant to become aware that one was too visible, especially as a Jew.

The absence of breasts established the "true" identity of N. O. Body. This absence signaled that Baer was not "passing" as a woman, that he was "really" a man. Yet the question of whether a Jewish male was a "real" man was one of the most contested as-pects of the "Jewish Problem." Baer's genitalia would not have been circumcised, because he was categorized as a female. Did this make him more of a man, even with ambiguous genitalia? The question of "passing" as anything but a Jew does not arise, for here gender seems to dominate the discourse of race until one examines the idealized body that the male author of the autobi-ography describes as his own. Baer became a senior figure in the Berlin Jewish community in the Weimar period, and in 1938 was able to immigrate to Palestine, where he died.

The male-to-female sexual surgery of Einar Wegener and the female-to-male transformation of Karl Baer, of course, focus on the transformation (surgical or otherwise) of the genitalia as the sign that makes the psyche happy. Recently a counterexample has been given of a male child, John, castrated at eight months be-cause of an accident during circumcision, who never became comfortable with his sexual role as a "Joan" and had a phallo-plasty once the earlier operation was revealed to him.[52] Yet the breasts, as the primary "visible" secondary sexual characteristic that defines the "female" in Western social interaction, are not in-consequential in defining sexual identity. John/Joan's breasts were not sufficient to redefine his identity and make him happy. The countertales of sexual surgery are also enlightening.

In Mark Rees's autobiography (1996) of his life as a female-to-male transsexual, the central theme remains the unhappiness of being in a body that does not seem to be one with the "soul."[53] Following his surgery, Rees founded Press for Change, the major transsexual lobbying group in Great Britain. According to his own account, Rees was a masculine-looking woman, and this ambiguity also led to unhappiness: "My unhappiness at home, at Art School and out in the street where every passer-by was a potential taunter, and the isolation all this engendered, drove me ever deeper into depression" (p. 27). Her physician's rejection of transsexual surgery led to further unhappiness: "What I did know was that the concern to avoid mutilation of the body was resulting in a mutilation of the mind" (p. 63). Hormone therapy and psychotherapy were undertaken, but without any success: "I was still 'in the wrong body.' Neither hormones nor psychotherapy had proved any use in 'curing' me." (p. 69). The hormone therapy, however, did enable her to begin her transformation. It caused her to stop menstruating and lowered her voice: "Within a few weeks my voice was changing enough for people to ask what was wrong with my throat" (p. 86). The voice, in its designation as male or female, also marks the body. It is no wonder that both voice/speech therapists and surgeons have devoted attention to the aesthetic surgery of the voice.[54] (One can note here the analogous problem of the racialized voice. Nineteenth-century medicine claimed that Jews spoke with a specific Jewish accent because of the musculature of the Jewish face and nose.)[55]

The central icon for this unhappiness was what Rees early in the autobiography calls "the battle of the Bra" (pp. 16 ff.). When she was fourteen, her mother bought her a brassiere, which became a sign of the unhappiness her breasts caused her. Her sexual maturity as a woman was signified by her breasts, and she "in the privacy of my room . . . pummeled my hated breasts with fury" (p. 16). The hormone therapy she undertook reduced the size of her breasts so that she was able to abandon "the hated bra," but she still had "nipples and breasts too large for a man" (p. 86). She disguised them by wearing heavier clothing until she had a bilateral mastectomy four years after beginning hormone therapy (p. 112). Her mastectomy, which made her transformation visible on her body, signaled the beginning of the "real" transformation in the autobiography.

The account stressed that her mother met at the hospital "a slight young man with a scarred chest" (p. 113), who had undergone a similar procedure. This scarring marks the new body of the transsexual male. Chapter 18, in which the bilateral mastectomy is described, is the core of the autobiography. In it, the actual transformation from unhappy to happy, from ill to healthy, occurs:

> My breasts were gone and the only scars were about three or four inches long which were almost under my arms. I was very pleased. In the years before this surgery I had wondered how I might react at this moment. Would I be shouting for joy that I'd lost a despised part of my body? In the event it wasn't like that at all.
>
> Immediately after the surgery I'd become accustomed to having a flat chest. In a way it were as if my breasts had never existed. They had been a bad dream and I'd woken up. Yet even though there was no sense of euphoria, I did feel that something alien had gone from me and I was becoming more normal. (p. 117)

Her transformation makes her into a scarred but happier person who understands that such procedures cannot be a cure-all: "for the majority [of transsexuals] a role change releases them into a new and fuller life" (p. 104). The breasts, more than the penis, are the sign of her transformation, of her joining the other category, now (in)visible in her masculinity, because her breasts had been the external, visible sign that had marked her unhappiness. Now she can "pass."

Analogous to Rees's account is the autobiography of Paul Hewitt, who, unlike Rees, described herself as an attractive woman who "wanted to step out of my female skin all of my life."[56] She stressed that she was not a genetic hermaphrodite having both XY and XX chromosomes (p. 93). (This is the latest genetic translation of Hirschfeld's fascination with the biological boundaries of sexual identity.) What defined her "skin" was this "foreign body with breasts" (p. 9). Hewitt's obsession with her breasts was all-consuming. She bound her breasts with yards of cloth, and this act was "vital to my state of mental well-being" (p. 116). She viewed her "flattened breasts with contempt" (p. 128). Her breasts defined her in a set of dichotomies: "I was brought up to believe in a black-and-white world, to believe in extremes: right and wrong; male and female; God and Satan; football and netball" (p. 18). And, one can add, with breasts and without breasts. This need to think in dichotomies is pervasive in her account. Hewitt went into the locker room following a football game as a man: "Then a colleague with Big Daddy's frame took off his shirt to reveal saggy breasts. What am *I* worrying about, I thought to myself." (p. 255) Yet the obsession with breasts, not as an anomaly on a man's body, but as a sign of her female identity, is at the very core of her narrative.

Indeed the entire narrative focuses on being able to have a double mastectomy. Her focus on this procedure was "not a whim" (p. 25). She "could not bear to see my own breasts" (p. 193). When asked, "'Why exactly do you want this operation, Paul?'" she replied, "'Because I'm a man, and men don't have boobs'" (p. 219). She intended to have her breasts removed then her uterus, and perhaps have "plastic surgery to construct an artificial penis" (p. 25). The order of these procedures is important. The breasts are removed for psychological reasons (to stop her sensing her body as that of a female): "I must transform the body I have so it fits as closely as possible my image of myself" (p. 43). Her uterus would then be removed "as a way of protecting against the risk of ovarian cancer" (p. 25). Finally, she would have the phalloplasty, perhaps, as a way of enabling her to urinate standing up and have sex (again following her order). Hewitt provides a detailed account of the process of creating male genitalia (including "prosthetic testes made out of silicone"), but observes that this "revolts me" (p. 90). She sees such surgery as "a high price to pay for unrealistic manhood" (p. 236). One quality of the body that does need alteration is the quality of the voice. In the case of female-to-male transsexuals (unlike in the reverse case), the hormone therapy does lower the voice somewhat (p. 91). Her goal is not to "'pass' as a male" but to "fulfill my own expectations" (p. 159).

At puberty her breasts seemed to have suddenly marked her body as that of a woman: "I had no breasts to speak of, but I had awoken with a huge pair from hell which seemed to have appeared overnight. I remember thinking I must have fallen victim to some bizarre genetic experiment" (p. 52). Her (nonidentical) twin sister did not experience this sense of the bizarre changes of her body, according to Hewitt. Hewitt's breasts were "the body parts which a monster has designed" (p. 265). After a long battle with the National Health Service, she eventually went to Belgium and had her breasts amputated at a private hospital. In recovery she looked down and "for the first time in twenty-seven years I saw the real Paul, the man I had been searching for and thought I would never find" (p. 285). Hewitt's discovery of her transsexual identity in the absence of her breasts defines the role of the transgender aesthetic surgery which enables her to "pass" now as a "real man."

The removal of the breast signifies the transformation of the female into the male. And yet there are other variations on this theme. With the generalized problems of implants, including the improved silicone implants available by the 1980s, there are cases of male-to-female transsexuals developing extended and/or drooping breasts. In 1989 the first case of *reduction* mammaplasty in a male-to-female transsexual was undertaken using a combination of conventional resection and implant change surgery.[57]

The central question asked by surgeons remains how successful their undertakings really are, which does not mean whether the techniques of the surgery are successful. Although there are extensive discussions of this matter, it is the psychological results of the surgery that stand at the center of the discussions of success. In a 1989 paper on the "prediction of regrets in postoperative transsexuals," the investigators discovered that "none of the 61 homosexual females or 36 homosexual males regretted surgery, compared to 4 of the 14 heterosexual males: a significant difference."[58] (In this context *heterosexual males* means heterosexual male-to-female transsexuals.) The questions covered both vaginoplasty and mastectomies.

The unsuccessful cases were defined as those in which unhappiness with sexual identity remained. Thus one patient stated that "surgery had failed to produce the coherence of mind and body she had been seeking" (p. 44). The authors concluded that it was not women's social role that made those transgendered females unhappy with their new bodies, rather it "was the failure of surgical sex reassignment to satisfy some *ineffable* impulse peculiarly associated with heterosexual dysphoria" (p. 45). An earlier paper commented that, postoperatively, female-to-male transsexuals were "found [to have] increased body satisfaction with increased amount of surgical reassignment."[59] Thus the more procedures, the happier the person: the most contented group had had mastectomies plus hysterectomies plus phalloplasties. It was found that internal procedures such as hysterectomies had a positive impact on the "transsexual's body image even though the outward appearance of the body was not changed in any way" (p. 462). Happiness is measurable in terms of the invisibility of individuals according to their own self-representation. It is the necessary self-deception of transsexual surgery that links it to other forms of aesthetic surgery. Like the identity of other aesthetic surgery patients, the transsexual's identity is linked to the ability of the individual to "pass." "Passing," according to the Web page compiled by Diane Wilson, a male-to-female transsexual, www.lava.net/~Egender, is "the ability to be accepted as a member of one's gender of choice. Yes, choice can be a loaded word; none of us 'chose' to be what we are, but we do choose how we deal with it." Autonomy has its limits.

Thus the question of the meaning ascribed to the breast and the validation of one's new body comes to be part of a complex web of meaning as to what masculinity or femininity is and how the body can or cannot be transformed to enable the individual to "pass" within a new identity. In every case, the inability to enter into the "appropriate" category is marked by clear signs from the members of that category about the inauthencity of the individual. Silence marks the individual's ability to "pass," and "passing" is the means to validate the new body. "Happiness" results only when there is a silent acceptance of a new identity.

THE FIRST CUT IS THE DEEPEST

The technique for repairing infant male circumcision provoked Johann Friedrich Dieffenbach to denounce "beauty surgery" in the 1840s. In the past decade there has been a resurgence of interest in decircumcision as aesthetic surgery in the United States. Such procedures are seen as restoring the body to its original, essential masculine form. The United States is the only nation in the world that circumcises the majority of its newborn males for nonreligious reasons. Although the number of infant male circumcisions dropped from 64.5 percent in 1979 to a low of 58 percent in 1988, it climbed back to 60 percent in 1992.[60] A 1997 survey noted a general decrease in the number of infant males circumcised in the United States. Immediately after World War II, about 80 percent of all American newborn males were circumcised, but the numbers have declined since then. The 1997 figures show that 81 percent of white men in America today have been circumcised, compared to 65 percent of African Americans and 54 percent of Latinos.[61] (A more precipitous decline occurred when the British National Health Service refused to pay for infant male circumcisions in the 1950s.) Circumcision defines the "exotic" male body, at least in gay culture. Whereas it is "in" to be "cut" among gay circles in Germany, it is "in" to be "uncut" in gay circles in New York City. The various attacks on circumcision have created a small industry for medical as well as nonmedical decircumcision procedures.[62]

Although many of the objections to infant nonritual circumcision stress its expense as the most frequently undertaken but medically unnecessary surgical procedure, the image of the duplicitous and dangerous Jew evoked by Dieffenbach also reappears in these debates. In Europe even today, circumcision defines the "Jew," and the "Jew" defines circumcision. The rationales against infant male circumcision consider it a form of "child abuse," a charge widely made at the close of the twentieth century by public figures such as the German psychoanalyst Alice Miller., long a resident of Switzerland, broke with traditional psychoanalysis over the issue of the reality of trauma as the origin of neurosis. Like Sándor Ferenczi at the end of his life, she argued that Freud was wrong in having abandoned the seduction theory. In her 1988 book *Banished Knowledge: Facing Childhood Injuries* she argued that *"crimes against children represent the most frequent of all types of crime"* (her emphasis). "Child abuse" encompasses all adult violence against children's bodies, "the actual physical mutilation of small children," and leads to a devastating critique of "the cruel mutilation of children's sexual organs."[63] Her argument here is clear: circumcision (male and female) is child abuse; child abuse turns abused children into child abusers; they then circumcise their children, who. . . . These are the most recent transmutations of the charges of ritual murder and ritual abuse lodged against those who are seen as the arch-circumcisers, the Jews, over the past millennia. The circumcised body is read as the dangerous body; the form of the body provides insight into the character of the circumcised male.

The University of Chicago sociologist Edward O. Laumann released a study of circumcision based on a sample of 1,410 men aged eighteen to fifty-nine, who had been interviewed in 1992 as part of his National Health and Social Life survey.[64] His findings were that circumcised men appeared "slightly more likely" than noncircumcised males to contract a sexually transmitted disease during their lifetimes because they were sexually more adventurous. He added that such men also seem to have a longer and more intense sexual life. This elaborates on the stereotype of the hypersexuality of Jewish males, which underlies their desire to marry non-Jews, according to Dieffenbach's contemporaries. In Laumann's sample, the circumcision rates were: 87 percent for sons of mothers who were college graduates, 81 percent for non-Hispanic white men, 65 percent for black men, and 54 percent for Hispanic men. As expected, the rate was highest among Jewish men—96 percent. However, the extremely small number of Jews (twenty-five), the only men who would have been ritually circumcised, determined the reading of the practice. Laumann's comment that circumcision is no longer a "religious marker" in the United States is certainly true; but the reverse is not true. The Jew is still defined by his sexuality. Following this logic, Jewish men were the sexually most adventurous of all the cohorts defined by Laumann. This argument was a "biological" but not necessarily a "racial" one.

Laumann claimed that circumcision blunts sexual sensitivity and that such reduction of sensitivity (rather than racial proclivity) makes the Jews hypersexual. Here he seemed to follow John R. Taylor at the University of Manitoba, whom he does not cite. Taylor claims that the small sheath of foreskin tissue removed during circumcision is filled with extremely sensitive nerve endings and mucus membrane cells and its removal permanently blunts erotic stimulation.[65] Sexual experimentation of all kinds results. Given the claim of an increase in sexually transmitted diseases of all kinds, these researchers read sexual experimentation as pathological. It is little wonder that Laumann's answer is to cite a 1990 paper on the reconstruction of the foreskin as a sign of the "significant movement against the circumcision of infants and the reversing of circumcision in adult men."[66] Laumann places the circumcised male in an anomalous position.

Given such demonization of circumcision, today's desire for the repair of the foreskin has to do with a restoration of the body into its imagined ideal state for medical and aesthetic reasons. Thus, in a letter to the editor of the *New Republic*, Richard De-Seabra, the director of the National Organization of Restoring Men (NORM), claimed that "foreskin restoration provides a definitive physical function, unlike breast reconstruction, for example, which offers only an aesthetic function. Also, foreskin restoration is hardly an ideology, it's a desire."[67] The desire of these men is to alleviate their unhappiness with their bodies: "Like many other middle-aged American men, Jim Bigelow was circumcised at birth, but he never felt happy about it. 'I often prayed that God would give my foreskin back to me.'"[68] An intact body assures a happy psyche.

The American tensions concerning circumcision are not unknown in the Jewish community in the United States. Unlike non-
Jews, most Jews circumcise their infant male children not for
hygienic but for ritual purposes. There had been a successful attempt among some nineteenth-century Rabbinic commentators
to defend Jewish ritual circumcision as a form of hygiene and,
therefore, as proof of Judaism being what Kant called a "rational
religion." But for Jews today circumcision is a ritual, not a medical practice. It is done because of divine command, not because
of human rationale. Recently there has been a resurgence of the
debate about infant male circumcision that had marked the first
generation of reformed Jewish thinkers in the 1840s. The most
radical of these, Samuel Holdheim, had unsuccessfully advocated the abolition of infant male circumcision as a sign of the
modernity of Jewish belief.[69] The image of circumcision as a form
of barbaric bloodletting dominated this discussion in the nineteenth century. It appeared in the rationale for the ritual murder
accusations in the 1890s, that Jews ritually slaughter non-Jewish
children for their blood. The argument ran: if the Jews will do this
to their own children, imagine what they will do to ours! At the
end of the twentieth century the accusation has resurfaced in the
identification of circumcision as a form of child abuse. In 1998
the Jewish anticircumcision crusader Ronald Goldman mustered
the contemporary American arguments against all infant male
circumcision.[70] He argued that the rationales for circumcision—
the maintenance of Jewish identity, physical conformity among
Jews, and health benefits—are either overstated or nonexistent.
Central to Goldman's argument are the notions of the cruelty of
circumcision as a surgical practice and of the resultant long-term
psychological as well as physiological effects on the adult Jewish
male. Jews should not circumcise their male children because it
makes them dysfunctional adults. The implication of Goldman's
stance is that the preservation of the foreskin in children will remedy such problems in adult men and, he adds in an appendix,
eliminate anti-Semitism, because anti-Semitism is caused by the
anxiety of non-Jews who see what Jews do to their children and
fear being mutilated by the Jews.

The first procedure for contemporary, elective foreskin restoration appeared in 1963, in an article by the South African surgeon Jack Penn (1909–96).[71] Penn's patient was a white male with "marked psychological disturbance due to his circumcision." He "was normal in every other way." Penn "degloved" the penis by cutting the skin at its base and pulling it up to form the new foreskin. With his new foreskin, Penn's patient was "completely rehabilitated psychologically." The cure was psychotherapeutic: the "happiness" of the patient was reconstituted along with his foreskin. There was no longer any chance of his being seen as "primitive."

The decircumcision debate has continued in South African culture, where the meaning of circumcision is now read quite differently in the light of the function of adult male circumcision within Xhosa society. Under apartheid, South African physicians, including Jewish surgeons, began to think of decircumcision as an answer to the "primitive," and (imagined) visible circumcised body.[72] Alec Russell, writing from Lusikisiki, Eastern Cape, reflected the anticircumcision feelings of the dominant culture in the new South Africa when he observed that members of the "Xhosa tribe have headed off into the bush for an agonizing initiation into manhood at the hands of an *ingcibi* (traditional surgeon) wielding a spear or a knife. The mutilations and deaths that followed the inevitable slips of the hand were traditionally dismissed as a sign that the victim had not been destined to reach manhood."[73] Such views would indeed make circumcision of all types dangerous and primitive acts. This reflects the deep division within the African National Congress concerning circumcision. Those Xhosa members who were circumcised, such as Nelson Mandela, opposed this connection between modernization and the opposition to circumcision.

Between 1977 and 1990, several further surgical methods were devised for decircumcision.[74] Among the American groups in the 1990s advocating the end of medical circumcision and, almost always, advocating decircumcision are INTACT, NOCIRC, NOHARMM, NORM, and RECAP (Re-cover a Penis). In addition there is a magazine, *Uncut*, devoted to the subject.[75] The claim is that decircumcision ameliorates psychological suffering:

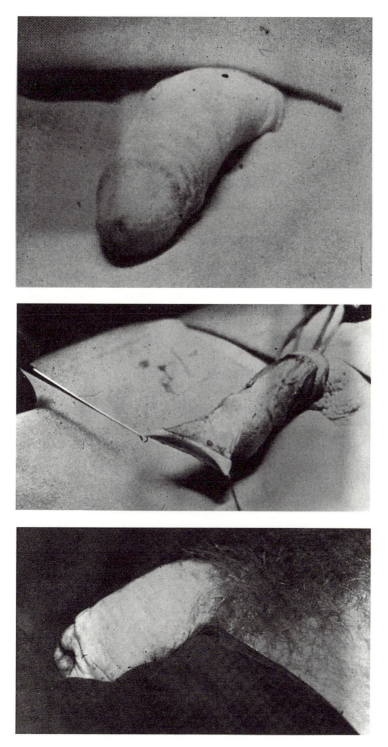

Jack Penn's decircumcision procedure.

Whether [circumcision] leaves psychological scars has long been debated. But clearly some circumcised men will go to great lengths to get a "new" foreskin. Dr. Donald M. Greer, a plastic surgeon at the University of Texas Health Science Center in San Antonio, has performed about 30 foreskin reconstructions since 1982. The cosmetic surgery involves transplanting skin from the scrotum onto the penis in four separate operations in a year. The operation, Greer says, eased the "psychic turmoil" his patients felt over their missing part.[76]

This anxiety drove at least one activist to attempt to reconstruct his own foreskin, a situation analogous to the small number of women who mutilated themselves in order to remove breast implants in the 1990s.[77] The desire to "pass" as healthy and whole in order to be happy remains central to all of the ideologies of the body.

Throughout its history, aesthetic surgery has striven to join the mainstream of medicine by promising patients uniquely effective therapies for becoming happy, healthy, and whole. In all these efforts there has lurked an additional promise, the dream of a renewed, perhaps even eternal youth, or at least its appearance. Before concluding our exploration of aesthetic surgery's remarkable role in modern culture, let's consider its attempts to fulfill that promise of youth.

CHAPTER NINE

Dreams of Youth and Beauty

BEAUTY AND AGE

$\mathcal{O}$F THE SIZE and shape of body parts come to be a measure of the boundary between the erotic and the unerotic, the perceived age of the body comes to have analogous importance.[1] How does one "pass" as "young"? Age was understood by the Enlightenment as a disease analogous to "fat." The aged body is unaesthetic, unerotic, and pathological. This was an Enlightenment trope, even haunting Wolfgang Amadeus Mozart's (1756–91) *The Magic Flute* (1791). When Papagena, disguised as an old woman, tempts her promised mate, Papageno, the effect is comic. Only when she is transformed back into her youthful self does she become erotic for both the audience and Papageno. One earlier stage of this boundary between youth (and the erotic) and age as its antithesis can be found in the construction of the images of the Jewish *synagogia* as the ancient, shriveled crone, who is always juxtaposed to the Christian *ecclesia*, who is young and beautiful. A ridge boundary between youth and age is not universally present across cultures and across history, but at the turn of the twentieth century, the number of individuals who desired to "pass" as youthful began to increase. Medicine began to strive to fulfill patients' desire and make them more youthful.[2] What had been the stuff of myth became the material of the clinic and laboratory.

There are two classic models of overcoming age. The first is the model of rejuvenation—the complete transformation of the aged body into a youthful one.[3] The second is the model of aesthetic surgery—returning the body to the semblance of youthfulness through specific surgical procedures.[4] They compete with one another in the popular imagination. In the twentieth century, both provide, through the institutions of medicine, means to fulfill the quest to "pass" as young (no matter how defined).

The desire for rejuvenation in the West is as old as myth. Did Ponce de Léon really find the fountain of youth? One doubts it. But Charles Édouard Brown-Séquard (1817–94), the noted nineteenth-century physiologist, believed that he had. Born in Mauritania (Mauritius), the child of an American sea captain and a French mother, Brown-Séquard made major discoveries in the endocrine system. "Rejuvenation" research became a subfield of endocrinology and led to the craze for "organotherapy" in the 1920s. When the "testosterone" patch for male impotence made the cover of *Time* magazine in 1996 and the development of Viagra, a specific drug against impotency, in the spring of 1997 shot its maker's stock into the stratosphere, one can measure the public interest in this model of rejuvenation. Indeed physicians now treat aging with human growth hormone, boasting: "'We're not about growing old gracefully. We're about *never* growing old."[5] What is vital is that the origin of the model of rejuvenation lies decades after Friedrich Henle (1809–85) discovered the "ductless glands" in 1841 and Claude Bernard (1813–78) described their internal secretions in 1855. The claims of rejuvenation built upon this knowledge of the workings of the endocrine systems, but they took on active force only with the development of aesthetic surgery.

In 1889, as a professor in Paris, Brown-Séquard proposed that the weakness of aging in men was the "gradual diminishing action of the spermatic glands" and, when he too began to weaken at age seventy-two, he injected himself with mixture of canine semen and blood from the testicular vein.[6] He was rejuvenated, at least by his own accounts. He restored his sexual potency and was able to move more freely and more youthfully. Brown-Séquard's account prompted a large number of experiments with rejuvenation. At the end of the century in Paris, Serge Avramovitch Voronoff (1866–1951) began to implant entire testicles and claimed that he could literally turn an aging ram into a vigorous buck. In moving to human subjects, Voronoff employed monkeys as donors, given the paucity of young men willing to donate testicles.[7] Forty-three patients received testicle grafts from (equally unwilling) monkeys. One must note that whereas Brown-Séquard was an endocrinologist, Voronoff was primarily a surgeon. As the chief surgeon at the Russian Hospital in Paris, he joined with Hippolyte Morestin during World War I to undertake reconstructive, orthopedic work and in the 1930s became the head of the reconstructive section at the French military hospital at Cannes.[8]

Eugen Steinach (1861–1944), the Austrian physiologist, was much better known in the United States than Voronoff.[9] Steinach claimed that the interstitial cells of the testicles ("the puberty gland") provided the key to eternal youth. When castrated animals had sex glands reimplanted in them, they seemed to become hypermasculine or hyperfeminine, according to his criteria of evaluation. In November 1918, Robert Lichtenstern, a Viennese urologist, undertook the first "Steinach" operation. He performed a unilateral vasectomy, severing the *vas deferens,* and claimed to see the increased youthfulness in his male patient. Blood pressure dropped, hemoglobin count increased as did body weight, skin became softer, and muscular strength improved. He believed that he was causing the older male body to be flooded with the secretions of the "puberty gland." Most important, according to Steinach, there was an increased general sense of happiness.

One of Steinach's most famous patients, at least indirectly, was Sigmund Freud. After Freud developed cancer of the jaw, he underwent a "Steinach" operation in 1926 to improve his chances of recuperation through rejuvenation.[10] Freud turned himself over to the urologist Viktor Blum for the procedure. Later Freud, in comments to Ernest Jones, claimed that the operation had absolutely no benefit in ameliorating his condition.[11]

In 1920 Freud had already dismissed the idea that an alternative "Steinach" operation could be effective as a "cure" for "male homosexuality by treating the patient's alleged hermaphroditic condition."[12] This "Steinach" operation was a surgical alternative to the procedures of transgender surgery that were just beginning to transform males (defined as homosexuals) into women. Steinach and his colleagues had surgically treated male homosexuals, whom they diagnosed as "hermaphrodites," by castrating them and transplanting into them "healthy," heterosexual testes. The procedure aimed to increase the patients' "masculinity." Freud noted that "it would be premature, or a harmful exaggeration, if at this stage we were able to indulge the hopes of a 'therapy' of inversion." No therapy for "inversion" could be effective, in Freud's view, if it was an attempt to cure the psyche by operating on the body.

Freud's earlier collaborator Wilhelm Fliess, completely estranged from him since 1904, undertook a similar attack on Steinach at roughly the same time, denying that one could alter the basic bisexuality of all human beings through the manipulation of the endocrine system. He refuted the view, which he ascribed to Steinach, that "beard and voice, breasts and buttocks; not to speak even of the psyche" are simply products of the "sexual glands."[13]

Steinach's procedure, which was intended to "cure" aging, was also seen as a surgical intervention to "cure" male homosexuality. It was an answer to the aesthetic restructuring of the external body in order to alter the psyche. Here the alteration was understood as being a change of the "essential" inner self, the endocrinological "self," and therefore the procedure altered the internal nature of the body in order to make the psyche "happy." That the treatment of "inversion" through transplant surgery using the model of the "hermaphrodite" would be attempted is not surprising, given the presuppositions of transgender surgery in the 1920s.

Surgical rejuvenation in males was paralleled by the use of X-ray treatments for the rejuvenation of the ovaries of women. This technique was developed in Vienna by Guido Holzknecht (1872–1931). Surgical procedures had seemed to be much less effective in rejuvenating women. Voronoff could not even suggest the use of monkey gland transplantations for women and he offered his female clients the following consolation: "The mortality statistics of every land prove that women live much longer than men. Hence they already have the advantage of us and consequently may still wait a few more years before the experiments in the course of development bring them the remedy which is to intensify and prolong their existence."[14] Voronoff stressed rejuvenation as a masculine project.

The major link between rejuvenation and aesthetic surgery was Max Thorek (1880–1960), the founder of the International College of Surgeons and surgeon in chief at the American Hospital in Chicago, who spent four years working on rejuvenation through transplants. Following the work of Voronoff, Thorek experimented with elective surgery, implanting monkey glands in a number of patients. By 1923, however, he had turned against rejuvenation, stating that "the term 'rejuvenation,' which is promiscuously used by certain medical men, is wrong and misleading. It gives the layman the idea that old men and women can become young again."[15] Indeed, Thorek suggested that what was undertaken was a "reactivation" (p. 189), because "no organ, or set of organs can be returned, by any method known so far, to a juvenile state when pathologic changes have made inroads on the structures and rendered them senile, in the accepted form of the term."[16] "Reactivation" is closer in tone to the notions of youth presented in the aesthetic surgery of his day. Youthfulness can only be mimicked through rejuvenation. One cannot really be young if one has aged, but one can "pass" as young.

In her novel *Black Oxen* (1923) Gertrude Atherton (1857–1948) worked out precisely such a fantasy.[17] Written at the peak of the American discussion about rejuvenation, *Black Oxen* provides a model for the imagined advantages and contingent problems of the process of total physical (and, therefore, psychological) transformation. Central to Atherton's representation of rejuvenation in this novel is the fact that, although the procedure was developed by older men for older men, the protagonist, Countess Zattiany, is an older woman. In Atherton's imagination, she has already undergone a series of transformations (following Henry James's model of the American woman). She was an American named

Mary Ogden who moved to Europe, married a man with a title, and after World War I returned rejuvenated to New York. She is the epitome of transmutation, indeed, in the novel she becomes everything to everyone. She is the representation of the essentially mutable female at the beginning of the age of aesthetic surgery. We first see her at the theater (the quintessential site of transformation)—through the eyes of members of the audience for whom she is a great European beauty of unknowable age: "In spite of its smooth white skin and rounded contours above an undamaged throat, it was, subtly, not a young face" (p. 5). She has been restored and now literally looks like a younger cousin, which is who she claims to be. She reveals that her "cousin" is now hospitalized in Vienna. "She took growing old very hard" (p. 47). Her own contemporaries doubt her authenticity as well as her story. They see her as a confidence person who is attempting to benefit from an accidental resemblance to their distant friend. They refuse to allow her to "pass." In attempting to discover who she really is, they uncover the fact of her rejuvenation.

For Atherton's audience (as well as for her characters), the resuscitation of the erotic has great significance. And the "erotic" here is contrasted with the barren. This model of rejuvenation was in its essence for Atherton (and her character) one of individual and racial renewal: "Civilization had heaped its fictions over the bare facts of nature's original purpose, imagination lashing generic sexual impulse to impossible demands for the consummate union of mind and soul and body. Mutuality! When man was essentially polygamous and woman essentially the vehicle of the race" (p. 56). The question of the racial intent of rejuvenation is powerfully stated in the novel.

In rejuvenation the Countess's lover sees the conflict of youth and age inverted—the aged, rather than losing power, would have perpetual control through their eternal youth. This would have positive social results: "The threat of overpopulation—for man's architectonic powers were restored if not woman's; to say nothing of his prolonged sojourn—would at last rouse the lawmakers to the imperious necessity of eugenics, birth control, sterilization of the unfit, and the expulsion of undesirable races. . . .

Human nature might attain perfection" (p. 180). Such perfection is only possible with the restoration of the reproductive function of the body at the imagined peak of youth. This was the thrust of the discussions that followed the announcement in April 1997 by Richard Paulson, chief of the infertility clinic at the University of Southern California, that Arceli Keh, a sixty-three-year-old patient, had given birth following hormone therapy and in vitro fertilization using a donated egg fertilized by her husband's sperm. The possibility of reproductive rejuvenation caused extraordinary consternation among medical ethicists throughout the world. The realization of such fantasies of total rejuvenation became an anathema.

The countess's friends, once told the secret, see themselves as "human even if we are old and ugly" (p. 135) and strongly identify with their friend. They become the sanctioning body that validates her undertaking. They also represent a new America that accepts the scientific domination of Europe: "I have been told that America never takes up anything new in science until it has become stale in Europe" (p. 135). Here the rejuvenation of the European scientific prowess provides a medium for individual change, but equally important, it becomes a sign of the modern.

What is it that Gertrude Atherton's protagonist actually imagines will change, besides the ability to breed better and purer citizens? The Countess desires the "re-energizing [of] my worn out mind and body" (p. 137). The order here is vital. Her psyche needs to be rejuvenated through the rejuvenation of the body. The intervention is a physical intervention, though she "explained in the simplest language she could command the meaning and the function of the ductless glands. . . . In women the slower functioning of the endocrines is coincident with the climacteric, as they have been dependent for stimulation upon certain ovarian cells. . . . I was a promising subject, for examination proved that my organs were healthy, my arteries soft; and I was not yet sixty" (p. 138). Her ovaries are exposed to X rays, and she begins to transform. After a month "it seemed to me that an actual physical weight that had depressed my brain lifted, and I experienced a decided activity of mind and body, foreign to both for many years" (p. 140). This is a means of affecting the psyche through the transformation of the body. Of course, the body too must be treated, but that is the purview of the beauticians. She has beauty treatments for her skin and looks forward to a decade of youthful happiness.

In this fictive world there is no longer any place for aesthetic surgery: "Beauty doctors gnashed their teeth, and plastic surgeons looked forward to the day when they must play upon some other form of human credulity" (p. 215). "Credulity," because all they can do is to remedy the externals of the body, not truly change the psyche. The promise of "happiness" through rejuvenation also eludes the protagonist. At the end of the novel she is unable to accept her new younger body and her much younger lover, who wishes to marry her and have a child with her. This was as undesirable in 1923 as in 1997. But in 1923, not having a child was seen as defining the New Woman, who desired her freedom; in 1997, having a child at the age of sixty-three was seen as an act against nature. The Countess is appalled by the notion that such a marriage would turn her back into an American (with the pejorative psychological meaning that has been evident throughout the volume). Transformations, at least in the Roaring Twenties, make no promise of happiness.

Late twentieth-century "cyberfiction" continues to imagine the complete transformation of the body. Bruce Sterling's (1954–   ) novel *Holy Fire* (1996) provides a cyberfiction account of rejuvenation in the future.[18] His fantasy of the late twentieth century is still a fantasy of total rejuvenation and restoration after the model of Gertrude Atherton. Such procedures are intended to replace aesthetic surgery in the culture of a dystopic Palo Alto of the future: "The Beautiful People have always been particularly eager to seize on any artifice of youth. Fifty years ago, people of this sort had been medical pioneers. Their primitive techniques, the biomedical cutting edge during the 2030s and 2040s, were hopelessly dated and crude. Now they truly looked the role of pioneers: very scarred and tired and hardscrabble" (p. 21). The scarring marks the past attempts at perfecting rejuvenation; it is clear from the tone of the novel that even the "most modern" techniques are inherently flawed, as they attempt to reach a perfection of the human body that is tied to an aesthetic and ideology of youth that Sterling sees as corrosive. In Sterling's imaginary future, the newest rejuvenating procedures are analogous to a literal rebirth. His protagonist, Mia Ziemann, represents the next generation desiring rejuvenation. As in Atherton's novel, making the central figure a woman stresses the erotic (read: reproductive) nature of such revitalizations.

To undertake this transformation the protagonist "would be fetally submerged in a gelatinous tank of support fluids. Her internal metabolic needs would be supplied through a newly attached umbilical. The hair and skin had to go. . . . All commensal organisms in the human body had to be destroyed" (p. 57). As in the rejuvenation of the body and the "race" at the close of Stanley Kubrick's *2001* (1968), the body becomes a fetus and is then reconstructed from the inside out. It is a form of death and resurrection that effects the psyche as much as the body. There are changes in mental processes such as "culture shock, anomie, postoperation letdown, a few hints of bipolar disorder. Plus good oldfashioned human mulish impatience" (p. 61). All of these are associated with postoperative aesthetic surgery. In this world, the psyche may be mapped "on a cellular level" yet "we can throw medical terms at the soul, but we can't box it up. We can't simply give people their identity the way we might give an injection; in the end people have to find their own souls," states her physician (p. 61). Happiness of the soul remains beyond the character's grasp and indeed, the entire novel after her transformation becomes a relentless and pointless search for "happiness" throughout the world.

The transformed body provides a mask of youthfulness, but it does not provide a resolution of the problems that confront the character or her world. The old problems are the new problems. The permanence of the new body does not change the erotic: "It's even worse now that women's bodies last forever," says one female character. "'Women never learn! Men contemplate beauty, but we have to *be* beauty. So the female is always the other, and we're never the center'" (p. 137). Gertrude Atherton's "New

Woman" answers this cry in *Black Oxen* by remaining autonomous, rejecting love for power at the end of the novel. This does
not make her any happier in her new body than the rejuvenation
in *Holy Fire* makes Mia.

The alternative to Sterling's nightmare is a future dystopia
dominated by aesthetic surgery. This is played out in John Carpenter's film *Escape from L.A.* (1996), in which a postmillennial
Beverly Hills is peopled entirely by "surgical failures." Like the
cinematic tradition of representing the half animal–half human
victims on H. G. Wells's (1866–1946) *Island of Dr. Moreau* (1896),
based of the aesthetic surgery of the 1890s, the deformed and unreal bodies represent a society gone mad and expressing its insanity through aesthetic surgery. When one enters "L.A." (a West
Coast mirror image to Carpenter's image of New York as a maximum security prison in his *Escape from New York* [1981]), one is
immediately seized and taken to the former Beverly Hills Hotel,
now a filthy hospital run by a fright-masked chief surgeon and
his blood-spattered assistants. They use the newcomers for spare
body parts to keep the surgically addicted inhabitants in "L.A."
alive. The horror is made comic when the surgeon examines the
body of a captive woman and, touching her breasts, exclaims,
"My God, they're real!" All other bodies are composite bodies.
The idea that sections of the body are "real" means that we have
left the world of a total rejuvenation of the body and descended
into the dystopia of aesthetic surgery. In the world of rejuvenation everything is "real" or at least seems real.

Rejuvenation remains a scientific undertaking, which over the
past century has become part of the science of genetics and of cellular regeneration. The desire to resuscitate and restore the body
to an original state seems never to vanish. It remains keyed to the
idea that youthfulness (and immortality) are paths to happiness.
The idea of a transplantation or a formula or a treatment that will
transform the body back into its "authentic" youthful state, remains the hope of many. In 1995, at the seventy-fourth annual
meeting of the American Association of Plastic Surgeons in San
Diego, D. M. Brown, A. L. Lantieri, N. M. Kania, and R. K. Khouri
presented what they claimed was the reversal of skin aging: evi-

dence of an aging factor. They claimed that the degenerative changes present in old skin could be reversed by transplanting the skin flap from an old animal to a younger animal. These findings suggested to them that the manifestations of skin aging were reversible and that this reversal was mediated by factors present in a young host.[19] Rejuvenation of the skin, however, is more closely allied to the theory of aesthetic surgery. It will provide a new "younger" skin rather than a resuscitated organism. This skin, one supposes, will make the patient happy. Not quite testicular transplantation, but close enough.

Closely related to the desire for "rejuvenation" is the idea of cloning, which has been a permanent part of the Western imagining of the ability (or inability) to perpetuate life across generations.[20] The health of the race, as Atherton would have defined it, could be improved by cloning identical copies of perfect people, each one beginning the life cycle over again and thus assuring continual youth. One central aspect of rejuvenation, the seeming permanence of identity even in the transformed body, is echoed in the fantasies of cloning. The clones seem (through the use of the model of "organic memory") to have the rudimentary memories of the original prototype. Clones are thus rejuvenated selves, able to live anew in identical bodies and with seemingly identical identities.

The anxiety about cloning as a form of rejuvenation is a permanent part of modern Western culture after the Shoah. Aldous Huxley (1894–1963) peoples his novel *Brave New World* (1946) with people developed through embryo splitting (called "bokanovskification").[21] Huxley used the image of the Nazi desire (and attempt) to create a new race of Germans in their *Lebensborn*, the breeding ground of the Master Race, and in the thought experiments of their biologists. Taking it one step further, Huxley imagined a world in which there were classes of eternally young people, always replacing one another. He separated his Gammas, Deltas, and Epsilons from the higher-class Alphas and Betas not just by economic status but also by biologically engineered physical and intellectual traits. The world is inhabited by identical people who remain young forever because they are replaced with identical copies as they age. Such states perpetuate themselves using perpetual rejuvenation as a form of slavery.

Woody Allen's parody of this tradition of the dangerous clone in *Sleeper* (1973) has him kidnap the severed nose of a Big Brother–like dictator before it can be cloned to oppress the world once more. Allen's relation of politics and cloning parallels that in Huxley's novel. The experiences of the Third Reich come to be a sublimated part of all modern discourses on cloning and thus rejuvenation. In Ben Bova's 1976 novel *Multiple Man,* no one knows whether a clone or the real president sits in the Oval Office when several exact copies of the U.S. president are found dead.[22] In Nancy Freedman's 1973 book *Joshua, Son of None,* the clone is a real president, John F. Kennedy.[23] All of these are not only novels about cloning but about the potential collapse of Western democracy through the agency of scientific evil. Yet all deal with adult copies rather than true "clones." One central text for the implications of contemporary cloning has its origins, as does Aldous Huxley's text, in images of the Third Reich: Ira Levin's novel and Franklin J. Schaffner's 1978 film *The Boys from Brazil* with Gregory Peck, Laurence Olivier, James Mason, Lilli Palmer, and Steve Guttenberg. In the novel and film, latter-day Nazis under the direction of the mad Nazi scientist Adolf Mengele unsuccessfully conspire to produce ninety-four clones of Adolf Hitler.[24] Here the clone provides the potential of the rejuvenation of the Nazis and their world through the creation of youthful copies rather than adult simulacra.

All of these dystopic fantasies of perpetual rejuvenation through cloning came to an odd type of fruition while I was writing this chapter. In the third week of February 1997, it was announced that Ian Wilmut, working in a private Scottish laboratory, had cloned a lamb from a cell of an adult sheep. She was named "Dolly" after the buxom country-music star Dolly Parton—because the cell came from the mother's udder.[25] The project was to create a youthful sheep. Calling the clone "Dolly" ironically set this apart from the model of aesthetic surgery and placed it on a different level from "mere" surgical change. It was an indicator of the power of "authentic" change as opposed to surface change. At least in choosing to name the sheep "Dolly," the scientists stated their intent to see the cloning as a "real breast implant" rather than mere silicone.

Wilmut's claim of success came at the conclusion of a long series of attempts to create "identical" organisms. The first practical model was suggested in 1938 by German embryologist Hans Spemann (1869–1941), who is often called the "father of modern embryology."[26] Working in Nazi Germany, with its own fantasies of breeding a "master race," he proposed what he called a "fantastical experiment": to remove the nucleus from an egg cell and put into its stead a nucleus from another cell. It was only in 1952 that two American scientists, Robert Briggs and T. J. King, used very fine pipettes to suck the nucleus out of a frog egg and replace it with one removed from a body cell of an adult frog. Eighteen years later the British developmental biologist John Gurdon inserted nuclei from advanced toad embryos rather than from adult tissue. The toad eggs developed into tadpoles, but died before becoming adults. In 1984, Steen Willadsen, a Danish embryologist working in Texas, succeeded in cloning a sheep using a nucleus from a cell of an early embryo. Wilmut was apparently able to use a cell from a fully-grown animal, fulfilling the Western fantasy of what "real" clones were—the youthful replication of the adult self.

Dolly's existence raised a series of concerns, virtually all articulated through the literary tradition mentioned above (especially by evoking *The Boys from Brazil*). Thus Patrick Dixon, an expert in the ethics of genetic engineering, called the sheep clone "a Frankenstein's monster and a short step from Hitler's dream of creating a master race."[27] We no longer have Gertrude Atherton's desire for the revitalization of the race through rejuvenation and eugenics. Dixon "warned of the dangers of human clones—like the plot of the film *The Boys from Brazil* in which boy copies of Hitler are created from one of his hairs." He added: "Imagine what Hitler would have done if he had access to this technology. By the end of the war, there could have been 50 to 100 children who were the image of Hitler.'" What one can also imagine (as of the date of the writing of this paragraph) is that the entire force of science could be turned to the reproduction of younger copies of our older selves. This is not merely the joy of the continuation of the "race," but the ultimate fantasy of the eugenic manipulators—a "perfect" world of "perfect" people, each person not merely made in his or her own image but actually "perfect" ever-younger selves. As Robert Coles has noted: "It tempts our narcissism enormously because it gives a physical dimension to a fantasy that one can keep going on through the reproduction of oneself."[28] And this is a fantasy of rejuvenation, with all of the Faustian echoes—remaining eternally young by cloning oneself as one's own child.

American culture has earlier parallels in literary fantasy to the modern concerns about rejuvenation and aesthetic surgery. There are two nineteenth-century tales by Nathaniel Hawthorne (1804–64) that present both alternatives to the transformation of the body as corrosive and as destructive. "Dr. Heidegger's Experiment" (1837) tells of an exercise in rejuvenating the body with water from the Fountain of Youth gone horribly wrong.[29] Hawthorne has his Dr. Heidegger invite four "melancholy old creatures," three men and a woman who "was a great beauty in her day," to drink from a carafe of water from the Fountain of Youth. The water first revives a pale, dried flower, whose color turns "a deepening tinge of crimson." The crimson of the flower, like the crimson of the birthmark, is a sign of the vitality of blood. When the four try the water, they gradually become younger and the old eroticism, which bound the three men to the woman, reappears. The "gray, decrepit, sapless, miserable creatures" become "young!" The woman looks into a mirror "to see whether some long-remembered wrinkle or crow's-foot had indeed vanished." They leap about the room and dance, knocking over the carafe of water, and they begin again to age. The lesson learned by the doctor who watched them is that youth is a poor substitute for the wisdom of age, but the four friends go off to search for the Fountain of Youth.

Hawthorne's account of "The Birth-Mark" (1846), which we discussed earlier, reflects the failure of an aesthetic procedure to alter one aspect of the body. The husband's obsessive attention to his wife's facial "imperfection," the birthmark, causes her death. His eventual "cure" for the birthmark is a tincture of the "Elixir of Immortality," "a liquid that should prolong life for years—perhaps interminably—but that . . . would produce a discord in nature, which all the world, and chiefly the quaffer of the immortal nostrum, would find cause to curse." The tincture lightens the "crimson mark," and the lighter it grows, the more feeble his wife becomes, until she dies. Hawthorne condemns both rejuvenation and aesthetic surgery as failures, playing on older Faustian notions of the necessary failure of both rejuvenation and reconstruction to make the human being "happy."[30]

The alternative model of aesthetic surgery, which Max Thorek finally advocated, was the surgical intervention to change the surface of the body, to change the face so that age seemed to vanish. Thorek's preoccupation with the face (as in his 1946 book on medical physiognomy and in his 1947 book on the techniques of photography) stressed notions of symmetry as defining the aesthetic.[31] All of this interest seems to have come out of his fascination with the rebuilding of faces and bodies after the seeming failure of his attempts at rejuvenation in the 1920s. As he wrote in his autobiography: "The beauty business keeps pace with the times."[32] And the techniques of aesthetic surgery of the aging face had been highly developed by the 1920s. It had begun, as had psychoanalysis, with the suggestions of a patient, and it had begun only after other forms of aesthetic surgery were well established.

The first accounts of aesthetic surgery for aging came in the first decade of the twentieth century. In 1901, according to his much later account, the surgeon and cultural historian Eugen Holländer (1867–1932) undertook the first rhytidectomy or "face-lift" on a Polish aristocrat.[33] Holländer's narrative is vital to understanding the role that patients played in initiating treatment by aesthetic surgeons. For just as Jacques Joseph's patients came to him with complaints about their (or their children's) ears or nose, they also made suggestions as to how these problems should be corrected. It was, of course, the surgeon's role to work out the specific techniques, the incisions, and to visualize the results by evoking aesthetic models.

In Holländer's case, the situation was somewhat different but even more exemplary, because the woman who came to him made very specific suggestions. She came with a drawing that illustrated to her surgeon how, if facial skin were removed at the front of the ear, the nasolabial fold and the corners of the mouth would be tightened. Holländer initially did not want to undertake this, but was compelled through "feminine persuasion" to do so. (The physician maintained the line between "real" medicine and "mere" cosmetics at this moment.) He removed small amounts of skin at the hairline and behind the ear and was able to make some limited changes on the upper face, which he considered "inferior" but made his patient happy. (In retrospect, he understood his procedure as an operation on the psyche and therefore as "real" medicine.)

In 1906 Erich Lexer (1867–1938) undertook a similar procedure on an actress. His patient had been pulling up the skin of her face by taping her forehead at night and drawing it tight with rubber bands over the top of her skull. This caused her skin to stretch, creating transverse folds above her zygomatic arches, but also provided a model for how a corrective procedure could be undertaken. Lexer removed S-shaped incisions of skin at the temples, behind the ears and at the hair-line. According to Lexer the result was a success.[34]

The number of facial procedures meant to "cure" the appearance of age and to enable individuals to "pass" increased after the beginning of the century. In Chicago, Charles Conrad Miller (1880–1950) by 1906 had developed procedures for the removal of "bag-like folds of eyelid skin."[35] Similar procedures had been suggested as early as Celsus, but were either the reconstruction of a missing eyelid (which, like the missing nose, was seen as a form of punishment) or the removal of a *palpebrae laxioris*, relaxed lid, as the folds of skin were understood to impair vision.[36] Johann C. G. Fricke (1790–1841) introduced the "modern" term *blepharoplasty* in 1829. Numerous approaches to the reconstruction

of both the upper and lower eyelid followed. But Miller's procedure in 1906 was self-consciously aesthetic. Miller is often given
credit for having developed the first rhytidectomy, which was
then copied by other surgeons of his day. Miller's career was typical for many of the early aesthetic surgeons, as patients (and their
families) constantly harassed him when procedures failed to deliver the expected changes in appearance and they could not
"pass." Eventually he gave up aesthetic surgery and turned to
general surgery—feeling that it was "more satisfying to cure disease than to satisfy vanity."[37]

In Paris, following the lead of Holländer and Lexer in listening
to their patients, Suzanne Noël began to excise excess skin in
order to tighten the face and remove wrinkles.[38] She began in
1912 when an actress returned from America (perhaps from a session with Miller in Chicago) and showed her the results of the
procedures that she had undergone there. The social stigma of
such procedures in Paris was clear: "Women have their operations and do not talk about it," Noël wrote. Silence here is also a
mark of consent. Although it is evident that she began by operating on what she described as desperate cases, such as a woman
abandoned by her husband, she quickly had clients who were
motivated by their "love of finery and beauty." In 1912, Jacques
Joseph developed a procedure for the tightening of sagging
cheeks (ptosis), which initially left a small scar in front of the ear.
He modified this (as he did with virtually all of his procedures)
to eliminate the scar.[39] In 1919 Raymond Passot, a student of
Morestin, developed a procedure for the removal of the double
chin. Such procedures continued through to the 1970s with numerous small improvements on the placement of incisions and
the removal of tissue.[40] But alternatives, such as estrogen therapy
(from the world of rejuvenation), had begun to take their place as
part of facial surgery.

The face-lift came to be a standard surgical procedure to change
the surface of the body through the tightening of the skin. The
aesthetic surgeons of the 1920s evoked the idea of rejuvenation of
the spirit. Charles Willi wrote in 1926 concerning subcutaneous
fat injections: "A lady enters the studio with a permanent frown,

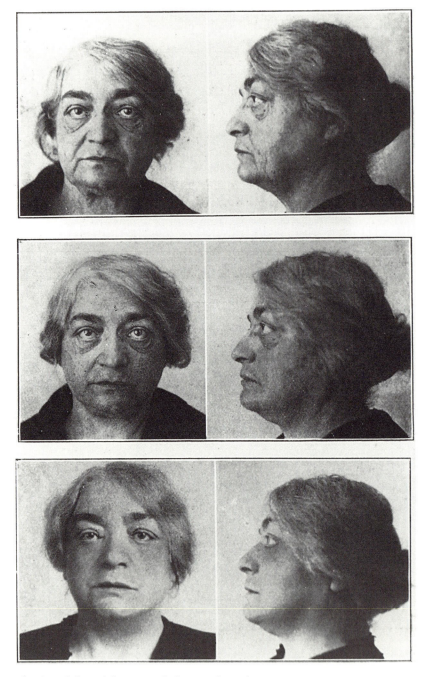

The face-lift and (*next page*) the resulting happy patient.

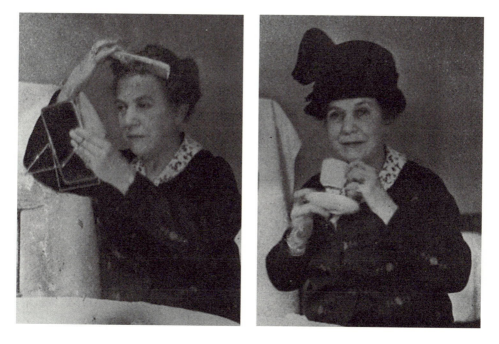

and a few minutes later the frown has disappeared for ever; she entered with two naso-labial lines cut as with a knife between her cheek and nose, a needle-prick and the furrows are filled for ever; she enters with wrinkles that suggest old age, she goes out a young unwrinkled woman. There is no pain, there is no danger, it is an instantaneous and painless rejuvenation. Nor is it possible to detect that hand of man and not hand of Nature has effected the transformation."[41] The anxiety about scarring is real in the world of the aesthetic surgeon, for it is the invisibility of the procedures that validates one's appearance. People cannot "pass" if they are scarred in such operations.

Charles Conrad Miller stressed that "signs of maturity in women must go. Featural surgeons can do much to perpetuate youthful contour, but usually it cannot be accomplished without a good deal of scarring, for most of the surgical steps which accomplish these effects require the excision of rather large segments of integument."[42] The acceptance of scarring (and the development of procedures that hide or mask or reduce scarring) became part of the history of facial surgery, including the history

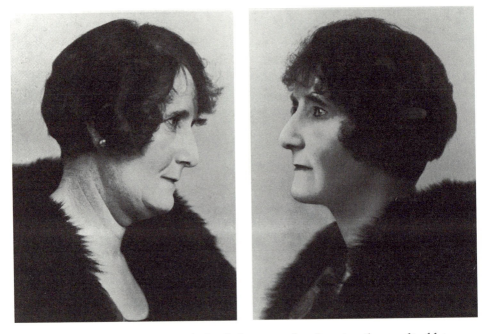

Charles Willi's "before and after" photographs, showing the result of fat injections after a week's treatment.

of the rhinoplasty and rhytidectomy. The scars must be reduced and the patient must be able to "pass" so that there can be a restitution "[of] her peace of mind and continued happiness," as J. Howard Crum said in 1928.[43] According to Crum, such happiness is universal, transcending "the triumph of feminism [which] would relegate beauty to a back seat so far as its importance in a woman's life was concerned" (p. 9). It was not for men alone: "women enjoy the sight of a pretty face, so long as prettiness is not rendered annoying by obvious self-complacency" (p. 10). The New Woman in the 1920s needed to be beautiful and to see beauty about her.

For women, aesthetic surgery is psychological therapy. This becomes a trope in contemporary fiction concerning healing and gender. Philip Roth, in his novel *American Pastoral* (1997), his paean to American life and the pain caused by becoming American, has Dawn Levov, the non-Jewish wife of his Jewish protagonist "Swede" Levov, see aesthetic surgery as a cure for her soul.[44] Not quite believing that surgery can transform the American soul as acculturation has transformed his family's psyche, Roth's "Swede," whose all-American good looks provide him social status and an insider position in spite of his ethnic identity, turns to the family doctor to ask about aesthetic surgery for his wife. The Jewish doctor, Shelly Salzman, comments: "You don't know how many women come to me who've been through a terrible trauma and they want to talk about something or other, and what turns out to be on their mind is just this, plastic surgery. The emotional and psychological implications can turn out to be something" (p. 353). After the face-lift in Switzerland, Swede falls into commonplaces about its effect: "Erased all that suffering. He gave her back her face" (p. 298). And his wife writes to her Swiss aesthetic surgeon: "I feel it's taken me these twelve months to recover from the surgery. I believe, as you said, that my system was more beaten down than I had realized. Now it is as if I have been given a new life. Both from within and from the outside. When I meet old friends I have not seen for a while they are puzzled as to what happened to me. I don't tell them" (p. 188). In this world, it is the woman who deals with trauma through aesthetic surgery; men only seem to soldier through without help—but clearly, according to Roth, only on the surface. For the true unhappiness of Swede's life is revealed only when the narrator begins to unravel the trauma beneath his placid features.

In the representation of clinical practice, men too have and need aesthetic surgery of the face: "Modern business demands it, social circles cater to it, and domestic relations are enhanced by it," as J. Howard Crum comments.[45] Indeed, in 1944 "the proportions as to sex [were] about ten females to one male."[46] Again, the "mental attitude" is changed by the aesthetic surgeon. "Happiness is a mental condition to be acquired by constant practice and effort. . . . Your face will tell the world the condition of your mental state. The plastic surgeon can smooth away the effect of past worries, hatreds, and sorrows. After these signs and marks have been erased it then depends upon the patients as to whether they will permit themselves to revert to their former conditions. . . . The ideal is, of course, a happy combination of perfect form together with a reflected glory of a harmonious inner self or life. The first may be the result of the plastic surgeon's skill but the latter must be developed entirely by the patient."[47] By the 1970s this view of the purpose of rhytidectomies had been slightly rephrased: "We have always known that inner psychic and spiritual changes bring about a new external radiance, but we are now discovering that the process also works in reverse: Change the external appearance—restore the lost years—of a person struggling continually against indifferent or negative social reactions, and the inner light that has died within begins to glow once more."[48] Twenty years later, the language of "rejuvenation" reappears in the discourse of the face-lift. "Rejuvenation" is a term now used by aesthetic surgeons to describe "minor" procedures used to revitalize appearance. This is opposed to "reincarnation" procedures such as face-lifts. A startling 208,000 such small interventions, known as "lunch hour" procedures, such as botox (botulism toxin), fat, and collagen injections were performed in 1995, compared to 63,000 face-lifts.[49] All aim at the "happiness" of the client by enabling them to "pass" as young and erotic. (One can add here that with the anxiety about BSE ["mad cow disease"], the use of injectable animal collagens has been put into question in Europe.[50] Mad cows do not happy clients make.)

As the number of patients desiring a more youthful appearance increases, high and popular culture still stresses the ephemeral nature of the "happiness" acquired through aesthetic surgery. In Fay Weldon's *The Life and Loves of a She-Devil* (1983), Ruth, described on the book's jacket as a "lumbering, clumsy woman, over six feet tall, with a jutting jaw topped by spouting moles," revenges herself on her petite (and beautiful) rival by destroying her life and then having aesthetic surgery so that she can literally assume her physical presence.[51] Having lost her husband to Mary Fisher, a writer of romances, Ruth ruminates: "I look at my face in the bathroom mirror. I want to see something different." (p. 44) She eventually turns to the aesthetic surgeons Mr. Ghengis and Mr. Roche, who claim they can alter everything "but the hands.

They remain as evidence of our heredity and our past" (p. 174). Mr. Roche is a sham surgeon, "having started life as a garage mechanic" who "realized that the human body was no more than a machine" and, with the help of forged qualifications, moved to California "when the boom in genetic engineering began" (p. 173). Aesthetic surgery remains problematic, for there is always the risk of "keloid scarring: puckering and wrinkling. A terrible mess! If it happens there is nothing we can do about it" (p. 202). Ruth's nose is straightened, her face lifted, her jaw reduced in size, her ears are pinned back, "loose skin from beneath the arms would be tucked and fat removed from shoulders, back, buttocks, hips and belly." Her legs would be shortened, her vagina tightened. He even "drew back her clitoris to heighten his patient's sexual response" (p. 219). The cost was $1,430,000, and the procedures took two years. A new person seems to have been created. One surgeon comments that the sexual surgery is "an interference with the essential self," to which his colleague replies: " 'There is no such thing as the essential self. . . . It is all inessential and all liable to change and flux, and usually the better for it" (p. 219). Having copied her rival's body, Ruth assumes her life after she dies, reclaiming her husband, her rival's home (and even her rival's mother!). There is no way of actually becoming her rival. She remains, as the last, bitter line in the novel has it "a lady of six foot two, who had tucks taken in her legs. A comic turn, turned serious" (p. 240). This is as dark a dystopia of aesthetic surgery as Atherton's or Sterling's view of rejuvenation or Huxley's of cloning. In a world that stresses authenticity and autonomy, the impossibility of both existing simultaneously leads to a dismissal of all transformations (in fiction) as a sign of vanity. The novel was filmed in 1989 with Roseanne Barr as Ruth and Meryl Streep as Mary Fisher. Roseanne Barr went on to have massive aesthetic surgery in 1994 that virtually rebuilt her face and body. This was a lived experience, not merely a role in a film. Is her new body more authentic than the new body of the character she played?

Aesthetic surgery seems in our collective literary fantasy not to provide the sort of rejuvenation that will make us "happy" by allowing us to "pass." Literature remains surprisingly "moral" when it sees individuals believing they can cross boundaries from the unerotic to the erotic, from the unhappy to the happy. Yet the explosion in the numbers and kind of rhytidectomies over the past ninety years illustrates the difference between the collective literary consciousness and group responses.

There is a hint of the complexities of rejuvenation and cloning still present within the fantasy of aesthetic surgery. In Mary Higgins Clark's *Let Me Call You Sweetheart* (1995) the plot of the murder mystery begins with an accidental meeting in the office of Charles Smith, an aesthetic surgeon.[52] In the course of the novel we learn that he has rebuilt the face and body of his daughter, "who was not a pretty girl" (p. 134), into that of a beauty with "high cheekbones, straight nose, exquisitely shaped pouty lips, luminous eyes, arched brows" (p. 6), and, of course, a totally "rebuilt" character: "within a year of the operation Suzanne had capped the transformation with her total change of personality" (p. 163). After she is murdered, Charles then proceeds to "re-create" (p. 213) his daughter's face by operating on a number of young women. They are made to look like his dead daughter through the "now very sophisticated" work of the aesthetic surgeon (p. 105). In the novel Clark calls this a "Pygmalion fantasy" (p. 163), in which the doctor worships his creation as a work of art come to life, a theme well known in the surgical literature in the image of the aesthetic surgeon as sculptor. When he sees his daughter's dead body, he feels as "Michelangelo would have felt had he seen his *Pietà* broken and defaced" (p. 260). This modern variation on Mary Shelley's (1797–1851) *Frankenstein* (1818) has the mad doctor cloning his dead daughter over and over again through surgery. He created and re-created his daughter both as father and as surgeon. Such fantasies must turn out badly and they do, much as in other such fictions. Duplicating the body is represented as an immoral act in the public fantasies about aesthetic surgery, but even more so, the notion of rebuilding the character and turning individuals into "happy" people is dismissed as potentially leading to madness and death.

The only true clones that science could actually have examined (before Dolly) were identical twins. What happens when twins age? The German aesthetic surgeon, Wolfgang Mühlbauer, examined the problem of aesthetic surgery on identical twins.[53] Here the cloning did not deal with offspring but with a version of the infamous twin studies that dominated German biology (and then American psychiatry) from the 1920s to the 1950s. Mühlbauer recounted his experiences with four different sets of twins who desired to have aesthetic surgery. Both of the twins in each pair shared the same problem. The pair of twin women aged fifty-two who desired rhytidectomies also insisted that all of the natural asymmetries be erased so that they would look more like one another. The idea of becoming more like the twin while also looking younger is a type of rejuvenation through aesthetic surgery. (The dominant twin "believed that she looked older than her sister," which she was by five minutes. Is this dysmorphophobia?) Such surgery stresses the anxiety we feel when only part of us (our twin, our clone) can "pass," and we, as in the case of Mr. Hyde, remain ugly, primitive, and unerotic. Can rejuvenation or aesthetic surgery allow us to imagine ourselves as the "happier" twin? Only the clone really knows.

POST-AESTHETIC BODIES

If Jacques Joseph turned to Leonardo for the models he employed to remodel the faces of his patients, the work of the French performance artist Orlan at first glance seems to turn the tables on him.[54] Her medium is aesthetic surgery: "I am the first artist to use surgery as a medium and to alter the purpose of cosmetic surgery: to look better, to look young. 'I is an other' ('je est un autre'). I am at the forefront of confrontation."[55] She calls her project "The Reincarnation of Saint Orlan," and has undergone a series of aesthetic surgical operations since May 1987 to transform herself into a new being with a new identity. She desires a true metamorphosis. She has had bits and pieces of herself remodeled on the basis of the aesthetic ideal as represented in Western art. She now literally has the chin of Botticelli's *Venus*, the eyes of a

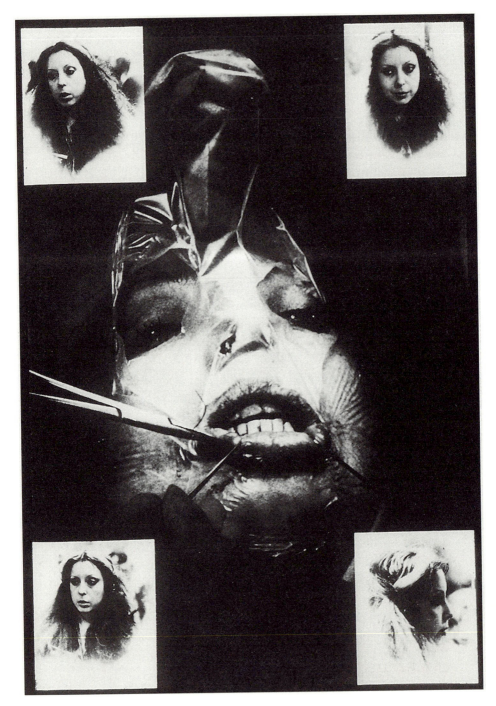

Orlan.

Fontainbleau *Diana,* the lips of Gustave Moreau's *Europa,* the nose of Jean-Léon Gérôme's *Psyche* and the brow of Leonardo's *Mona Lisa.*

The notion of the composite body as the perfect body is certainly unique neither to the history of art nor to the history of aesthetic surgery. The classical Greek sculptor Zeuxis, at least according to Pliny, selected five beautiful virgins to pose for him so that he could select the perfect body parts for an ideal image of Helen of Troy. This myth is also told of Apelles' portrait of Diana of Ephesus.[56] In modern art it is specifically continued in the use of the composite from the "portraits" of Arcimboldo (1527–93) to Salvador Dali's (1904–89) extraordinary war scene as a portrait of a soldier, which graced the cover of *Match* on October 12, 1939.[57]

Orlan's first aesthetic surgery as art was on May 30, 1987—her fortieth birthday. Eight more followed. On May 30, 1990, her forty-third birthday, Dr. Chérif Kamel Zahar performed liposuction on her face and thighs while she was under local anesthetic: "'I have given my body to Art.' After my death it will not therefore be given to science, but to a museum. It will be the centerpiece of a video installation."[58] Videos and stills of all of the procedures were made; closed-circuit television made a live audience possible; and the procedures were framed by readings and accompanied (at other sites) by dance. After a chin implant was introduced in the third procedure in July 1990, there was a change of surgeon. The art collector / aesthetic surgeon Dr. Bernard Cornette de Saint-Cyr undertook the fourth procedure. With his participation, the boundary between the surgeon as sculptor (the ideal of Joseph and Thorek) and the producer of the work of art vanished. Or perhaps Pierre Bourdieu was right after all when he observed that the "'subject' of artistic production and its product is not the artist but the whole set of agents who are involved in art, are interested in art, have an interest in art and the existence of art, who live on and for art, the producers of works regarded as artistic (great and small, famous—i.e., 'celebrated'—or unknown), critics, collectors, go-betweens, curators, art historians, and so on."[59] To which we can add, aesthetic surgeons.

Orlan subjects her body to increasingly complex aesthetic alterations—in spite of the public discussion about breast implants, she had *silicone* implants inserted near her temples to simulate bulges in the face of Leonardo's *Mona Lisa*. Her art, however, couples the Western obsession with "perfecting" the body through aesthetic surgery to "the modern love affair with the camera."[60] For if the "before and after" photographs are the epistemological essence of proof that aesthetic surgery enabled the patient to "pass," so too her art, captured in color stills and videotape, offers proof to the later viewer of her transformation. Her transformation into the Mona Lisa was undertaken in November 1993 by a feminist aesthetic surgeon, Dr. Marjorie Cramer, in New York City and was transmitted by satellite to Montreal, Banff, and Paris, where enthralled audiences watched it. The "before and after" portraits of the aesthetic surgeon have become art.

According to Orlan's own account, she does not intend to mimic the works of art she evokes. Rather she intends to use these bits and pieces of the aesthetics of the West to show the effect of exaggeration. Her new nose is "the largest nose which is technically possible" built on her face. The end product of the performance is more conventional. The concrete result of her art consists of a number of large color photographs of the artist: "Orlan, impeccably made-up and coifed, with the surgeon's cut-here crayon marks on her face; Orlan with a terrifying two-pointed implement probing her bloody nostril; Orlan with a flap of skin dangling behind her ear; Orlan with a large needle in her lip. Two images show Orlan six days after the doctor's ministrations, Orlan with hemorrhaged, blood-red eyes, and Orlan smiling, holding a bunch of narcissi."[61] The result of the surgery is an increased visibility, the scars of her surgery become signs of her art: "THIS IS ORLAN!!! A woman of privilege and power. She has had repeated cosmetic surgery and she leaves the hospital with REAL SCARS! Can I touch them? Can I touch you, Orlan?"[62] shouts Richard Schechner, the noted director, having just visited her latest performance.

Orlan observed: "'I have always considered my body as privileged material for the construction of my work. One can consider my work to be classical portraiture. Each operation is like a rite of passage,' she added. 'Art must disrupt our thoughts. It is not there to comfort us. It must take risks and be deviant.'"[63] But what can one actually use as the model for the aesthetic surgical procedure? "'The idea of taking somebody else's facial parts is absurd. You cannot take somebody else's eyes and put them in your eyes,' she says through a translator. 'It's the history behind the [character], not the face, that I'm taking.'"[64] It is the history of the character, of the meaning ascribed to the face, that she desires to evoke.

Orlan "grandly proclaims her work to be 'a fight against nature and the idea of God' and also a way to prepare the world for widespread genetic engineering."[65] This statement places Orlan's enterprise within the actual imagined sphere of aesthetic surgery as the improvement of the race. The Lamarckian fantasies of Jewish patients that their children's children would inherit the now (in)visible nose have become one with the fantasy of the infinitely improvable body. The aesthetic surgical operations Orlan has undergone since 1990 have transfigured her appearance to a greater or lesser degree. Her intent is eventually to create a new persona: "I will solicit an advertising agency to come up with a name, a first name, and an artist's name: next I will contract a lawyer to petition the Republic to accept my new identities with my new face. It is a performance that inscribes itself into the social fabric, a performance that challenges the legislation, that moves towards a total change of identity."[66] With her liposuction, a prosthesis inserted in her chin, silicone bumps like budding horns inserted in her forehead, and a huge prosthetic nose fitted, molded, screwed, affixed, or otherwise fashioned to her face, she desires to "pass" as a new person with a new character and a new history. She has transformed her operations into glittery televised performances, in which the wide-awake but benumbed artist reads selected texts to her audience, while the attendant surgery team go about their grisly work in gowns designed by Issey Miyake, Paco Rabanne, and other, lesser-known designers.

Is the final aim of Orlan's "project" a total self-transformation, or is it to "pass"? Isn't her desire to create a New Woman, remade in her own image—the anti-image of art? The new identity, which she will attempt to register with the official authorities, will be this new person. She will have become the new woman. Yet for all her exhibitionism and overt masochism, her desire is permanent invisibility—to become an exhibit like all other exhibits at an art gallery. (The idea for this series of actions came when she had a local anesthetic for an extrauterine pregnancy in 1978. She saw herself opened on the table "a kind of living, speaking autopsy."[67] This distance is the distance of the observer; she has become her own audience.)

Orlan's desire to turn surgery into art has other analogs. The art of Annie Sprinkle, exhibiting her vagina held open by a speculum, prefigured Orlan's exposure of her genitals on a closed-circuit monitor, held open by a speculum; her surgery project is certainly analogous to those of photographers, such as Matuschka, fascinated by their own and other women's mastectomies, but this is not merely a form of "feminist protest." Rather, performance groups such as "Jew Meat" (in San Francisco) have equally stressed the meaning of the ethnic male body. Circumcision has become performance. The rapid spread of infant male circumcision in the West as a form of prophylaxis means that this ritual practice (which led to complex responses on the part of Jews at the turn of the century) is read in new ways.

In post-apartheid South Africa, the decline of adult male circumcision has led to kidnappings of young men by circumcision societies for ritual purposes. The government is quite ambivalent about this. The attempts on Nelson Mandela's part to preserve circumcision stems from his identity as a Xhosa, a member of a tribe that circumcises its young men; his political allies in the African National Congress attempted to place limits on this procedure, labeling it a sign of "barbarism." This has made circumcision a hot political issue. The image of ritual Xhosa circumcision as South African art, however, makes the act into a form of aesthetic surgery.

The South African performance artist Richard Kilpert described his own attempt at turning another surgical procedure into art.[68] One of his students at the Dakawa Arts and Crafts Center under went his *abakwetha* ceremony and was ritually circum-cised. "luyanda sofisa had his black foreskin cut off at an unusu-ally sober ceremony behind sugarloaf hill. Traditionally the sev-ered and bloody prepuce has to be taken and buried some distance from the initiate's khaya, which by this stage is burning nicely, along with all childhood possessions." Kilpert removed the student's buried prepuce, and what followed is best told in his own words:

> with my purple and yellow prize i arrived at that fateful crit af-ternoon, armed with surgical steel, local anesthetic and a sewing kit from shell garage. i was going all the way. i was about to si-multaneously undo what some doctorfuck had done to me before i could kick back, comment on the retention of the child in Xhosa life and highlight some important misconceptions about race and gender generally (hell, i'll leave it to the critics) in the n[ew] s[outh] a[frica]. not to mention give myself a probable dose of hiv.

> as i said it got a bit messy and after cutting my penis where the ex-foreskin scar was, slipping on the now green-black appendage, and sewing myself up, I had lost a lot of blood and had to go to settlers hospital. . . . i now carry my splendid multiracial cock as a fin-de-siècle icon of racial and sexual equality, a veritable flag of international pride.

Given that the first contemporary surgical procedure for the re-constitution of the foreskin was developed by a South African, as we discussed earlier, it is striking that the aesthetic use of such a reconstruction comes to be a piece of multicultural performance art in the new South Africa. Such acts turn surgery into political and ethical statements, but only through the vehicle of irony. Can Kilpert now truly "pass" as a New South African? The new South African flag of red, white, green, yellow, and black, with its evo-cation of the richness of land and people, now has an analog in his penis. The ironic tone transforms the procedure, which has here purely ritual form, into an act that demands that the viewer or listener understand the desire to "pass" and the impossibility of its fulfillment.

Aesthetic surgery as art is not only the concern of the female. Yet Orlan's action is a self-conscious repudiation, according to her own statement, of patriarchal aesthetics, which dominate women and provide the idealized image for the aesthetic surgeon. She defends using aesthetic surgery: "Centuries ago, the life expectancy was 30 or 40. Now you can live up to 80 years. The inside usually feels younger than the outside does, so that there is something that is not pleasing to ourselves," she says. "Plastic surgery is like taking an antibiotic to avoid dying of some kind of infection. It helps yourself become more comfortable with who you are."[69] Aesthetic surgery becomes total rejuvenation.

The heroines of cyberfiction novels have now become "real" in Orlan's performance of the ballet of aesthetic surgery. The critics respond as if they are wired into the discourse of what aesthetic surgery is to remedy: "She may be brave—or stupid, or deeply troubled—she may be trying to slough her narcissism as she sloughs her skin, but Orlan, in losing one identity, aims to gain another. What then? Will she be happier, more fulfilled, a better artist?"[70] Or as the London art historian Sarah Wilson stated in an interview, Orlan is "an artist who can manage her own metamorphosis."[71] She writes elsewhere that Orlan "herself becomes master, perverts and challenges 'the beauty problem' and with a shocking literalism insists upon the knife and the cut."[72] Kathy Davis, the author of the best feminist study of aesthetic surgery, concurs: "Orlan is just an extreme example of what is basically the same phenomenon: women who have cosmetic surgery want to be 'their own Pygmalion.'"[73] Here too the notion of the aesthetic surgeon as sculptor has been transformed into the surgical patient as sculptor.

Given the evidently masochistic tendencies of Orlan's art (even before her aesthetic surgery project), is not one possible reading the identification with the aesthetic surgeon? Is her project not a metamorphosis into the (in)visible self, the new self, the happier self? The new identity she acquires is that of aesthetic sculptor of her own body. Such identification with the role of the physician would indeed make the masochist happy. Happiness remains the end goal of aesthetic surgery, whether it is the happiness of the psyche transformed or of the aesthetic impulse fulfilled.

An answer to Orlan's praise of aesthetic surgery can be found in a fascination with reconstructive surgery in the visual culture in the 1990s. The Massachusetts photographer Sage Sohier's "About Face" series, shown at the Friends of Photography Exhibition in San Francisco in 1996, documented a series of (for her) clearly reconstructive procedures. Consisting of four series and twelve single images of individuals with "facial tumors, . . . victims of accidents, or [with] congenital facial problems," she contrasts "her" patients with "those who 'elect' to have cosmetic surgery."[74] She sees her photographs as about "survival—and its costs." Thus one series documents in seven images the procedure for the reconstruction of the nose of a sixty-three-year-old woman who had a basal cell carcinoma removed from the base of her nose. The first four images detail the surgery, half hour by half hour; the subsequent three, the postsurgical recovery ending six months after the procedure. Another series details the surgery to improve the appearance of a woman who had suffered from jaw cancer. The first image is of her state before the reconstructive procedure, the next three document the procedure and the immediate postoperative state, and the final one is a family portrait with her daughter and granddaughter four weeks after surgery.

Sohier's project is to document the repair of the patients' faces and their return to the aesthetic norms. She employs the "before and after" model that dominates the history of the medical representations of facial surgery. Her photographs, in their generous form, 14 × 14 inches, have the studied quality of portrait photography attendant on the tradition in aesthetic surgery. Thus the final family portrait mentioned above uses almost a visual cliché of family "happiness" to define both the success of the procedure and also the difficult future for someone with a severely disfigured face without the support of the family. Sohier sees this as a "'re-birth' or re-emergence of the person at the end of the surgery, and in the days and weeks following." Her own interest in this question came from her mother's experience of anxiety at being seen as a "cripple" after an iatrogenic infection in her knee following surgery.

Anxiety about appearance haunts Sohier's images. She undertakes a "documentary" approach to enable "viewers [to be] reminded both of the fragility of the human condition, and of the amazing ability of the body to heal itself and of individuals to regain—sometimes even strengthen—their sense of self." The reviewer of the San Francisco show saw Sohier's work as "gruesome but life-affirming. The surgery she documented (at the Massachusetts Eye and Ear Infirmary) aims to reshape faces after operations to remove cancers and other tumors have left hideous scars. The goal is to let the patients feel good about their appearance and live normal lives."[75] Happiness is the goal and surgery is the means of achieving it. Representing this happiness through art should have a moral lesson for the observer. It points toward the overcoming of adversity, and yet the overall effect of such images harkens back to the use of similar photographs from Jacques Joseph's clinic in the antiwar literature of the 1920s. Its moral effects result from the idea that the deformation of the face is the most horrible thing that can happen to the body. The unhappiness is that of the observer, rather than that of the patient. Sohier must set these patients apart from those who merely elect to change their appearance for vanity's sake, because the latter's deformations seem unnoticeable to her. "Real" deformity demands "real" identification in this worldview, and provides "real" happiness. And it is real, as in the "before and after" images, because it can be represented.

The fantasies about the transmutation of the body and the psyche in the West are legion. Kiss a frog and . . . But the realization of such fantasies in the operating theater of the aesthetic surgeon has more complex implications for our sense of who we are and who we can become (or not become). The body as art and art as the basis for understanding the body echo the commonplace about art being the locus of truth and goodness. All of these myths become real in our world, and we, as patients and physicians, act as if they can become real—and, therefore, are real. The ongoing cultural history of aesthetic surgery is thus the history of art and beauty and danger and change. In other words, it is a history of the modern with all its contradictions and complexities.

"Passing" as Human

*A*FTER SURGERY becomes art, art becomes surgery. What more is left to imagine? The transformability of the individual was the promise of the Renaissance and became the political platform of the Enlightenment. Change has now become the mantra of modernity. And it is an idea of transformation closely linked to the power we attribute to art. This was especially true at the beginning of the era of aesthetic surgery. Rainer Maria Rilke's (1875–1926) poem of 1908 evoked the "Torso of an Archaic Apollo," with its perfect, idealized male body:

> Yet his torso glows: a candelabrum set
> before his gaze which is pushed back and hid,
>
> restrained and shining. Else the curving breast
> could not thus blind you, nor through the soft turn
> of the loins could this smile easily have passed
> into the bright groin where the genitals burned.[1]

You can become the perfection of the work of art. Imaging such a classical ideal leads the poet to command the reader in the final line: *"You must change your life."*

In the age of Rilke, the viewers of the archaic torso of Apollo could not only model their aesthetic sense on the seemingly ageless beauty of classical art, they could literally rebuild their bodies to mimic its fragmentary perfection. The desire of Enlightenment thinkers such as Thomas Jefferson to make the world over into an idealized Greece has given way to the poet's command that we must change our lives because we have seen (and now can become?) the perfect soul as well as the perfect body of the work of art.

We now march off into the next millennium knowing that we will become better, we must become better, we shall become better. We can change our bodies and our lives. We will fit ourselves into society by restructuring our bodies to make our souls happy. We imagine the world outside of ourselves as a happier place than our inner world. For the acquisition (not merely the pursuit) of happiness—or at least the absence of sadness—is the great promise of our post-Prozac world. Aesthetic surgery is one of the means by which we believe we can accomplish this goal.

Happiness in our modern world is in part defined by the desire to vanish into the world beyond ourselves where there is no difference. We want to become happy *like everyone else* and thus be *absolutely unique* in our happiness. This contradiction is at the *heart of the matter* (which is the phrase Sigmund Freud scribbled in the margins of his books when he believed he had found the central truth in his reading). The heart of the matter in aesthetic surgery is the common human desire to "pass."

"Passing" is the other side of the coin of our persistent and constant need to generate stereotypes in order to organize the world. When we walk down the street we immediately, instantly, and without much thought (it seems so natural) categorize everyone we see. We see them and we need to recognize them. Are they friend or foe, dangerous or benign, to be avoided or to be approached? Our categories seem to be real in our world. They are rooted, we think, in the natural categories of our world and our society. The screaming man on the corner looks dangerous, acts dangerous, must be dangerous—and we respond with fear, a fear generated by the category through which we have organized our impressions of him. We cross the street and hurry on. And yet when we reach the corner, we see that he is shouting out an advertising slogan and trying to give passersby free samples. What was terrifying is now benign; we have to reorganize our world and we do so effortlessly and elegantly. Our testing of reality shows us that our categories are malleable and are constantly in need of reshaping and recalibrating.

And yet there are moments when the desire for one's own sense of uniqueness is such that everyone appears different, dangerous, absurd. The California artist Ashley Bickerton notes: "When it comes to 'passing,' sometimes you do your damnedest just to feel part of your own species. Genetic similarities, mental biopro-grams, and common language are no guarantees. Some days when walking the streets of this great hissing metropolis, my mind boggles at the perverse explosion of absurd bipedal pri-mates who wrap their shameful nakedness in comical drapes." [2] Belonging and not belonging, desiring to belong and fleeing from it, map our sense of the world. And the categories of belonging that we desire or fear are part of our common fantasies about how the world must be organized.

Our vocabulary of fantasy images represents the world. We ac-cumulate these images through our history, our culture, our soci-ety. They are, however, rooted in a basic dichotomy of seeing—a dichotomy that divides the "good" from the "bad." Our illusion, born of our most infantile experiences, is that the "good" is "good" not because it is benign but because we believe we can control it; the "bad" represents those aspects of the world that we believe lie outside of our control. This is the grandiosity of the in-fant who truly believes at one moment that she or he is the world. Only the experience of the inability to control that world disrupts the infant's sense of control, and that disruption becomes the model for all that we imagine we fear. *"You must change your life."*

The desire to "pass" is an attempt to recuperate that infantile split between the "good" and the "bad" aspects of the world, a split that becomes central to our means of organizing the world. "Passing" is a means of trying to gain control. It is the means of restoring not "happiness" but a sense of order in the world. We "pass" in order to regain control of ourselves and to efface that which is seen (we believe) as different, which marks us as visible in the world. Relieving the anxiety of being placed into a visible, negative category, aesthetic surgery provides relief from imagin-ing oneself as a stereotype. This is the origin of the happiness gen-erated by aesthetic surgery. The happiness of the patient is the fantasy of a world and a life in the patient's control rather than in the control of the observer on the street. And that is not wrong. This promise of autonomy, of being able to make choices and act upon them, does provide the ability to control the world. It can (and does) make people happy.

This is an illusionary but necessary claim of happiness. The fantasy of "passing," unlike the fantasy of controlling the world, focuses on a single, limited aspect—a nose too large, hair too sparse, a breast too small. Changing that has symbolic significance for the individual, for the body that we change is itself a symbolic body rather than a real body. It is the body generated through the act of visual stereotyping and organizing the world. It may seem that surgeons are operating on the material of the body, but they (and we) know better: they are reshaping our fantasies of ourselves. The new nose may resolve those fantasies for the moment or forever, or may lead us to demand even more proof of our control over our bodies. But the vocabulary of images is always shifting, and we try to escape being stereotyped by fixing our faces and our bodies at a specific moment in time. *"You must change your life."*

Each individual has had to learn again and again that the symbolic body, as much as the "real" material body, is always collapsing, always promising to slide into oblivion. The symbolic body, our fantasy of fitting into the world, of being unseen, unrecognized, unstereotyped, needs constant reinforcement. Robert Frost (1875–1963) understood that "something there is that doesn't love a wall / That sends the frozen-ground-swell under it, / And spills the upper boulders in the sun." This symbolic body is solid, real, and yet constantly in collapse, like Frost's wall, which "makes gaps even two can pass abreast," and constantly needs rebuilding. "The gaps I mean, / No one has seen them made or heard them made, / but at spring mending-time we find them there."[3] We need such reinforcement in our active fantasies about the body. The gaps appear and we must silently mend them or have them mended for us. One of the sites for the management of our bodily fantasies over the past hundred years has been aesthetic surgery.

We turn to medicine, the realm that deals with the collapse of the material body, to find our specialists. The doctors are our agents in dealing with what Mark C. Taylor has called "the unavoidable betrayal of the body."[4] This betrayal is the natural dissolution of the body, which appears to rupture and destroy our normal healthy state. Taylor also notes that the "most insidious diseases are those which leave no apparent trace, diseases that are silent, invisible, sometimes even casting a semblance of health." But what of those "diseases" of the soul, the disease created by our sense of our selves rather than by the agent of disease and decay. How is the sense of self to be restored into that state "silent, invisible, sometimes even casting a semblance of health," which is the end product of aesthetic surgery? The alteration of our fantasies about our bodies makes us happy and therefore healthy.

Our invisibility marks our desire to return to that ideal state in which we had control of the world. William Butler Yeats (1865–1939) has his "A Woman Young and Old" fantasize:

> If I make the lashes dark
> And the eyes more bright
> And the lips more scarlet,
> Or ask if all be right
> From mirror to mirror,
> No vanity's displayed:
> I'm looking for the face I had
> Before the world was made.[5]

It is the desire for control, for the face that existed "before the world was made," before we came to recognize that we were thrown into the world, never its master, that lies at the heart of "passing." Mortality is the ultimate proof of this lack of control over the world, but real history, real politics can have much the same effect. Becoming aware that one is marked through one's imagined visibility as aging, or inferior, or nonerotic, concepts that become interchangeable, can make one long for the solace of that original fantasy of control. And we need to find a means by which we can be transformed into that ideal that we now believe ourselves to desire. The reality of prejudice, of being seen as different, can mark us as deeply as our sense of the growing visibility of our own mortality. *"You must change your life."*

The authenticity of our transformation is vouched for by the physician's role in our society, even though we are not in any sense patients. When we turn to the physician, we demonstrate our autonomy and abdicate it simultaneously. Ours is the most modern of worlds, in which we seek new methods to do what we have felt we needed to do forever. We are not those looked upon and judged; we look upon and judge. In a caricature, Ralph Waldo Emerson (1803–82) portrayed "man" as a pair of eyes riding on a set of legs. We are seeing animals who organize our world by sight and create visual categories that provide meanings for us in this most confusing of worlds. Therefore we re-create ourselves and become, as Rilke demanded, different. *"You must change your life."* It is the promise and curse of the modern world.

NOTES

PREFACE

1. On the history of the nose, see Harold M. Holden, *Noses* (Cleveland: World, 1950), dedicated to "My Teacher, Dr. Jacques Joseph"; Alfred David, "An Iconogaphy of Noses: Directions in the History of a Physical Stereotype," in Jane Chance and Andrew O. Wells Jr., eds., *Mapping the Cosmos* (Houston, Tex.: Rice University Press, 1985), pp. 76–94; Sharon Romm, comp., *Noses by Design*, prepared in cooperation with the National Museum of American History, Medical Sciences Division, and coordinated by Barbara Melosh (Washington, D.C.: National Museum of American History, 1986); and Paul Barolsky, *Michelangelo's Nose: A Myth and Its Maker* (University Park: Pennsylvania State University Press, 1990). On the more general history of physiognomy, see the recent social and cultural histories by Claudia Schmölders, *Das Vorurteil im Leibe: Eine Einführung in die Physiognomik* (Berlin: Akademie Verlag, 1995) and her edited volume, *Das exzentrische Blick: Gespräch über Physiognomik* (Berlin: Akademie Verlag, 1996), which includes many of the "classic" texts. A general volume to which I contributed is Rüdiger Campe and Manfred Schneider, eds., *Geschichten der Physionomik: Text-Bild-Wissen* (Freiburg I. Br.: Rombach, 1996).

2. Robert Kleck, "Physical Stigma and Nonverbal Cues Emitted in Face to Face Interaction," *Human Relations* 21 (1968): 19–28.

3. Charles Darwin, *The Descent of Man and Selection in Relation to Sex* (New York: D. Appelton, 1897), p. 575.

4. Alfred C. Haddon, *The Study of Man* (New York: G. P. Putnam's Sons, 1898), p. 69.

5. Oswald Spengler, *Der Untergang des Abendlandes* (1918–22; rpt., Munich: Beck, 1981), p. 135.

6. Richard Sennett, *The Fall of Public Man* (New York: Norton, 1974), p. 171.

7. Blair O. Rogers, "John Orlando Roe—not Jacques Joseph—the Father of Aesthetic Rhinoplasty," *Aesthetic Plastic Surgery* 10 (1986): 63–88, quotation on p. 70.

8. The literature on the history of the face that is relevant to this study ranges from studies of facial pathology such as Willard L. Marmelzat's "Daviel on the 'Noli-Me-Tangere': A Lost Chapter in the History of Cutaneous Cancer of the Face," *Journal of the History of Medicine and Allied Sciences* 4 (1949): 188–95, to the history of fashion such as Fenja Gunn's *The Artificial Face: A History of Cosmetics* (Melbourne: Wren, 1973).

9. George M. Trevelyan, *Clio: A Muse and Other Essays Literary and Pedestrian* (London: Longmans, Green, 1913), p. 9.

CHAPTER ONE
JUDGING BY APPEARANCES

1. On the history of aesthetic surgery, see Otto Hildebrand, *Die Entwicklung der plastischen Chirugie* (Berlin: August Hirschwald, 1909); Karl Kassel, *Geschichte der Nasenheilkunde*

von ihren Anfängen bis zum 19. Jahrhundert (1914; rpt., Hildesheim: Olms, 1967); Maxwell Maltz, *Evolution of Plastic Surgery* (New York: Froben Press, 1946); George Bankoff, *The Story of Plastic Surgery* (London: Faber and Faber, 1952); Pierre-François Grigaut, *La chirurgie esthétique et plastique* (Paris: Presses universitaires de France, 1962); Allan Ragnell, *The Development of Plastic Surgery in Stockholm in the Last Decennium* (Stockholm: Acta chirurgica Scandinavica. Supplementum 348, 1965); Frank McDowell, ed., *The Source Book of Plastic Surgery* (Baltimore: Williams & Wilkins, 1977); Antony F. Wallace, *The Progress of Plastic Surgery: An Introductory History* (Oxford: Willem A. Meeuws, 1982); M. Eberle, *Die Geschichte der Lippenplastik* (Diss., Freiburg i. Br., 1982); Joachim Gabka and Ekkehard Vaubel, *Plastic Surgery, Past and Present: Origin and History of Modern Lines of Incision* (Munich: S. Karger, 1983); Mario González-Ulloa, ed., *The Creation of Aesthetic Plastic Surgery* (New York: Springer, 1985); Jerome P. Webster, "The Story of a Plastic Surgery Library," *Proceedings of the Charaka Club* 12 (1985): 14–24; Willard L. Marmelzat, "History of Dermatologic Surgery: From the Beginnings to Late Antiquity," *Clinics in Dermatology* 5 (1987): 33–43; Lenore Wright Anderson, "Synthetic Beauty: American Women and Cosmetic Surgery" (Ph.D. diss., Rice University, 1989); John Camp, *Plastic Surgery: The Kindest Cut* (New York: Henry Holt, 1989); June Thurber Cox, "Cultural Images of the Body: An Inquiry into the History of Human Engineering" (Ph.D. diss, University of California, Berkeley, 1990); D. J. Reisberg and S. W. Habakuk, "A History of Facial and Ocular Prosthetics," *Advances in Ophthalmic Plastic and Reconstructive Surgery* 8 (1990): 11–24; A. Faga and L. Valdatta, "Plastic Surgery in the Early Nineteenth Century: Notes on the Collections in the University of Pavia's Museum of History," *Plastic and Reconstructive Surgery* 86 (1990): 1220–26; Heinz-Peter Schmiedebach, Rolf Winau, and Rudolf Häring, eds., *Erste Operationen Berliner Chirugen 1817–1931* (Berlin: De Gruyter, 1990), pp. 131–78; Anne Marie Balsamo, "Reading the Gendered Body in Contemporary Culture, 1980–1990 (Body Building, Feminist Theory)" (Ph.D. diss., University of Illinois, Urbana-Champaign, 1991); B. Haeseker, "1891–1991: The Centenary of Innovative Reconstructive Hand Surgery by Carl Nicoladoni," *British Journal of Plastic Surgery* 44 (1991): 306–9; Erwin Haas, *Plastische Gesichtschirurgie* (Stuttgart: Georg Thieme Verlag, 1991); August Lange, "Die Rhinoplastik im 'Goettingischen Taschenkalendar auf das Jahr 1805': eine Bemerkung zur Geschichte der Nasenwiederherstellung," *Würzburger medizinhistorische Mitteilungen* 9 (1991): 345–50; Robert Scheer, *The Cosmetic Surgery Revolution: An Objective Guide to Understanding Your Cosmetic Surgery Choices* (Los Angeles, Calif.: Summit Pines Press, 1992); M. Bernklau, *Über die historischen Entwicklung der rekonstruktiven Gesichtschirugie in der Zeit von 1800 bis 1950* (Diss., Giessen, 1992); A. C. Elias, "A Case of Cheiloplasty—1864," *Journal of Oral and Maxillofacial Surgery* 50 (1992): 998–99; Sharon Romm, *The Changing Face of Beauty* (St. Louis: Mosby Year Book, 1992); Willard L. Marmelzat, "Bits of History, Bits of Mystery: A Historical Review of Chemical Rejuvenation of the Face," in Robert Kotler, ed., *Chemical Rejuvenation of the Face* (St. Louis: Mosby Year Book, 1992), pp. 33–39; Noëlle Châtelet, *Trompe-l'oeil: Voyage au pays de la chirurgie esthétique* (Paris: Belfond, 1993); Kurt Kristen, "Zur Geschichte der Kieferchirugie dargestellt am Beispiel der Rehabiliationen von Trägern einer Lippen-Kiefer-Gaumenspalte," *Sitzungsberichte der Heidelberger Akademie der Wissenschaften* (1993–94): 33–47; Albino Comelli, *Da narciso al narcisismo: Storia e psicologia del corpo: Costume, medicina, estetica* (Trento: Reverdito, 1993); David M. Reifler, ed., *The American Society of Ophthalmic Plastic and Reconstructive Surgeons (ASOPRS): The First Twenty-Five Years: 1969–1994; History of Ophthalmic Plastic Surgery: 2500 B.C.–A.D. 1994* (Winter Park, Fla.: American Society of Ophthalmic Plastic and Reconstructive Surgery, 1994); Peter Proff, "Möglichkeiten der Plastisch-Rekonstruktiven und Tumor-Chirurgie in der frühbyzantinischen Medizin," in Josef Domes et al., eds., *Licht der Natur: Medizin in Fachliteratur und Dichtung* (Göppingen: Kümmerle, 1994), pp. 307–28; Christoph Weisser, "Die Nasenersatzplastik nach Heinrich von Pfalzpaint: Ein Beitrag zur Geschichte der plastischen Chirurgie im Spätmittelalter mit Edition des Textes," in Joseph

Domes et al., eds., *Licht der Natur: Medizin in Fachliteratur und Dichtung* (Göppingen: Küm-merle, 1994), pp. 485–506; Elizabeth G. Haiken, "Body and Soul: Plastic Surgery in the United States, 1914–1990" (Ph.D. diss., University of California, Berkeley, 1994); Elizabeth G. Haiken, "Plastic Surgery and American Beauty in 1921," *Bulletin of the History of Medicine* 68 (1994): 429–53; M. G. H. Bishop, "The Making and Re-making of Man, 1: Mary Shelley's 'Frankenstein' and Transplant Surgery," *Journal of the Royal Society of Medicine* 87 (1994): 749–51; Kathy Davis, *Reshaping the Female Body: The Dilemma of Cosmetic Surgery* (New York: Routledge, 1995); S. Furlan and R. F. Mazzola, "Alessandro Benedetti, a Fif-teenth-Century Anatomist and Surgeon: His Role in the History of Nasal Reconstruction," *Plastic and Reconstructive Surgery* 96 (1995): 739–43; Walter Hoffmann-Axthelm et al., *Die Geschichte der Mund-, Kiefer- und Gesichtschirurgie* (Berlin: Quintessenz Verlag, 1995); Anne Balsamo, *Technologies of the Gendered Body: Reading Cyborg Women* (Durham, N.C.: Duke University Press, 1996); Peter Paul Brunner, *Die Entwicklung der Knochenplastik am Un-terkiefer im Ersten Weltkrieg* (Zurich: Juris, 1996). Following the completion of this manu-script, a revision of Elizabeth Haiken's excellent study of aesthetic surgery in the United States appeared under the title *Venus Envy: A History of Cosmetic Surgery* (Baltimore: Johns Hopkins University Press, 1997). Her altered title points toward a focus on gender, which is, however, not the center of her work. See also the essay by Kathy Davis, "Pygmalions in Plastic Surgery," *Health* 2 (1998): 23–40, and the literary monograph by Tim Armstrong, *Modernism, Technology and the Body: A Cultural Study* (Cambridge, Eng.: Cambridge Uni-versity Press, 1998), pp. 75–183.

2. "Technological Advances Lead Many to Undergo Smaller Procedures in Facial Plas-tic Surgery, New Survey Shows," *PR Newswire*, October 8, 1996.

3. Charles Siebert, "The Cuts That Go Deeper," *New York Times Magazine*, July 7, 1996, pp. 6, 20.

4. "Technological Advances."

5. The best overview of Talcott Parsons's representation of illness and the patient re-mains Bryan S. Turner's "Sickness and Social Structure: Parsons's Contribution to Med-ical Sociology," in Robert J. Holton and Bryan S. Turner, eds., *Talcott Parsons on Economy and Society* (London: Routledge, 1986), pp. 107–42. See Talcott Parsons and Renee Fox, *Ill-ness, Therapy and the Modern Urban American Family* (Indianapolis: Bobbs-Merrill, 1967).

6. On the psychological and social construction of the body, see Stephen Kern, *Anatomy and Destiny: A Cultural History of the Human Body* (Indianapolis: Bobbs-Merrill, 1975); Jean Maisonneuve and Marilou Bruchon-Schweitzer, *Modèles du corps et psychologie esthétique* (Paris: Presses universitaires de France, 1981); Pedro Laín-Entralgo, *El cuerpo humano* (Madrid: Espasa Calpe, 1987); Marilou Bruchon-Schweitzer, *Une psychologie du corps* (Paris: Presses universitaires de France, 1990); Barbara Duden, *The Woman beneath the Skin: A Doctor's Patients in Eighteenth-Century Germany*, trans. Thomas Dunlap (Cambridge, Mass.: Harvard University Press, 1991); Efrat Tseëlon, *The Masque of Feminity: The Presen-tation of Woman in Everyday Life* (London: Sage, 1995); Jon Stratton, *The Desirable Body: Cul-tural Fetishism and the Erotics of Consumption* (Manchester: Manchester University Press, 1996); Susan Bordo, *Twilight Zones: The Hidden Life of Cultural Images from Plato to O. J.* (Berkeley and Los Angeles: University of California Press, 1997).

7. See the ongoing debate as mirrored in R. L. Simon and T. S. Hill, "Facial Plastic Surgery: Subspecialty Helps Otolaryngology Define Its Boundaries," *Otolaryngology—Head and Neck Surgery* 115 (1996): 1–14.

8. "Dentist Will Part with Hair Work," *The Bulletin* (Bend, Ore.), December 8, 1996, p. B4. The dentist in question had participated in a forty-hour anesthesia training program and "said he has been trained in cosmetic surgery and should be allowed to perform those pro-cedures." "'I've had excellent results,' he said. 'My patients are happy. I've never had a suit. Nobody's hinted at it.'"

9. Gary M. Kaplan, "Putting on a Happier Face: Business People and Cosmetic

Surgery," *Nation's Business* 74 (August 1986): 40; "Body Work," *U.S. News & World Report* 117 (October 17, 1994): 15; *Wall Street Journal,* January 15, 1997, p. 1.

10. Oliver Bennett, "Welcome to the Hotel Cardiac Bypass . . . ," *The Independent,* October 13, 1996, p. 3; Mungo Soggot, "South Africa; Germans under SA's Scalpels?" *Africa News,* January 31, 1997; Alexandra Williams, "Butchered for Beauty: How Cut-Price Cosmetic Surgery Packages to Poland End In Agony," *Sunday Mirror,* March 30, 1997, p. 14; Rachel Sarah, "Cosmetic Surgery Business Gets Lift," *Prague Post,* July 19, 1995.

11. Guy de Chauliac (d. 1368), perhaps the most important surgeon of his time, defined the role of surgery as threefold: *solvit continuum* (separating the fused), *iungit separatum* (connecting the divided), and *exstirpat superfluum* (removing the extraneous). See Guy de Chauliac, *Chirurgia magna,* ed. Gustav Keil (Darmstadt: Wissenchaftliche Buchgesellschaft, 1976), p. 3.

12. Marie-Christine Pouchelle, *The Body and Surgery in the Middle Ages,* trans. Rosemary Morris (New Brunswick, N.J.: Rutgers University Press, 1990).

13. Gaspare Tagliacozzi (1554–90) made the distinction between *chirurgia curtorum (per insitionem)* (surgery healing by grafts) and *chirurgia decoratoria* (beauty surgery). All references are to Gaspare Tagliacozzi, *La chirurgia plastica per innesto,* trans. and ed. Werner Vallieri. Bologna. Università. Cattedra di storia della medicina. Vita e opere di medici e naturalisti, 3 (Bologna: n. p., 1964), and the standard monograph on him by Martha Teach Gnudi and Jerome Pierce Webster, *The Life and Times of Gaspare Tagliacozzi, Surgeon of Bologna 1545–1599* (Milan: U. Hoepli; New York: H. Reichner, 1950).

14. Hildebrand, *Entwicklung der plastischen Chirurgie,* p. 8.

15. Philippe Frédéric Blandin, *Traite d'anatomie topographique, ou anatomie des régions du corps humain, considerée spécialement dans ses rapports avec la chirurgie et la médecine opératoire* (Paris: Germer-Baillière, 1834). The term *autoplasty* had reasonably wide acceptance, even in the United States, where Thomas Mütter wrote *Cases of Deformity of Various Kinds, Successfully Treated by Plastic Operations* (Philadelphia: Merrihew and Thompson, 1844). See Gustave Aufricht, "The Development of Plastic Surgery in the United States," *Plastic and Reconstructive Surgery* 1 (1946): 3–26.

16. P. J. Desault, *Oeuvres chirurgicales: ou, Tableau de sa doctrine & de la pratique dans le traitement des maladies externes,* 3 vols. (Paris: C. V. Desault . . . [et al.], 1798–99).

17. Carl Ferdinand von Graefe, *Rhinoplastik; oder, Die Kunst den Verlust der Nase organisch zu ersetzen, in ihren früheren Verhältnissen erforscht und durch neue Verfahrungsweisen zur höheren Vollkommenheit gefördert* (Berlin: Realschulbuchhandlung, 1818).

18. Eduard Zeis, *Handbuch der plastischen Chirurgie* (Berlin: G. Reimer, 1838). All citations from this will be from the translation by T. J. S. Patterson, *Zeis' Manual of Plastic Surgery* (Oxford: Oxford University Press, 1988).

19. Robert M. Goldwyn, *The Patient and the Plastic Surgeon* (Boston: Little, Brown, 1991), p. 54.

20. Johann Friedrich Dieffenbach, *Die operative Chirurgie,* 2 vols. (Lepizig: F. A. Brockhaus, 1845), 1:515.

21. The originary position of Dieffenbach in most histories of reconstructive surgery is striking. According to this narrative, he is the "Altmeister der plastischen Chirugie" who frees the field for the first time from its baneful association with the syphilitic and makes it into a "real" surgical specialty during the period of the establishment of such fields. See Hoffmann-Axthelm et al., *Geschichte der Mund-, Kiefer- und Gesichtschirurgie,* p. 234, for the latest use of this trope.

22. See my "Cultural and Socio-economic Background," in Larry Millikan and Lawrence Charles Parish, eds., *Global Dermatology* (New York: Springer, 1994), pp. 20–27, as well as John Thorne Crissey and Lawrence Charles Parish, *The Dermatology and Syphilology of the Nineteenth Century* (New York: Praeger, 1981); and Joachim J. Herzberg and

Gunter W. Korting, eds., *Zur Geschichte der deutschen Dermatologie: zusammengestellt aus An-lass des XVII. Congressus Mundi Dermatologiae, 24.–29. Mai, 1987* (Berlin: Grosse Verlag, 1987).

23. Hermann Klencke, *Diatetische Kosmetik; oder, Gesundheits- und Schönheitspflege der äusseren Erscheinung des Menschen; eine Volkschrift* (Leipzig: Kummer, 1875).

24. See the very title of the central bodybuilding journal, *Der Kulturmensch: Zeitschrift für körperliche und geistige Selbstzucht, unter Mitwirkung hervorragender Ärzte und Ästhetiker, sowie namhafter Mitarbeiter aus den Gebieten des Sports, der Nahrungsmittellehre, der Toiletten-chemie und Bekleidekunst* (1904–5), which continued from 1906 to 1914 under the better-known title *Körperkultur*. The quotation is from "Wortungetüme," *Der Kulturmensch* (October 15, 1904): 19–20, quotation from p. 20.

25. Physicians such as Edmund Saalfeld (1862–1930) helped popularize the field by writing pragmatic handbooks on medical cosmetology. Edmund Saalfeld, *Lectures on Cosmetic Treatment: A Manual for Practioners,* trans. J. F. Halls Dally (London: Rebman, 1911), pp. 106–7. This is a translation of Saalfeld's *Kosmetik, ein Leitfaden für praktische Ärzte* (Berlin: Springer, 1908). See also Ignaz Saudek, *Kosmetik; ein kurzer Abriss der ärztlichen Ver-schönerungskunde* (Leipzig / Berlin: B. G. Teubner, 1915) and Fritz Juliusberg, *Leitfaden der Kosmetik für Ärzte* (Berlin / Vienna: Urban & Schwarzenberg, 1922). Saalfeld's small hand-book on the topic, which first appeared as a series of essays in 1892, was widely translated and read. The initial response to this field was profound skepticism, as it usurped the label *cosmetic* used by the "'beauty specialist' or other quacks." As the London surgeon P. S. Abraham noted in his introduction to the English edition of Saalfeld's book: "When Dr. Saalfeld sent me his little book, and asked me to find him an English publisher, if I thought it suitable for translation, I must confess that I was at first a little staggered at the title 'Kos-metik'" (p. xiv). Only when he was assured that it was not a "vulgar advertisement" did he agree to translate the book, and thence medical cosmetology developed in Great Britain. P. Josef Eichhoff (1855–1914) and Heinrich Paschkis (1849–1923) continued this tradition of physician-authored handbooks, and produced major cosmetological hand-books for physicians as well as the lay public. See P. Joseph Eichhoff, *Praktische Kosmetik fur Ärzte und gebildete Laien* (Leipzig: Deuticke, 1892), and Heinrich Paschkis, *Kosmetik fur Ärzte* (Vienna: Alfred Holder, 1893). Most dermatologists of the time credited the latter with putting the field onto a "scientific" footing. See Max Joseph, *A Short Handbook of Cosmetics,* trans. D.J.G. (London: William Heinemann, 1914), p. vi. The cosmetological work of Samuel Jessner (1859–1929) was aimed specifically at the treatment of skin and hair symptoms of syphilitics. He dealt with the use of soap and cosmetics as additional means of "aesthetic" therapy. For the aesthetic surgeons, this field seemed closely identified with their own goals. See Samuel Jessner, *Lehrbuch der Haut- und Geschlechtsleiden einschliesslich der Kosmetik,* 2 vols. (Leipzig: Curt Kabitsch, 1920), 1:427–45; see also Jessmer's *Kom-pendium der Hautkrankheiten einschliesslich der Syphilide und einer kurzen Kosmetik. Für Studierende und Ärzte* (Würzburg: A. Stuber, 1900).

Certainly the term *cosmetic surgery* was well in place by 1912, when the Berlin sur-geon/historian Eugen Holländer (1867–1932) wrote his overview of "cosmetic surgery." Eugen Holländer, "Die kosmetische Chirugie," in Max Joseph, ed., *Handbuch der Kosmetik* (Leipzig: Veit, 1912), pp. 670–712. Max Joseph was a Berlin-based dermatologist.

At virtually the same moment, in 1911, those surgeons advocating the adoption of "cos-metic" procedures and evidently at home in both the American and German surgical worlds, such as Frederick Strange Kolle (1871–1929), were able to make a clear distinction between reconstructive and "cosmetic" rhinoplasty. Frederick Strange Kolle, *Plastic and Cosmetic Surgery* (New York: D. Appleton, 1911), chapter 15 (Rhinoplasty), pp. 339–447; chapter 16 (Cosmetic Rhinoplasty), pp. 448–70.

Martin Gumpert (1897–1955), who played a major role in the development of aesthetic surgery during the Weimar Republic, edited a handbook of medical cosmetics in 1931, by which time "cosmetic" surgery played a central role. Martin Gumpert, *Die gesamte Kosmetik, Entstellungsbekampfung: ein Grundriss fur Ärzte und Studierende* (Leipzig: Thieme, 1931). Compare Jean Ann Graham and Albert M. Kligman, eds., *The Psychology of Cosmetic Treatments* (New York: Praeger, 1985). Gumpert's handbook grew out of his work in a clinic for people with deformities, and covered not only surgical but also psychological and social questions raised by medical cosmetics. Indeed, by this point handbooks of cosmetic dermatology presented surgical procedures to enable disfigured people to mask their appearance and "pass" as healthy. Thus, in A. Buschke, Alfred Joseph, and Werner Birkenfeld, *Leitfaden der Kosmetik für die Ärtzliche Praxis* (Berlin: De Gruyter, 1932), the first ninety-six pages deal with the more traditional preparations, while pages 97–215 deal with surgical procedures. Yet as late as the early 1930s, when Eugen Holländer published the standard surgical overview of the field, he referred to it as "plastic (cosmetic) surgery." Eugen Holländer, "Plastische (Kosmetische) Operation: Kritische Darstellung ihres gegenwärtigen Standes," in Georg Klemperer und Felix Klemperer, eds., *Neue deutsche Klinik: Handwörterbuch der praktischen Medizin mit besonderer Berücksichtigung der inneren Medizin, der Kinderheilkunde und ihrer Grenzgebiete,* 11 vols. (Berlin: Urban & Schwarzenberg, 1928–32), 9:1–17. The boundary between the two aspects of this field remained clear and yet flexible. The ambiguity evident at the establishment of the field lies at the heart of the anxiety about aesthetic surgery even today.

26. Maurice Henry Collis, *The Aesthetic Treatment of Hare-Lip: With a Description of a New Operation for the More Scientific Remedy of This Deformity* (Dublin: J. Falconer, 1868).

27. Harold Gillies, *The Development and Scope of Plastic Surgery,* the Charles H. Mayo lecture for 1934 (Chicago: Northwestern University, 1935), p. 26.

28. Jacques W. Maliniak, *Sculpture in the Living: Rebuilding the Face and Form by Plastic Surgery* (New York: Romaine Pierson, 1934), p. 193. On the case of Henry Junius Schireson, who operated on Fanny Brice and was denounced as "King of Quacks" in the American Medical Association's popular medical journal, see Robert Maris, "King of Quacks," *Hygeia* 22 (1941): 414–15.

29. Eric Jameson, *The Natural History of Quackery* (London: Michael Joseph, 1961), pp. 88–90. See also Roy Porter, *Health for Sale: Quackery in England, 1660–1850* (Manchester: Manchester University Press, 1989).

30. On the beauty myth, see Gerald R. Adams and Sharyn M. Crossman, *Physical Attractiveness: A Cultural Imperative* (Roslyn Heights, N.Y.: Libra, 1978); Lois W. Banner, *American Beauty* (Chicago: University of Chicago Press, 1983); Robin Tolmach Lakoff and Raquel L. Scherr, *Face Value: The Politics of Beauty* (Routledge & Kegan Paul, 1984); Hillel Schwartz, *Never Satisfied: A Cultural History of Diets, Fantasies, and Fat* (New York: Free Press, 1986); Wendy Chapkis, *Beauty Secrets: Women and the Politics of Appearance* (Boston: South End Press, 1986); Sabra Waldfogel, "The Body Beautiful, the Body Hateful: Feminine Body Image and the Culture of Consumption in Twentieth-Century America" (Ph.D. diss, University of Minnesota, 1986); Arthur Marwick, *Beauty in History: Society, Politics, and Personal Appearance* (London: Thames and Hudson, 1988); Camille Paglia, *Sexual Personae: Art and Decadence from Nefertiti to Emily Dickinson* (New Haven: Yale University Press, 1990); Naomi Wolf, *The Beauty Myth: How Images of Female Beauty Are Used against Women* (New York: W. Morrow, 1991); Sara Halprin, *Look at My Ugly Face: Myths and Musings on Beauty and Other Perilous Obsessions with Women's Appearance* (New York: Viking, 1995); Kaz Cooke, *Real Gorgeous: The Truth about Body and Beauty* (London: Bloomsbury, 1995); Nancy Friday, *The Power of Beauty* (New York: Harper Collins, 1996); Richard Sartore, *Body Shaping: Trends, Fashions, and Rebellions* (Commack, N.Y.: Nova Science Publishers, 1996); and Frida Kerner Furman, *Facing the Mirror: Older Women and Beauty Shop Culture* (New York: Routledge, 1997).

31. Marc Lagarde, *Les injections de paraffine, leurs applications en chirurgie générale, en oto-rhino-laryngologie, en ophtalmologie, art dentaire et en esthétique* (Paris: Rousset, 1903); V. Micheli-Pellegrini and G. M. Manfrida, "Rhinoplasty and Its Psychological Implications: Applied Psychological Observations in Aesthetic Surgery," *Aesthetic Plastic Surgery* 3 (1979): 299–319, quotation from p. 300. See G. Baudrand, *La chirurgie esthétique et le droit* (Poitiers: Société française d'imprimerie et de librairie, 1938).

32. Goldwyn, *Patient and the Plastic Surgeon,* p. 54.

33. Susanne S. Warfield, *Esthetician's Guide to Working with Physicians* (Albany, N. Y.: Milady Publishers, 1996).

34. See my *Health and Illness: Images of Difference* (London: Reaktion Books, 1995).

35. Thus, no other surgical subspecialty has as complex historical research tools as Frank McDowell, ed., *The McDowell Indexes of Plastic Surgical Literature,* 5 vols. (Baltimore: Williams & Wilkins, 1977–81).

36. Michel Foucault, *The History of Sexuality,* vol. 1, *An Introduction,* trans. Robert Hurley (New York: Vintage, 1980), p. 146.

37. Sanford Gifford, "Cosmetic Surgery and Personality Change: A Review and Some Clinical Operations," in Robert M. Goldwyn, ed., *The Unfavorable Result in Plastic Surgery: Avoidance and Treatment* (Boston: Little, Brown, 1972), p. 30.

38. See Owen and Sarah Wangensteen, *The Rise of Surgery: From Empiric Craft to Scientific Discipline* (Minneapolis: University of Minnesota Press, 1978), pp. 275–326. On the historical context of general surgery as it applies to the history of aesthetic surgery, see Christopher Lawrence, ed., *Medical Theory, Surgical Practice* (London: Routledge, 1992); P. B. Adamson, "Surgery in Ancient Mesopotamia," *Medical History* 35 (1991): 428–35; Ulrich Trohler, " 'To Operate or Not to Operate?: Scientific and Extraneous Factors in Therapeutical Controversies within the Swiss Society of Surgery, 1913–1988," *Clio Medica* 22 (1991): 89–113; Martin Duke, *The Development of Medical Techniques and Treatments: From Leeches to Heart Surgery* (Madison, Conn.: International Universities Press, 1991); Pouchelle, *Body and Surgery in the Middle Ages;* J. Thompson Rowling, "The Rise and Decline of Surgery in Dynastic Egypt," *Antiquity* 63 (1989): 312–19; Daniel de Moulin, *A History of Surgery, with Emphasis on the Netherlands* (Dordrecht: Nijhoff, 1988); Mark Ravitch, *A Century of Surgery: The History of the American Surgical Association* (Philadelphia: Lippincott, 1981); Ben Barker-Benfield, "Sexual Surgery in Late Nineteenth-Century America," *International Journal of Health Services* 5 (1975): 279–98; *Surgery in America: From the Colonial Era to the Twentieth Century,* 2d ed., ed. A. Scott Earle (New York: Praeger, 1983); Noble S. R. Maluf, "Use of Veins in Surgery: A History," *Sudhoffs Archiv für Geschichte der Medizin und der Naturwissenschaften* 67 (1983): 50–73; A. L. Wyman, "The Surgeoness: The Female Practitioner of Surgery, 1400–1800," *Medical History* 28 (1984): 22–41; and Gert H. Brieger, "Medicine and Surgery in 1909," *Transactions and Studies of the College of Physicians of Philadelphia* 7 (1985): 17–25

39. Excerpted in Gert H. Brieger, ed., *Medical America in the Nineteenth Century: Readings from the Literature* (Baltimore: Johns Hopkins University Press, 1972), pp. 198–200.

40. Throughout this book I shall be using the terms *happy* and *unhappy* (and their variants) in quotation marks. This signals not merely the construction of mental health categories out of a philosophical discourse of "happiness," but also that the use of the term is actually taken from the psychological and surgical literature on the topic. "Happiness" is often contrasted with "psychologically distressed." See Robert M. Goldwyn's discussion of "happiness as an objective," in his *Patient and the Plastic Surgeon,* p. 62, and P. Marcus, "Psychological Aspects of Cosmetic Rhinoplasty," *British Journal of Plastic Surgery* 37 (1984): 313–18, especially p. 315.

41. On the history of happiness, see Stephen A. White, *Sovereign Virtue: Aristotle on the Relation between Happiness and Prosperity* (Stanford, Calif.: Stanford University Press, 1992);

Maximilian Forschner, *Über das Glück des Menschen: Aristoteles, Epikur, Stoa, Thomas von Aquin, Kant* (Darmstadt: Wissenschaftliche Buchgesellschaft, 1993); Danielle Büschinger, ed., *L'idée de bonheur au Moyen Âge: Actes du colloque d'Amiens de mars 1984* (Göppingen: Kümmerle, 1990); Jan Lewis, *The Pursuit of Happiness: Family and Values in Jefferson's Virginia* (Cambridge, Eng.: Cambridge University Press, 1983); and Alan O. Ebenstein, *The Greatest Happiness Principle: An Examination of Utilitarianism* (New York: Garland, 1991).

42. Immanuel Kant, "What is Enlightenment?" in Lewis White Beck, ed., *On History* (Indianapolis: Bobbs-Merrill, 1963), p. 3.

43. Autonomy is a contested concept in modern American thought. See David Riesman, Nathan Glazer, and Reuel Denney, *The Lonely Crowd: A Study of the Changing American Character* (New Haven: Yale University Press, 1950); Robert N. Bellah et al., *Habits of the Heart: Individualism and Commitment in American Life* (Berkeley and Los Angeles: University of California Press, 1985); and Willard Gaylin and Bruce Jennings, *The Perversion of Autonomy: The Proper Uses of Coercion and Constraints in a Liberal Society* (New York: Free Press, 1996).

44. Richard Sennett, *The Fall of Public Man* (New York: Norton, 1974), p. 68.

45. Ibid., p. 90.

46. Adalbert G. Bettman, "The Psychology of Appearances," *Northwest Medicine* 28 (1929): 182–85, quotation on p. 182.

47. George L. Mosse, *The Image of Man: The Creation of Modern Masculinity* (New York: Oxford University Press, 1996).

48. On the German case, which actually defines the field for the first time, see Claudia Huerkamp, *Der Aufstieg der Ärzte im 19. Jahrhundert* (Göttingen: Vandenhoek & Ruprecht, 1985) (on Prussia); Arleen Marcia Tuchman, *Science, Medicine and the State in Germany: The Case of Baden, 1815–1871* (New York: Oxford University Press, 1993); and Annette Drees, *Die Ärzte auf dem Weg zu Prestige und Wohlstand: Sozialgeschichte der württenbergischen Ärzte im 19. Jahrhundert* (Münster: F. Coppenrath, 1988).

49. Maxwell Maltz, *Doctor Pygmalion: The Autobiography of a Plastic Surgeon* (New York: Thomas J. Crowell, 1953), pp. 5–6.

50. Daniel Kevles, *In the Name of Eugenics* (New York: Alfred A. Knopf, 1985), p. 267.

51. This conjuncture has already been suggested in sociology by Marcia Bayne-Smith, ed., *Race, Gender, and Health* (Thousand Oaks, Calif.: Sage, 1995), and in literary studies by Valerie Smith, "Reading the Intersection of Race and Gender in Narratives of Passing," *Diacritics* 24 (1994): 43–57, and Melanie Levinson, "'To Make Myself for a Person': 'Passing' Narratives and the Divided Self in the Work of Anzia Yezierska," *Studies in American Jewish Literature* 13 (1994): 2–9.

52. Not "passing" is being too visible. It is being perceived as too different by those constructing the social boundaries. "Passing" is simply being visible as a member of a different cohort. Willard Gaylin notes that African Americans who seek aesthetic surgery because they are "ashamed of 'black' features" show a desire to "belong to a group, to be acceptable, to be lovable [which] is psychologically equated with being worthy, safe, and secure." Gaylin and Jennings, *Perversion of Autonomy*, p. 171. "Passing" is not being "invisible." Thus the "unattractive" is, for example, eternally differentiated from the "attractive" as a separate category of social organization. This becomes a "medical" problem once the "unhappiness" that results from being unattractive is defined as a psychopathic phenomenon.

53. Dr. med. A. G., "Menschliche Schönheit," *Kraft und Schönheit* 1 (March 1901): 2–3, quotation on p. 3.

54. Judith Walzer Leavitt, *Typhoid Mary: Captive to the Public's Health* (Boston: Beacon Press, 1996).

55. A. Burgdorf and C. Burgdorf, "A History of Unequal Treatment: The Qualifications

of Handicapped Persons as a 'Suspect Class' under the Equal Protection Clause," *Santa Clara Lawyer* 15 (1975): 875–910.

56. Lawrence Hayworth, *Autonomy* (New Haven: Yale University Press, 1986), p. 46.

57. Thomas Scanlon, "A Theory of Freedom of Expression," *Philosophy and Public Affairs* 1 (1972): 204–26, quotation on p. 215.

58. Isaiah Berlin, *Four Essays on Liberty* (London: Oxford University Press, 1969), p. 131.

59. See Max Weber, *The Theory of Social and Economic Organization,* trans. and ed. Talcott Parsons and A. M. Henderson (New York: Free Press, 1947), pp. 130–32; 324–29.

60. William Armand Lessa, *Landmarks in the Science of Human Types* ([New York:] Brooklyn College Press, 1942), p. 1.

61. See the excellent history of the physiognomy of the criminal by Claudia Schmölders, "Das Gesicht des Angeklagten: Über physiognomisches (Ver)Urteilen," *Rechtshistorisches Journal* 15 (1996): 205–36.

62. On the history of the representation of aesthetic surgery in the cinema, see Stuart C. Callé and James T. Evans, "Plastic Surgery in the Cinema, 1917–1993," *Plastic and Reconstructive Surgery* 93 (1994): 422–33.

63. See the discussion in Haiken, "Body and Soul," pp. 248ff.

64. *New York Times,* February 19, 1997, p. A10.

65. A. G. Schuring and R. E. Dodge Jr., "The Role of Cosmetic Surgery in Criminal Rehabilitation," *Plastic and Reconstructive Surgery* 40 (1967): 268–70.

66. *San Francisco Examiner,* July 13, 1921, section 18, p. 1.

67. *New York Times,* April 8, 1927, section 22, p. 6.

68. On the history of this concept, see Oliver Brachfeld, *Inferiority Feelings in the Individual and the Group,* trans. Marjorie Gabain (Westport, Conn.: Greenwood, 1972), p. 203.

69. "Penis Implant Surgeon Jailed," *The Herald* (Glasgow), September 15, 1994, p. 6.

70. Brian Wallis, "Black Bodies, White Science: Louis Agassiz's Slave Daguerreotypes," *American Art* 9 (1995): 39–61.

71. Thomas Walkington, *The Optick Glasse of Hvmors, or the Touchstone of a Golden Temperature, or the Philosophers Stone to Make a Golden Temper: Wherein the Foure Complections Sanguine, Cholericke, Phlegmaticke, Melancholicke are Succinctly Painted Forth, and Their Externall Intimates Laide Open the Purblind Eye of Ignorance It Selfe, by Which Euery One May Iudge of What Complection He is, And Answerably Learne What is Most Sutable to his Nature* (London: Imprinted by John Windet for Martin Clerke, 1607), p. 34v.

72. Ann Japenga, "Face-Lift City: Palm Springs, California," *Health* 7 (March 1993): 46.

73. R. W. Connell, *Masculinities* (Berkeley and Los Angeles: University of California Press, 1995), p. 50.

74. Gifford, "Cosmetic Surgery and Personality Change," p. 31.

75. "Technological Advances."

76. In the United Kingdom in 1995 sixty-five thousand people underwent aesthetic surgery; ten thousand of them were women who had their breasts enlarged. Face-lifts were the second most common procedure for women, whereas men were most likely to have nose jobs. The common age for surgery in the United Kingdom dropped from 50–55 to 40–48 years. Nicki Pope and Paul Nuki, "Cosmetic Surgery Tops Santa's List," *Sunday Times,* December 22, 1996, p. 4. Even so, the overall acceptance of aesthetic surgery in the United Kingdom is less than in the United States. In a survey of women in 1995, only 6 percent answered that they would be interested in having aesthetic surgery. Among those interested in having aesthetic surgery, the following procedures were considered a possibility: fat removal (liposuction) 29 percent, eyelid revision 20 percent, face-lift 16 percent, nose job 11 percent, breast enlargement 9 percent, breast reduction 9 percent. Janet Knight, "Women's Problems," *Daily Mirror,* April 25, 1995, p. 6. That same year, 13 percent of British men expected to have aesthetic surgery at some stage. "Men Fail to Shape Up in

Survey," *The Herald* (Glasgow), June 11, 1996, p. 4. Although aesthetic surgery in the United Kingdom is not yet on the level of the United States, it is clear that modern Britain is becoming an "aesthetic surgery" culture with a future parity of the genders also possible, as is the case in the United States.

77. Simona de Logu, "Plastic Surgery Gets Boost in Brazil," *Reuters,* December 6, 1996.

78. Amaranta Wright, "In Argentina, Cosmetic Surgery Tops Popular Conversation Topics," *Dallas Morning News,* May 26, 1996.

79. Kimberly Ellena Bergman, "Women's Ideas about Beauty (Physical Attractiveness)" (Diss., California School of Professional Psychology, Los Angeles, 1990).

80. John Woodforde, *The History of Vanity* (Stroud: Alan Sutton, 1992).

81. Bankoff, *Story of Plastic Surgery,* p. 165.

82. Lionel Trilling, *Sincerity and Authenticity* (Cambridge, Mass.: Harvard University Press, 1972). See Michael Shortland, "Setting Murderous Machiavel to School: Hypocrisy in Politics and the Novel," *Journal of European Studies* 8 (188): 93–119.

83. Friedrich Nietzsche, *Twilight of the Idols,* trans. R. J. Hollingdale (Harmondsworth: Penguin, 1972), p. 77.

84. Alfred Berndorfer, "Aesthetic Surgery as Organopsychic Therapy," *Aesthetic Plastic Surgery* 3 (1979): 143–46, quotation on p. 146.

85. Wallace, *Progress of Plastic Surgery,* pp. 97–98.

86. Blair O. Rogers, "The First Pre- and Post-Operative Photographs of Plastic and Reconstructive Surgery: Contributions of Gurdon Buck (1807–1887)," *Aesthetic Plastic Surgery* 15 (1991): 19–33.

87. S. M. Kalick, "Aesthetic Surgery: How It Affects the Way Patients Are Perceived by Others," *Annals of Plastic Surgery* 2 (1979): 128–34.

88. Kolle, *Plastic and Cosmetic Surgery,* chapter 18 (Case Recording Methods), pp. 491–97.

89. Christian A. Peterson, *The Creative Camera Art of Max Thorek* (Chicago: Dr. Max Thorek Memorial Foundation, 1984).

90. Pierre Bourdieu et al., *Photography: A Middle-brow Art,* trans. Shaun Whiteside (Stanford, Calif.: Stanford University Press, 1990).

91. Salvador Castañares, "Ethics in Aesthetic Surgery," *Aesthetic Plastic Surgery* 1 (1977): 209–12, quotation on p. 211.

92. Elizabeth Morgan, *The Complete Book of Cosmetic Surgery: A Candid Guide for Men, Women, and Teens* (New York: Warner, 1988), pp. 45–64, quotation on p. 52. Compare M. Eugene Tardy and Robert Brown, *Principles of Photography in Facial Plastic Surgery* (New York: Thieme Medical Publishers; Stuttgart: Georg Thieme Verlag, 1992).

93. Bruce J. Crispin, Edmond R. Hewlett, Young Hwan Jo, Sumiya Hobo, and David S. Hornbrook, *Contemporary Esthetic Dentistry: Practice Fundamentals* (Tokyo: Quintessence, 1994), p. 11.

94. See, for example, H. Becker's letter, "The Computer and Truth," *Plastic and Reconstructive Surgery* 94 (1994): 896–97.

95. Robert M. Goldwyn, "The Missing Postoperative Photograph and Other Evasions," *Plastic and Reconstructive Surgery* 92 (1993): 943–44. Goldwyn introduces what is certainly the most extensive illustrated representation of reconstructive surgery, Burt Brent, ed., *The Artistry of Reconstructive Surgery: Selected Classic Case Studies,* 2 vols. (St. Louis: C. V. Mosby, 1987). The volumes begin with the sentence, "Plastic surgery is an art form." (1:xiii)

96. See Stanley B. Burns, "The Nude in Medical Photography: A Historical Perspective, with Modern Legal Ramifications," *Journal of Biological Photography* 64 (1996): 15–26; M. Peres, D. Teplica, and Stanley B. Burns, "Nudity in Clinical Photography: A Literature Review and the Quest for Standardization," *Journal of Biological Photography* 64 (1996): 3–13; and B. Jones, "Ethics, Morals, and Patient Photography," *Journal of Audiovisual Media in Medicine* 17 (1994): 71–76.

97. *Journal of Health and Hospital Law* 23 (1990): 249.

98. Benjamin Gelfant, *Cosmetic Plastic Surgery: A Patient's Guide* ([Vancouver]: Flapartz Press, 1997), p. 13.

CHAPTER TWO
VICTORY OVER DISEASE

1. All quotations are from Louisa M. Alcott, *Little Women* (Boston: Roberts Brothers, 1868) and *Little Women, Part Second* (Boston: Roberts, 1869) (later called *Good Wives*). See Ann B. Murphy, "The Borders of Ethical, Erotic, and Artistic Possibilities in *Little Women*," *Signs* 15 (1990): 562–85.

2. Samuel R. Wells, *New Physiognomy, or, Signs of Character: As Manifested through Temperament and External Forms, and Especially in "The Human Face Divine"* (1866; rpt., New York: American Book Company, 1871), p. 211.

3. Daniel Shealy, "'Families Are the Most Beautiful Things': The Myths and Fact of Louisa Alcott's March Family in *Little Women*," in Susan R. Gannon and Ruth Anne Thompson, eds., *The Child and the Family: Selected Papers from the 1988 International Conference of the Children's Literature Association, College of Charleston, Charleston, South Carolina, May 19–22, 1988* (New York: Pace University, 1989), pp. 65–69.

4. Cited from the unpublished manuscript in Charles E. Horton, Hugh H. Crawford, and Jerome E. Adamson, "John Peter Mettauer—America's First Plastic Surgeon," *Plastic and Reconstructive Surgery* 27 (1961): 268–78, quotation on p. 277. See also Deborah Kuhn McGregor, *Sexual Surgery and the Origins of Gynecology: J. Marion Sims, His Hospital, and His Patients* (New York: Garland, 1990), for a sense of the nineteenth-century American context.

5. John Dryden, quoted in William Hay, *Deformity: An Essay* (London: Printed for R. and J. Dodsley . . . and sold by M. Cooper, 1755), p. 7.

6. All quotations are from Nathaniel Hawthorne, *Tales and Sketches* (New York: The Library of America, 1982), pp. 764–80.

7. See Barbara Eckstein, "Hawthorne's 'The Birthmark': Science and Romance as Belief," *Studies in Short Fiction* 26 (1989): 511–19.

8. Nikolai Gogol, *Diary of a Madman and Other Stories*, trans. Ronald Wilks (New York: New American Library, 1972), p. 56. The identification of Gogol's character's dilemma with "the enormous popularity which rhinoplasty enjoys today" makes a mid-twentieth-century association seemingly self-evident for Paul Friedman, "The Nose: Some Psychological Reflections," *The American Imago* 8 (1958): 337–50, quotation on p. 337.

9. Dr. v. Klein, "Über Rhinoplastik," *Heidelberger Klinische Annalen* 2 (1826):103–11.

10. Claude Quéntel, *History of Syphilis*, trans. Judith Braddock and Brian Pike (London: Polity, 1990), p. 21.

11. Jonathan Hutchinson, *Syphilis* (London: Cassell & Co., 1887), pp. 458–60. On the history of congenital syphilis, see J. D. Oriel, *The Scars of Venus: A History of Venereology* (London: Springer, 1994), pp. 57–70.

12. All quotations are from Gaston Leroux, *The Phantom of the Opera*, introduction by Max Byrd (New York: New American Library, 1987), here, p. 9. See also the discussion in Slavoj Zizek, "Grimaces of the Real; or, When the Phallus Appears," *October* 58 (1991): 45–68, and Hinrich Hudde, "Ödipus als Detektive: Die Urszene als Geheimnis des geschlossenen Raums," *Zeitschrift für französische Sprache und Literatur* 86 (1976): 1–25.

13. *The Works of Voltaire*, 42 vols. (Akron, Ohio: Werner, 1904), vol. 1, *Candide*, pp. 73–74. See Jean Sareil, "Sur la généalogie de la vérole," *Teaching Language through Literature* 26 (1986): 3–8.

14. Quotation from Johann Friedrich Dieffenbach, *Chirurgische Erfahrungen, besonders*

über die Wiederherstellung zerstörter Theile des menschlichen Körpers nach neuen Methoden, 4 vols. (Berlin: Enslin, 1829–34), 3:39.

15. Quotation from the opening sentence of Robert F. Weir, "On Restoring Sunken Noses without Scarring the Face," *New York Medical Journal* 56 (1892): 449–54, reprinted in Frank McDowell, ed., *The Source Book of Plastic Surgery* (Baltimore: Williams & Wilkins, 1977), pp. 136–46, quotation on p. 136. As one notable French surgeon stated at the very beginning of the twentieth century: "In the majority of cases, [saddle nose] is an indication of congenital syphilis, and it is easy to understand how heavily the mark of the so-called 'shameful disease' weighs upon those afflicted. The unfortunate and often innocent victim feels himself branded before the world." Cited in George Sava, *Beauty from the Surgeon's Knife* (London: Faber and Faber, 1939), p. 164.

16. Robert Gersuny, "Über einige kosmetische Operationen," *Wiener medizinische Wochenschrift* 53 (1903): 2253–58, quotation on p. 2253. On Billroth and Gersuny, see Erna Lesky, "Die Entwicklung der wissenschaftlichen Kosmetik in Österreich," *Ästhetische Medizin* 9 (1960): 199–210.

17. Cited from McDowell, *Source Book*, p. 147.

18. Julius Preuss, *Biblisch-talmudische Medizin: Beiträge zur Geschichte der Heilkunde und der Kultur überhaupt* (Berlin: S. Karger, 1911), pp. 339–41.

19. James Welwood, trans., *Socratic Discourses by Plato and Xenophon* (London: J. M. Dent, 1913), pp. 177, 189.

20. M. de Montaigne, *Essays* (London: Penguin Books, 1958), p. 336.

21. Svetlana Alpers, *The Making of Rubens* (New Haven: Yale University Press, 1995), p. 123.

22. See Cicero, *De Fato,* cited by Thomas Cooper, "Observations Respecting the History of Physiognomy," *Memoires of the Literary and Philosophical Society of Manchester* 3 (1790): pp. 414–15.

23. J. Jadassohn, ed., *Handbuch der Haut- und Geschlechtskrankheiten,* 23 vols. (Berlin: Julius Springer, 1931), 23:399–400.

24. J. F. Dieffenbach, *Die operative Chirugie,* 2 vols. (Leipzig: Brockhaus, 1845), 1:312–92, on plastic surgery of the nose. In-text citations are to this work. See also Richard Lampe, *Dieffenbach* (Leipzig: J. A. Barth, 1934); Wolfgang Genschorek, *Wegbereiter der Chirurgie: Johann Friedrich Dieffenbach, Theodor Billroth* (Leipzig: S. Hirzel, 1982); U. Ulrich and C. Lauritzen, "Johann Friedrich Dieffenbach, 1792–1847: 'Vater der plastischen Chirurgie' in Deutschland," *Deutsche medizinische Wochenschrift* 117 (1992): 1165–67; F. E. Mueller, "Der Chirurg Johann Friedrich Dieffenbach und sein Einfluss auf die Entwicklung der Plastischen Chirurgie," *Chirurgie* 63 (1992): 127–31; and H. Wolff, "Das chirurgische Erbe: zum 200. Geburtstag von Johann Friedrich Dieffenbach," *Zentralblatt für Chirurgie* 117 (1992): 238–43. On the institutional history of reconstructive surgery in Berlin, see Paul Diepgen and Paul Rostock, eds., *Das Universitätsklinikum in Berlin: Seine Ärzte und seine wissenschaftliche Leistung* (Leipzig: Barth, 1939) on Dieffenbach (pp. 66–80) and on Graefe (pp. 55–66); and Gerhard Jaeckel, *Die Charité: Die Geschichte eines Weltzentrums der Medizin* (Bayreuth: Hestia, 1963) on Graefe and Dieffenbach (pp. 231, 238–47).

25. See the bibliography in Thomas J. S. Patterson, *The Patterson Index of Plastic Surgery, 1864 A.D. to 1920 A.D.,* which is volume 3 of Frank McDowell, ed., *The McDowell Indexes of Plastic Surgical Literature,* 5 vols. (Baltimore: Williams & Wilkins, 1977–1981, here 1978), p. 456.

26. Weir, "On Restoring Sunken Noses," cited from McDowell, *Source Book*, p. 139.

27. James Israel, "Zwei neue Methoden der Rhinoplastik," *Archiv für klinische Chirugie* 53 (1896): 255–65. Also in McDowell, *Source Book*, pp. 151–55. On Israel, see Dagmar Hartung von Doetinchen and Rolf Winau, eds., *Zerstörte Fortschritte: Das Jüdische Krankenhaus in Berlin 1756–1861–1914–1989* (Berlin: Hentrich, 1989), pp. 106–12.

28. George H. Monks, "Correction, by Operation, of Some Nasal Deformities and Dis-

figurements," *Boston Medical and Surgical Journal* 139 (1898): 262–67, quotations on pp. 265, 262.

29. Harold Gillies, *The Development and Scope of Plastic Surgery,* the Charles H. Mayo lecture for 1934 (Chicago: Northwestern University, 1935), p. 8. He is paraphrasing his paper on this topic that made his reputation as an "aesthetic" surgeon: H. D. Gillies, "Deformities of the Syphilitic Nose," *British Medical Journal* 2 (1923): 977–79.

30. Charles H. Willi, *The Face and Its Improvement by Aesthetic Plastic Surgery* (London: Macdonald and Evans, 1955), p. 51.

31. On platinum implants, see Claude Martin, *Des résultats éloignés de la prothèse immédiate: Dans les résections du maxillaire* (Lyon: A. Storck; Paris: G. Masson, 1893). On ivory implants, see Benito Vilar-Sancho, "An Old Story: An Ivory Nasal Implant," *Aesthetic and Plastic Surgery* 11 (1987): 157–61.

32. Walter Hoffmann-Axthelm et al., *Die Geschichte der Mund-, Kiefer- und Gesichtschirurgie* (Berlin: Quintessenz Verlag, 1995), p. 225.

33. Cited by Blair O. Rogers, "Nasal Reconstruction 150 Years Ago: Aesthetic and Other Problems," *Aesthetic Plastic Surgery* 5 (1981): 283–327, here p. 290.

34. Byrom Bramwell, *Atlas of Clinical Medicine,* 3 vols. (Edinburgh: Printed by T. and A. Constable at the University Press, 1892–96).

35. All quotations are from Laurence Sterne, *The Life and Opinions of Tristram Shandy, Gentleman,* ed. Ian Campbell Ross (Oxford: Clarendon Press, 1983). See also Alfred David, "An Iconography of Noses: Directions in the History of a Physical Stereotype," in Jane Chance and R. O. Wells Jr., eds., *Mapping the Cosmos* (Houston: Rice University Press, 1985), pp. 76–97; and Robert G. Walker, "A Sign of the Satirist's Wit: The Nose in *Tristram Shandy,*" *Ball State University Forum* 19 (1978): 52–54.

36. Thomas Gibson, "The Prostheses of Ambroise Paré," *British Journal of Plastic Surgery* 8 (1955–56): 3–8, quotation on p. 3.

37. Donald F. Bond, ed., *The Tatler,* 3 vols. (Oxford: Clarendon Press, 1987), 3:317–22.

38. Marie Mulvey Roberts, "Pleasures Engendered by Gender: Homosociality and the Club," in Roy Porter and Marie Mulvey Roberts, eds., *Pleasure in the Eighteenth Century* (London: Macmillan, 1996), pp. 48–76, quotation on p. 63.

39. See, for example, Blair O. Rogers, "A Brief History of Cosmetic Surgery," *Surgical Clinics of North America* 51 (1971): 265–88, as well as Rogers's "Chronological History of Cosmetic Surgery," *Bulletin of the New York Academy of Medicine* 47 (1971): 265–302.

40. "Ex ejusdem lacerto detruncabat, ita ut nulla deformitas oris sequeretur." Ernst Gurlt, *Geschichte der Chirugie und ihrer Ausübung; Volkschirurgie, Alterthum, Mittelalter, Renaissance,* 3 vols. (Berlin: Hirschwald, 1898), 2:489.

41. Christoph Weisser, "Die Nasenersatzplastik nach Heinrich von Pfalzpaint: Ein Beitrag zur Geschichte der plastischen Chirurgie im Spätmittelalter mit Edition des Textes," in Josef Domes et al., eds., *Licht der Natur: Medizin in Fachliteratur und Dichtung* (Göppingen: Kümmerle, 1994), pp. 485–506.

42. All quotations are from Gaspare Tagliacozzi, *La chirurgia plastica per innesto,* trans. and ed. Werner Vallieri. Bologna. Università. Cattedra di storia della medicina. Vita e opere di medici e naturalisti, 3 (Bologna: n.p., 1964); and the standard monograph on Tagliacozzi by Martha Teach Gnudi and Jerome Pierce Webster, *The Life and Times of Gaspare Tagliacozzi, Surgeon of Bologna, 1545–1599* (Milan: U. Hoepli; New York: H. Reichner, 1950).

43. Gaspare Tagliacozzi, *Gasparis Taliacotli . . . De curtorum chirurgia per insitionem; libri dvo. In quibus es omnia, quae ad huius chirurgiae, narium acilicet, aurium, ac labiorum per inaitionem reataurandorum cum theoricen, tum practicen pertinere videbantur, clarissima methodo cumulatissime declarantur. Additis cutis traducis instrumentorum omnium, atque deligationum iconibus, & tabulis . . .* (Venetiis: Apud G. Bindonum iuniorem, 1597).

44. Revised translation from Giovanni Pico della Mirandola, "Oration on the Dignity

of Man," in Ernst Cassirer, Paul Oskar Kristeller, and John Herman Randall Jr., eds., *The Renaissance Philosophy of Man* (Chicago: University of Chicago Press, 1948), pp. 224–26. My emphasis. See also Stephen Jay Greenblatt, *Renaissance Self-Fashioning: From More to Shakespeare* (Chicago: University of Chicago Press, 1984).

45. Gustav Keil, "Zur Geschichte der plastischen Chirugie," *Laryngo-Rhino-Otologie* 57 (1978): 581–91, here p. 584.

46. Otto Hildebrand, *Die Entwicklung der plastischen Chirugie* (Berlin: August Hirschwald, 1909), p. 9.

47. John Bulwer, *Anthropometamorphosis: Man Transform'd: OR, The Artificiall Changling Historically Presented* (London: William Hunt, 1653), p. cv.

48. Margaret Pelling, "Appearance and Reality: Barber–Surgeons, the Body and Disease," in A. L. Beier and Roger Finlay, eds., *London 1500–1700: The Making of the Metropolis* (London: Longman, 1986), pp. 82–112, quotation on p. 94.

49. Bulwer, *Anthropometamorphosis*, p. cvii. This is paralleled by the long discussion about the nose of the black in the aesthetic theory of the eighteenth century. There the flattened nose is understood by many European thinkers, such as Lessing and Christoph Martin Wieland (1733–1813), as a sign of the comic nature of the black's aesthetic sensibility. It is comic precisely because blacks could possibly consider such a nose erotic.

50. Gurlt, *Geschichte der Chirurgie*, 2:496.

51. Matthaes Gothofredus Purmannus, *Großer und gantz neu-gewundener Lorbeer-Krantz oder Wundt-Artzney* (Frankfurt: M. Rohrlach, 1705), chapter 33, pp. 232–36.

52. I am indebted to the work of Ann Laura Stoler, *Race and the Education of Desire: Foucault's History of Sexuality and the Colonial Order of Things* (Durham, N.C.: Duke University Press, 1995), as well as to that of David Arnold, *Colonizing the Body: State Medicine and Epidemic Disease in Nineteenth-Century India* (Berkeley and Los Angeles: University of California Press, 1993). No commentator, however, has remarked on the transmission of rhinoplasty as a sign of the medical infiltration of the "homeland" and its physiognomy from the colonial sphere.

53. Reprinted in McDowell, *Source Book*, pp. 75–77.

54. Denys Forrest, *Tiger of Mysore: The Life and Death of Tipu Sultan* (London: Chatto & Windus, 1970), p. 33n. 3

55. One must remember that by the end of the sixteenth century in Europe, the missing nose was no longer the result (if it had ever been) only of violence, on or off the battle field or dueling ground. Even the cut-nose had come to have moral implications. All missing noses were signs of immorality. The legends of the "Oriental" cruelty associated with the nose came to be seen as a natural extension (and perhaps even a projection) of the European reading of the too-small nose. Thus, in the eighteenth century, the age of India, when Edward Gibbon (1737–94) recounted some of the legends told by the medieval historians of the early Christian emperor Constantine V, he stressed the moral context of these tales. The emperor, by the way, was called Copronymus (one who shits) by the chroniclers, but probably not to his face. His "lust confounded the eternal distinction of sex and species, and he seemed to extract some unnatural delight from the objects most offensive to human sense." He "scourged and mutilated" his own servants and loved to listen to the agony of those he tortured, and, oddly, "a plate of noses was accepted [by him] as a grateful offering." Gibbon indicates that the monks who spun these legends about the emperor were those whose worship of images the emperor abhorred and stopped because of his radical iconoclasm. The monks painted the most horrific portrait possible of the emperor, who died, according to them "stained . . . with the ulcers which covered his body; anticipated before his death the sentiment of hell-torturers." (As Heinrich Heine warned, never anger writers, for they, like Dante, can put you in a permanent literary Inferno.) In other words, he died marked by the signs of leprosy, the early parallel to syphilis, with all

of its moral implications. Among these signs of leprosy was his desire for human noses to replace the one he lost. Some modern commentators take Gibbon's tale as a statement of the reality of the practice of the amputation of noses in Byzantium. Edward Gibbon, *The Decline and Fall of the Roman Empire,* 3 vols. (New York: Modern Library, n.d.), 2:879. See also J. P. Remensnyder, M. E. Bigelow, and R. M. Goldwyn, "Justinian II and Carmagnola: A Byzantine Rhinoplasty?" *Plastic and Reconstructive Surgery* 63 (1979): 19–25.

56. Eduard Zeis, *Handbuch der plastischen Chirurgie* (Berlin: G. Reimer, 1838). All quotations from this work will be taken from the translation by T. J. S. Patterson, *Zeis' Manual of Plastic Surgery* (Oxford: Oxford University Press, 1988), p. 53.

57. Garland Cannon and Kevin R. Brine, eds., *Objects of Enquiry: The Life, Contributions, and Influences of Sir William Jones, 1746–1794* (New York: New York University Press, 1995).

58. To measure the medical world into which this procedure was adopted, see Susan C. Lawrence, *Charitable Knowledge: Hospital Pupils and Practitioners in Eighteenth-Century London* (Cambridge, Eng.: Cambridge University Press, 1996).

59. G. D. Singhal, G. N. Chaturved, and S. N. Tripathi, eds. and trans., *Fundamental and Plastic Surgery Considerations in Ancient Indian Surgery: Based on Chapters 1–27 of Sutrasthana of Susruta Samhita* (Varanasi, India: Singhal Publications, 1981), pp. 275–98. See Dharampal, comp., *Indian Science and Technology in the Eighteenth Century: Some Contemporary European Accounts* (Delhi: Impex India, 1971); J. P. Bennett, "Sir William Fergusson and the Indian Rhinoplasty," *Annals of the Royal College of Surgeons of England* 66 (1984): 444–48; D. J. Brain, "The Indian Contribution to Rhinoplasty," *Journal of Laryngology and Otology* 102 (1988): 689–93; as well as S. C. Almst, "History and Evolution of the Indian Method of Rhinoplasty," in G. Sanvenero-Rosselli, ed., *Fourth International Congress of Plastic and Reconstructive Surgery, Rome, October 1967* (Amsterdam: Excerpta medica, 1969), pp. 19–25.

60. Kaviraj Kunja Lal Bhishagratna, *The Susruta Samhita,* 3 vols. (Calcutta: n.p., 1907–16 [1918]), 1:152–54.

61. The implications of the surgery are broader. The Ayurveda system presupposes that most (if not all) illnesses are psychosomatic, seeing "the role of mind as visualized at all levels, i.e., constitutional, physiological, pathological as well as at the stage of the management of disease." Singhal, Chaturved, and Tripathi, *Fundamental and Plastic Surgery Considerations,* p. xxiv. In such surgery the line between aesthetic and reconstructive is blurred, as the reconstruction of the ripped earlobe restores its function but also remedies its appearance, and therefore restores the happiness of the individual. Thus such procedures fit elegantly into the ideology of the relationship between the "beautiful" and the "healthy" that dominated European thought in the Enlightenment. See John M. de Figueiredo, "Ayurvedic Medicine in Goa according to the European Sources in the Sixteenth and Seventeenth Centuries," *Bulletin of the History of Medicine* 58 (1984): 225–35. According to S. Mahdihassan, "The Concepts of Use and Beauty as Corresponding with Those of Reality and Appearance," *Bulletin of the Indian Institute of the History of Medicine* 22 (1992): 19–21, beauty and function are linked absolutely in the Ayurvedic system and in the meaning ascribed to the rebuilt nose. Ayurvedic psychology, which defined the repair of the nose as a restoration of the integrity of the entire body, and thus the balance of the mind, is accepted as part of the tradition of the restoration of noses. When this Indian technique was translated into the repair of the British nose, the Enlightenment reading that equated health and beauty was central in its acceptance as a legitimate form of surgery.

62. J. C. Carpue, *An Account of Two Successful Operations for Restoring a Lost Nose from the Integuments of the Forehead* (1816; rpt. Birmingham, Ala.: The Classics of Medicine Library, 1981).

63. Carl Ferdinand von Graefe, *Rhinoplastik; oder, Die Kunst den Verlust der Nase organ-*

isch zu ersetzen, in ihren früheren Verhältnissen erforscht und durch neue Verfahrungsweisen zur höheren Vollkommenheit gefördert (Berlin: Realschulbuchhandlung, 1818).

64. Julius von Szymanowski, "Zur plastischen Chirurgie," *Vierteljahrsschrift für die praktische Heilkunde* (Prague) 60 (1858): 127–56; see also Szymanowski's *Handbuch der operativen Chirurgie* (Braunschweig: Vieweg, 1870). The figures are cited in Joachim Gabka and Ekkehard Vaubel, *Plastic Surgery, Past and Present: Origin and History of Modern Lines of Incision* (Munich: S. Karger, 1983), p. 29.

65. Tribhovandas Motichand Shah, *Rhinoplasty: A Short Description of One Hundred Cases* (Junagadh: Sarkari, 1889); cited from McDowell, *Source Book,* pp. 121–27, quotation on p. 121.

66. Gillies, *Development and Scope of Plastic Surgery,* p. 2.

67. T. L. Pennell, *Among the Wild Tribes of the Afgan Frontier* (London: Seeley, Service & Co., 1927), pp. 191–93. Compare this with the Southeast Asian view recounted in Ann Laura Stoler, "Sexual Affronts and Racial Frontiers: European Identities and the Cultural Politics of Exclusion in Colonial Southeast Asia," in Ann Laura Stoler and Frederick Cooper, eds., *Tensions of Empire: Colonial Cultures in a Bourgeois World* (Berkeley and Los Angeles: University of California Press, 1997), pp. 198–237.

68. G. Pramod Kumar, "Back in Shape . . . with Her Scalpel," *The Hindu,* May 12, 1997, p. 26.

CHAPTER THREE
THE RACIAL NOSE

1. Peter Camper, *Über den natürlichen Unterschied der Gesichtszüge in Menschen verschiedener Gegenden und verschiedenen Alters,* trans. S. Th. Sömmerring (Berlin: Voss, 1792). See in this context Miriam Claude Meijer, "The Anthropology of Petrus Camper (1722–1789)" (Ph.D. diss., University of California, Los Angeles, 1991), and Stephen Jay Gould, *The Mismeasure of Man* (New York: W. W. Norton, 1996).

2. Lorenz Oken, *Lehrbuch der Naturphilosophie,* 3 vols. (Jena: Friedrich Frommann, 1811), 3:370–71.

3. Gotthold Ephraim Lessing, *Laocoön,* trans. William A. Steel (London: Everyman's Library, 1970), pp. 89ff.

4. Johann Caspar Lavater, *Physiognomische Fragment zur Beförderung des Menschenkenntnis und Menschenliebe,* 4 vols. (Leipzig: Weidmann, 1775–78). The most recent comprehensive introduction to Lavater is Ellis Shookman, ed., *The Faces of Physiognomy: Interdisciplinary Approaches to Johann Caspar Lavater* (Columbia, S.C.: Camden House, 1993). See also Karl Maurer, "Entstaltung: Ein beinahe untergegangener Goethescher Begriff," in Rudolf Behrens and Roland Galle, eds., *Leib-Zeichen: Körperbilder, Rhetorik und Anthropologie im 18. Jahrhundert* (Würzburg: Königshausen & Neumann, 1993), pp. 151–62; Liliane Weissberg, "Literatur als Representationsform: Zur Lektüre von Lektüre," in Lutz Danneberg et al., eds., *Vom Umgang mit Literatur und Literaturgeschichte: Positionen und Perspektive* (Stuttgart: Metzler, 1992), pp. 293–313; Richard Grey, "Die Geburt des Genies aus dem Geiste der Aufklarung: Semiotik und Aufklärungsideologie in der Physiognomik Johann Kaspar Lavaters," *Poetica* 23 (1991): 95–138, as well as Grey's "Sign and Sein: The *Physiognomikstreit* and the Dispute over the Semiotic Constitution of Bourgeois Individuality," *Deutsche Vierteljahrsschrift fur Literaturwissenschaft und Geistesgeschichte* 66 (1992): 300–332; and Michael Shortland, "Barthes, Lavater and the Legible Body," in Mike Gane, ed., *Ideological Representation and Power in Social Relations: Literary and Social Theory* (London: Routledge, 1989), pp. 17–53, as well as Shortland's "Power of a Thousand Eyes: Johann Caspar Lavater's Science of Physiognomical Perception," *Criticism* 28 (1986):

379–408. Of central importance in this is the work of Barbara Maria Stafford, "'Peculiar Marks': Lavater and the Countenance of Blemished Thought," *Art Journal* 46 (1987): 185–92. See as well Stafford's books: *Good Looking: Essays on the Virtue of Images* (Cambridge, Mass.: MIT Press, 1996); *Artful Science: Enlightenment, Entertainment, and the Eclipse of Visual Education* (Cambridge, Mass.: MIT Press, 1994); and *Body Criticism: Imaging the Unseen in Enlightenment Art and Medicine* (Cambridge, Mass.: MIT Press, 1991).

5. See my *On Blackness without Blacks: Essays on the Image of the Black in Germany*, Yale Afro—American Studies (Boston: G. K. Hall, 1982), pp. 19–34.

6. Winthrop D. Jordan, *White over Black: American Attitudes toward the Negro, 1550–1812* (Chapel Hill: University of North Carolina Press, 1968), p. 260n. See my *Difference and Pathology: Stereotypes of Sexuality, Race, and Madness* (Ithaca, N.Y.: Cornell University Press, 1985), pp. 131–50.

7. Camper, *Über den natürlichen Unterschied*, p. 62.

8. Lavater, *Physiognomische Fragment*, 3:98 and 4:272–74. This reference is cited (and rebutted) in Paolo Mantegazza, *Physiognomy and Expression* (New York: Walter Scott, 1904), p. 239.

9. Robert Knox, *The Races of Men: A Fragment* (Philadelphia: Lea and Blanchard, 1850), p. 134.

10. Camper, *Natürliche Unterschied*, p. 7.

11. See the standard racial anthropology of the Jew written during the first third of the twentieth century, Hans F. K. Günther, *Rassenkunde des jüdischen Volkes* (Munich: J. F. Lehmann, 1930), here pp. 143–49. These two quotations are taken from von Luschan and Judt.

12. Adam G. de Gurowski, *America and Europe* (New York: D. Appleton, 1857), p. 177.

13. Denis Diderot and Jean Le Rond d'Alembert, *Encyclopédie, ou dictionnaire raisonné des sciences, des arts et des métiers, par une société de gens de lettres*, 36 vols. (Geneva: Pellet; Neufchâtel: Société Typographique, 1778–79), 22:419–24, quotations on p. 420.

14. Charles Darwin, *The Descent of Man and Selection in Relation to Sex* (New York: D. Appleton, 1897), p. 579.

15. Robert Hichens, *The Unearthly* (New York: Cosmopolitan Book, 1926), p. 53.

16. F. Scott Fitzgerald, *The Great Gatsby*, ed. Matthew J. Bruccoli (New York: Scribner, 1992), pp. 73–76.

17. Frances Cooke Macgregor, *Transformation and Identity: The Face and Plastic Surgery* (New York: Quadrangle Press / New York Times Book Company, 1974), p. 99.

18. A summary of the literature on Jews and blacks is offered in the chapter "Die negerische Rasse," in Günther, *Rassenkunde des jüdischen Volkes*, here pp. 155–56.

19. John O. Roe, "The Deformity Termed 'Pug Nose' and Its Correction, by a Simple Operation," *The Medical Record* 31 (June 4, 1887): 621–23; reprinted in Frank McDowell, ed., *The Source Book of Plastic Surgery* (Baltimore: Williams & Wilkins, 1977), pp. 114–19, here, p. 114.

20. Robert F. Weir (1838–94) commented in the late nineteenth century on procedures developed by the Berlin surgeon James Israel (1848–1926), the chief surgeon of the Jewish Hospital in Berlin. Israel's procedures were developed to cure the saddle nose. Weir noted that "the scar . . . is the unavoidable result of this operation" and that the failure of the procedure sometimes "reproduces the deformity." Robert F. Weir, "On Restoring Sunken Noses without Scarring the Face," cited from McDowell, *Source Book*, p. 137.

21. John O. Roe, "The Correction of Nasal Deformities by Subcutaneous Operations: A Further Contribution," *Medical Record* 68 (1905): 1–7, quotation on p. 3.

22. Sir Charles Bell, *The Anatomy and Philosophy of Expression as Connected with the Fine Arts*, 3d ed. (London: John Murray, 1844), p. 20.

23. See my *Seeing the Insane* (Lincoln: University of Nebraska Press, 1996), pp. 188–89.

24. John O. Roe, "Correction of Nasal Deformities," p. 3.

25. Mary Cowling, *Artist as Anthropologist: The Representation of Type and Character in Victorian Art* (Cambridge, Eng.: Cambridge University Press, 1989), pp. 125–29. The image of the nose reproduced by Cowling from the physiognomic literature of the nineteenth century representing the Irish is identical with those in the "before" images reproduced by Roe.

26. John Beddoe, *The Races of Britain* (1885; rpt. Washington, D.C.: Cliveden Press, 1983), pp. 10–11. See Nancy Stepan, *The Idea of Race in Science: Great Britain, 1800–1960* (London: Macmillan, in association with St. Anthony's College, Oxford, 1982), p. 103.

27. Noel Ignatiev, *How the Irish Became White* (New York: Routledge, 1996).

28. Lewis Perry Curtis, *Apes and Angels: The Irishman in Victorian Caricature* (Washington, D.C.: Smithsonian Institution Press, 1971). For images of jaws and noses, see pp. 20f., 29f., and 45; and Richard Ned Lebow, *White Britain and Black Ireland: The Influence of Stereotypes on Colonial Policy* (Philadelphia: Institute for the Study of Human Issues, 1976).

29. Reinhard R. Doerries, *Iren und Deutsche in der Neuen Welt: Akkulturationsprozesse in der amerikanischen Gesellschaft im späten neunzehnten Jahrhundert* (Stuttgart: F. Steiner, 1986).

30. Samuel R. Wells, *New Physiognomy, or, Signs of Character: As Manifested through Temperament and External Forms, and Especially in "The Human Face Divine"* (1866; rpt. New York: American Book Company, 1871), p. 217.

31. Arthur G. Petit, *Mark Twain and the South* (Lexington: University Press of Kentucky, 1974), pp. 139–55, 207–10.

32. Walter White, "Has Science Conquered the Color Line?" *Negro Digest* (December 1949): 37–40, quotation on p. 37. On the problems associated with "passing as white" in America, see the older historical study by Joel Williamson, *New People: Miscegenation and Mulattoes in the United States* (1980; rpt. Baton Rouge: Louisiana State University Press, 1995), as well as the insightful new critical studies by Werner Sollors, *Neither Black nor White yet Both: Thematic Explorations of Interracial Literature* (New York: Oxford University Press, 1997), and Susan Gubar, *Racechanges: White Skin, Black Face in American Culture* (New York: Oxford University Press, 1997), pp. 13–25.

33. Blair O. Rogers, "John Orlando Roe—not Jacques Joseph—the Father of Aesthetic Rhinoplasty," *Aesthetic Plastic Surgery* 10 (1986): 63–88.

34. Sylvia Thompson, "Facing Up to a Face Lift," *Irish Times*, August 22, 1994, p. 10.

35. Curtis, *Apes and Angels*. For images of big, protruding ears, see pp. 49, 54, 63, 67, and 80.

36. Yetti Redmond, "Holding Back the Years," *Irish Times*, June 8, 1992, p. 8.

37. Ibid.

38. Edward Falces and John Imada, "Aesthetic Surgery in Asians," in Eugene H. Courtiss, ed., *Male Aesthetic Surgery* (St. Louis: Mosby, 1991), pp. 159–69, quotations on p. 159.

39. Eugenia Kaw, "Medicalization of Racial Features: Asian American Women and Cosmetic Surgery," *Medical Anthropology Quarterly* 7 (1993): 74–89, quotation on p. 74.

40. Günther, *Rassenkunde des jüdischen Volkes,* p. 217, with a summary of the literature on Jewish eyes.

41. M. Chien Chih Tzu Chu, *Nu Hsing Mei Yung Hsin Chih* (Taipei: Kuo chi tsun wen ku shu tien, 1995).

42. See my "Lam Qua and the Westernization of Medical Illustration in Nineteenth-Century China," *Medical History* 30 (1986): 57–69.

43. Y. Shirakabe, T. Kinusgasa, M. Kawata, T. Kishimoto, T. Shirakabe, "The Double-Eyelid Operation in Japan: Its Evolution as Related to Cultural Change," *Annals of Plastic Surgery* 15 (1985): 224–41.

44. See the discussion by Naoyuki Ohtake and Nobuyuki Shioya, "Aesthetic Breast Surgery in Orientals," in Nicolas G. Georgiade, Gregory S. Georgiade, and Ronald Rief-

kohl, eds., *Aesthetic Surgery of the Breast* (Philadelphia: W. B. Saunders, 1990), pp. 639–53, here p. 639.

45. Yukio Shirakabe, "The Development of Aesthetic Facial Surgery in Japan: As Seen through a Study of Japanese Pictorial Art," *Aesthetic Plastic Surgery* 14 (1990): 215–21.

46. Yoshikiyo Koganei, *Beiträge zur physische Anthropologie der Aino. I. Untersuchungen am Skelet; II. Untersuchungen am Lebenden. Mitteilungen aus der medizischen Facultät der kaiserlich-japanische Universität zu Tokio* 2 (1893).

47. Darwin, *Descent of Man*, p. 579.

48. T. Nishihata and A. Yoshida, "Augmentation Rhinoplasty Using Ivory," *Clinical Photography* 7 (1923): 8–10.

49. Frank Dikötter, *The Discourse of Race in Modern China* (London: Hurst, 1992).

50. Henry J. Schireson, *As Others See You: The Story of Plastic Surgery* (New York: Macaulay, 1938), p. 141.

51. Emiko Ohnuki-Tierney, *Illness and Culture in Contemporary Japan: An Anthropological View* (Cambridge, Eng.: Cambridge University Press, 1984), pp. 51–66.

52. Shizu Sakai, "The Impact of Western Medicine and the Concept of Medical Treatment in Japan," in Yoshio Kawakita, Shizu Sakai, and Yasuo Otsuka, eds., *History of Therapy: Proceedings of the 10th International Symposium on the Comparative History of Medicine—East and West* (Tokyo: Tanaguchi Foundation, 1990), pp. 157–71.

53. The meaning ascribed to the reconstructed face and its association with the "West" in modern Japan is also colored by the experience of the atomic bomb and the Hiroshima maidens. If the desire to "look American" through aesthetic surgery captured Japanese (and then Vietnamese) society from the 1950s to the 1970s, then it was paralleled in both cultures by the meaning of the scars of war and their reconstructive amelioration. In 1955 twenty-five women who had survived the dropping of the atom bombs at Hiroshima and Nagasaki were invited by a private goodwill group to receive cosmetic surgery at Mt. Sinai Hospital in New York. They became known in the United States as the "Hiroshima maidens." Much of the surgery undertaken on this group dealt with the reconstruction and re-building of the face, especially the eyelids and nose. Their images were widely circulated in periodicals such as *Life* magazine, and their scarred faces (and the desire of American medicine to recuperate them) became part of a shared American and Japanese understanding of the scarred face. 53. Disfigured by the American bombing, these faces were presented as the means by which Americans could now provide some recompense for the dropping of the first atomic bombs. The "happiness," however, seems to have been felt solely by the American physicians who performed the procedures and the public that paid for them. The results of the surgery were discussed with the women in a television interview forty years after the operation:

Michiko Yamoka: After the operation—
May Lee: [interviewing] Good. So you were happy.
Chiko Yamoka: Yeah, happy.
May Lee: [reporting] The treatments removed much of the physical scars, but Michiko's psychological wounds are still deep. Her most horrible memory is witnessing the death of her friends, which she says was her fault. (SHOW: NEWS 9:14 A.M. ET, CNN, August 5, 1995)

The "curative" power of the surgery was experienced more by the Americans who saw the correction of war wounds in the civilian population as a form of moral correction for the action of having dropped the first atomic bombs. Facial wounds came to have complex meanings in the attempt to reconstitute "happiness." In Japan the ability to change the *jibyo* of these individuals through aesthetic surgery seemed quite limited. The surgery may have made Michiko superficially "happy," but did not change her basic sense of her psychological damage. See Rodney Barker, *The Hiroshima Maidens: A Story of Courage, Compassion and Survival* (Harmondsworth: Penguin, 1986).

54. Ohtake and Shioya, "Aesthetic Breast Surgery in Orientals," p. 639.

55. Y. Mutou, "Augmentation Mammaplasty with the Akiyama Prosthesis," *British Journal of Plastic Surgery* 23 (1970): 58–62.

56. Kyoko Ishimara, "Young Women Turn to Plastic Surgery, But Is a New Face Really What They're Looking For?" *Nikkei Weekly,* December 28, 1992/January 4, 1993.

57. When Western commentators imagine the Japanese body, they idealize it as unscarred and as "Western." Thus Roland Barthes (1915–80), *L'empire des signes* (Geneva: A. Skira, 1970), fantasized about the Japanese actor Tetsuro Tanba's "Western" eyes in his 1970 study of Japanese culture. It may well be these (unoperated) eyes that came to serve as the idealized model for the contemporary Japanese face. These "Western" eyes also haunt the major shift in portraiture in postwar Japan, the *manga,* or illustrated comic book. The origins of modern *manga* can be found in the humorous illustrations of Katsushika Hokusai (1760–1849), who coined the term out of the Chinese ideograms *man* (involuntary and/or morally corrupt) and *ga* (picture). His imagery was rooted in the physiognomy of Japanese caricatures and used the conventions of representing the Japanese physiognomy as different from other "foreign" physiognomies.

58. Yoshiko Matsushita, "Mama, He's Making Eyes for Me . . . and a New Chin," *Asia Times,* May 19, 1997, p. 1.

59. One can add that precisely the same scenario can be played out in regard to young men in today's Japan. It seems clear that the shift in attitude toward aesthetic surgery is a generational one. In a recent issue of the teenage magazine *Bart* (March 10, 1997, pp. 98–103) there was an article on young men in their late teens undergoing cosmetic procedures that cost them as much as ¥350,000 for a nose job and ¥300,000 for an eyelid procedure. This essay, accompanied by "before and after" photographs, chronicled the masculine drive for "happiness" through the Western aesthetic alteration of the *too*-Japanese body.

60. The physiognomy of the contemporary *manga* (and the *anime,* the animated film), however, is rooted in the animated work of Ozamu Tezuka (1926–89) from the 1950s. Influenced by American animated cartoons, such as those of Walt Disney, Tezuka "developed some of the characteristics of *manga* . . . noting that he drew the princess with big, round eyes in exotic, foreign settings." "Manga's Appeal Not Limited to Japanese Fans," *Daily Yomiuri,* December 11, 1996, p. 3; see also Frederik L. Schodt, *Manga! Manga! The World of Japanese Comics* (Tokyo: Kodansha, 1986). In postwar Japan, such deracialized ("Western") eyes came to be representative of the physiognomy of the *manga* and were read as a way of imagining a new, exotic, and happy body. The *manga* in this tradition (especially those for girls) have depicted the characters as outrageously "Western." This is certainly related to the modern tradition of the "girls' opera" (known as "Takarazuka," after a city near Osaka), which represents a fictional "Western" (actually "nowhere") world with an all-female cast (with the male characters played by the young actresses). "Takarazuka" presents a world analogous to the Occidentalist girls' comics in Japan with "neutral" (read: Western) physiognomies. Recently there have appeared very "Japanese" *manga* and *anime,* such as those by Katsuhiro Otomo. His best-known work is *Akira,* a near-future science fiction in which Japanese characters are depicted with "Japanese" eyes.

61. Le Gia Vinh, "Study of Facial Dimensions in Vietnamese Young People: Their Application into Aesthetic and Plastic Surgery," *Anthropologie* 27 (1988): 113–15.

62. Nguyen Man Phuong, "Vietnam: As Confucianism and Socialism Erode, Crime Thrives," *Inter Press Service,* October 1, 1996.

63. Pascale Trouillaud, "More Vietnamese Going under the Beauty Knife," *Agence France Presse,* November 30, 1995, 08:14 Eastern Time.

64. Le Thang Long, "Vietnamese Men Line Up for a Nip and Tuck," *Agence France Presse,* June 7, 1996.

65. Dean Lokken, "Doctor Says Cosmetic Surgery Makes Gains in China," *U. S. News & World Report,* October 17, 1994.

66. "Blinded Woman Sues Beauty Parlor," United Press International, October 14, 1996, Monday, BC cycle.

67. Alison Dakota Gee, "The Price of Beauty," *Asiaweek,* August 2, 1996, p. 38.

68. United Press International, May 1, 1996, Wednesday, BC cycle.

69. Khoo Boo-Chai, "Plastic Construction of the Superior Palpebral Fold," *Plastic and Reconstructive Surgery* 31 (1963): 74. See also Khoo's "Augmentation Rhinoplasty in the Orientals," *Plastic and Reconstructive Surgery* 34 (1964): 81.

70. The beautiful as it is understood in contemporary Chinese culture remains the symmetrical. Indeed, it defines the beautiful for the clinical practice of aesthetic surgery. See X. Wang and Z. Zhang, "Three Dimensional Analysis of the Facial Lateral Region with Beautiful Appearance of Chinese and Its Clinical Value" [in Chinese], *Chung-Hua Kou Chiang i Hsueh Tsa Chih/Chinese Journal of Stomatology,* 30 (1995): 131–33 and 191. The search for happiness comes to be the search for the beauty present in the perceived symmetry of the Western face, or at least of the Asian face now reconfigured as neither Western nor too "Oriental." Naree Krajang, a Thai jazz singer, who had fat removed from her upper eyelids to make them look rounder and a nasal implant inserted in her "too-small" nose, stated that "Westerners have perfect figures, beautiful faces and shapes. . . . We want to be beautiful, like foreigners." Shiela McNulty, "Asians Bear the Knife for Western Look," *San Jose Mercury News,* February 21, 1995, p. A1. The foreigners, by implication, are truly happy, but would everyone want to be able to cross that border into the world of the beautiful, the happy, the healthy, and the well-to-do?

71. Claudia Kolker and Dai Huynh, "A Beauty of a Dispute," *Houston Chronicle,* September 8, 1996, p. 33.

72. Steve Glain, "Cosmetic Surgery Goes Hand in Glove with the New Korea," *Wall Street Journal,* November 23, 1993, p. A1.

73. Elaine T. Matsushita, "Americans, Too: For Asian Americans, as for Other Minorities, Full Assimilation into the American Mainstream Is a Bittersweet Process," *Chicago Tribune,* April 29, 1992, p. C6.

74. Laura Accinelli, "Eye of the Beholder," *Los Angeles Times,* January 23, 1996, p. E1.

75. Gish Jen, *Mona in the Promised Land: A Novel* (New York: Vintage, 1996).

76. Penny Colman, *Madam C. J. Walker: Building a Business Empire* (Brookfield, Conn.: Millbrook Press, 1994).

77. Blair O. Rogers, " The Role of Physical Anthropology in Plastic Surgery Today," *Clinics of Plastic Surgery* 1 (1974): 439–98; and W. E. Berman, "The Non-Caucasian (Ethnic or Platyrrhine) Nose," *Ear Nose Throat Journal* 74 (1995): 747–48 and 750–51.

78. Werner Sollors, "Theory and Ethnic Message," *MELUS: The Journal of the Society for the Study of the Multi-Ethnic Literature of the United States* 8 (1981): 15–17; and Sollors's collection *The Invention of Ethnicity* (New York: Oxford University Press, 1989).

79. M. L. Ettler, "Körperkultur und Zuchtwahl," *Politisch-Anthropologische Revue* 3 (1904/5): 624–29, quotations on pp. 635, 628.

80. Weir, "On Restoring Sunken Noses," cited from McDowell, *Source Book,* p. 139.

81. Jacques Joseph, *Nasenplastik und sonstige Gesichtsplastik, nebst einem Anhang über Mammaplastik und einige weitere Operationen aus dem Gebiete der äusseren Körperplastik: Ein Atlas und ein Lehrbuch* (Leipzig: C. Kabitzsch, 1931). All quotations are from the translation by Stanley Milstein: Jacques Joseph, *Rhinoplasty and Facial Plastic Surgery with a Supplement on Mammaplasty and Other Operations in the Field of Plastic Surgery of the Body* (Phoenix: Columella Press, 1987), p. 83.

82. The "negroid nose" is one seen as one of the categories that warranted surgical intervention in contemporary Brazil today. One does not want to be seen as "too black." See Aymar Sperli, "Exo-Rhinoplasty: A New 'Old Approach' in Aesthetic Rhinoplasty," and Edwaldo Bolivar de Souza Pinto, "Rhinosculpture: Treatment of the Nasal Tip, Columella, and Lip Dynamics," both in the online *Brazilian Journal of Plastic Surgery*, October 31, 1996 (www.plasticsurgery.org). Both of these essays list "negroid nose" as one of the nasal forms to be "repaired."

83. Jacques W. Maliniak, *Sculpture in the Living: Rebuilding the Face and Form by Plastic Surgery* (New York: Romaine Pierson, 1934), p. 55.

84. Schireson, *As Others See You*, p. 276.

85. Harry Laughlin Papers, Box C-2-1, Truman State University, Kirksville, Mo.

86. Jack Penn, *The Right to Look Human: An Autobiography* (Johannesburg: McGraw-Hill, 1974). See D. H. Walker, "The History of Plastic Surgery in South Africa," *Adler Museum Bulletin* 11 (1985): 6–11.

87. W. Earle Matory Jr., "Aesthetic Surgery in African-Americans," in Eugene H. Courtiss, ed., *Aesthetic Surgery* (St. Louis: Mosby, 1991), pp. 170–84, quotation on p. 174.

88. W. Earle Matory Jr. and Edward Falces, "Non-Caucasian Rhinoplasty: A Sixteen-Year Experience," *Plastic and Reconstructive Surgery* 77 (1986): 239–52.

89. Robert M. Goldwyn, *Beyond Appearance: Reflections of a Plastic Surgeon* (New York: Dodd, Mead & Co., 1986), pp. 200–201.

90. Patricia J. Williams, *The Rooster's Egg* (Cambridge, Mass.: Harvard University Press, 1995), pp. 238–39.

91. Jenny Choi, "New Thinking on Cosmetic Surgery: Keep Your Ethnic Identity," *Self*, December 1992, p. 43.

92. Elisabeth Rosenthal, "Ethnic Ideals: Rethinking Plastic Surgery," *New York Times*, September 25, 1991, p. C1.

93. Macgregor, *Transformation and Identity*, p. 92.

94. Harold E. Pierce, "Cosmetic Head and Face Surgery—Ethnic Considerations," *Journal of the National Medical Association* 72 (1980): 487–92. See also the earlier essay by R. S. Flowers, "The Surgical Correction of the Non-Caucasian Nose," *Clinics of Plastic Surgery* 1 (1977): 69–87.

95. Matory and Falces, "Non-Caucasian Rhinoplasty."

96. P. E. Grimes and S. G. Hunt, "Considerations for Cosmetic Surgery in the Black Population," *Clinics in Plastic Surgery* 20 (1993): 27–34, here p. 31

97. Thomas D. Rees, "Discussion of W. Earle Matory Jr. and Edward Falces, 'Non-Caucasian Rhinoplasty: A Sixteen-Year Experience,'" *Plastic and Reconstructive Surgery* 77 (1986): 252.

98. Maudlyne Ihejirka, "More Ordinary People Seeking Plastic Surgery," *Chicago Sun-Times*, March 30, 1997, p. 38.

CHAPTER FOUR
MARKS OF HONOR AND DISHONOR

1. George H. Monks, "Correction, by Operation, of Some Nasal Deformities and Disfigurements," *Boston Medical and Surgical Journal* 139 (1898): 262–67, here p. 262. For the context, see Antony F. Wallace, *The Progress of Plastic Surgery: An Introductory History* (Oxford: Willem A. Meeuws, 1982), p. 23.

2. Simon Louvish, *Man on the Flying Trapeze: The Life and Times of W. C. Fields* (New York: W. W. Norton, 1997).

3. Laurie Winslow, "Forum for Men to Stress Image," *Tulsa World*, February 25, 1997, p. A9.

4. Tom Bayles, "Woman Duped into Signing Away Rights to $381 Million Fortune," *Charleston Gazette*, March 6, 1997, p. 1A.

5. Cheryl Johnson, "The Mouse That Roared," *Star Tribune*, September 19, 1996, p. 4B.

6. John O. Roe, "The Deformity Termed 'Pug Nose' and Its Correction, by a Simple Operation," *The Medical Record* 31 (June 4, 1887): 621–23, reprinted in Frank McDowell, ed., *The Source Book of Plastic Surgery* (Baltimore: Williams & Wilkins, 1977), pp. 114–19, here p. 114.

7. Joseph Jacobs, *Studies in Jewish Statistics, Social, Vital and Anthropometric* (London: D. Nutt, 1891), p. xxxii.

8. Thomas Mann, "The Blood of the Walsungs," in *Death in Venice and Seven Other Stories*, trans. H. T. Lowe-Porter (New York: Vintage, 1989), pp. 289–316, quotation on p. 290.

9. Amos Elon, *Herzl* (New York: Holt, Rinehardt and Winston, 1975), p. 63.

10. Quoted from Konrad H. Jarausch, *Students, Society, and Politics in Imperial Germany: The Rise of Academic Illiberalism* (Princeton: Princeton University Press, 1982), p. 350. See also Jarausch's *Deutsche Studenten, 1800–1970* (Frankfurt a. M.: Suhrkamp, 1984), pp. 82–93, as well as Michael Kater, *Studentenschaft und Rechtsradikalismus in Deutschland, 1918–1933: Eine sozialgeschichtliche Studie zur Bildungskrise in der Weimarer Republik* (Hamburg: Hoffmann und Campe, 1975), pp. 145–62.

11. W[illiam] O[sler], "Berlin Correspondence," *Canada Medical and Surgical Journal* 2 (1874): 308–15, quotation on p. 310.

12. Jarausch, *Students*, p. 272.

13. Quoted by Peter Pulzer, *The Rise of Political Anti-Semitism in Germany and Austria* (London: Peter Halband, 1988), p. 246.

14. Ludwig Lévy-Lenz, *Erinnerungen eines Sexual-Arztes: Aus den Memorien eines Sexologen* (Baden-Baden: Wadi-Verlagsbuchhandlung, 1954), p. 460. See also Lévy-Lenz's *Praxis der kosmetischen Chirugie, Fortschritte und Gefahren* (Stuttgart: Hippokrates, 1954).

15. Friedrich Trendelenburg, *Die erste 25 Jahre der Deutschen Gesellschaft für Chirurgie: Ein Beitrag zur Geschichte der Chirurgie* (Berlin: Julius Springer, 1925), p. 197.

16. Stephan Mencke, *Zur Geschichte der Orthopädie* (Munich: Michael Beckstein, 1930), pp. 68–69.

17. Bruno Valentin, *Geschichte der Orthopädie* (Stuttgart: Georg Thieme, 1961), pp. 101–2.

18. Edward T. Ely, "An Operation for Prominence of the Auricles," *Archives of Otology* 10 (1881): 97; reprinted in McDowell, *Source Book*, pp. 346–49.

19. The traditional histories of reconstructive surgery do not cover Joseph's role in the history of aesthetic surgery. See, for example, Joachim Gabka and Ekkehard Vaubel, *Plastic Surgery, Past and Present: Origin and History of Modern Lines of Incision* (Munich: S. Karger, 1983), which mentions Joseph in passing but does not even supply his biography in its biographical appendix. The only comprehensive history of aesthetic surgery that discusses his role, without any social context, is Mario González-Ulloa, ed., *The Creation of Aesthetic Plastic Surgery* (New York: Springer, 1985), pp. 87–114.

20. Jack E. Davis and Horacio H. Hernandez, "History of the Aesthetic Surgery of the Ear," in González-Ulloa, ed., *Creation of Aesthetic Plastic Surgery*, pp. 115–35.

21. Hans F. K. Günther, *Rassenkunde des jüdischen Volkes* (Munich: J. F. Lehmann, 1930), p. 218.

22. Telemachus Thomas Timayenis, *The Original Mr. Jacobs* (New York: Minerva Publishing Co., 1888), p. 21. See Michael Selzer, ed., *"Kike!": A Documentary History of Anti-Semitism in America* (New York: World Publishing, 1972), plate 16.

23. William H. Luckett, "A New Operation for Prominent Ears Based on the Anatomy of the Deformity," *Surgical Gynecology & Obstetrics* 10 (1910): 635–37; reprinted in McDowell, *Source Book*, pp. 351–53, quotation on p. 351

24. All quotations are from the English translation of Heinrich Mann, *Man of Straw* (London: Penguin, 1984). The book was first published by Kurt Wolff in Berlin in 1918 as

Der Untertan. On the question of the reading of Jewish ears, see Itta Schedletzky, "Majestätsbeleidigung und Menschenwürde: Die Fatalität des Antisemitismus in Heinrich Manns Roman *Der Untertan,*" *Bulletin des Leo-Baeck-Instituts* 86 (1990): 67–81, here pp. 74–76. See also the images of the "Jewish ear" in *Die Macht der Bilder: Antisemitische Vorurteile und Mythen,* ed. Jüdisches Museum des Stadt Wien (Vienna: Picus, 1995), p. 173.

25. Alan Bullock, *Hitler and Stalin: Parallel Lives* (New York: Knopf/Random House, 1992), p. 537.

26. Alfred Berndorfer, "Aesthetic Surgery as Organopsychic Therapy," *Aesthetic Plastic Surgery* 3 (1979): 143–46, quotation on p. 143.

27. John R. Baker, *Race* (New York: Oxford University Press, 1974), p. 238.

28. Jacques Joseph, "Über die operative Verkleinerung einer Nase (Rhinomiosis)," *Berliner klinische Wochenschrift* 40 (1898): 882–85. All quotations are from Jacques Joseph, "Operative Reduction of the Size of a Nose (Rhinomiosis)," trans. Gustave Aufricht, *Plastic and Reconstructive Surgery* 46 (1970): 178–81, here p. 178; reproduced in McDowell, *Source Book,* pp. 164–67. See also Paul Natvig, *Jacques Joseph: Surgical Sculptor* (Philadelphia: W. B. Saunders, 1982), pp. 23–24; C. Walter and D. J. Brain, "Jacques Joseph," *Facial Plastic Surgery* 9 (1993): 116–24; S. Milstein, "Jacques Joseph and the Upper Lateral Nasal Cartilages," *Plastic and Reconstructive Surgery* 78 (1986): 424.; D. J. Hauben, "Jacques Joseph (1865–1934)," *Laryngologie, Rhinologie, Otologie* 62 (1983): 56–57; T. Gibson and D. W. Robinson, "The Mammary Artery Pectoral Flaps of Jacques Joseph," *British Journal of Plastic Surgery* 29 (1976): 370–76; and Paul Natvig, "Some Aspects of the Character and Personality of Jacques Joseph," *Plastic and Reconstructive Surgery* 47 (1971): 452–53. On the general history of rhinoplasty, see Blair O. Rogers, "A Chronological History of Cosmetic Surgery," *Bulletin of the New York Academy of Medicine* 47 (1971): 265–302; Blair O. Rogers, "A Brief History of Cosmetic Surgery," *Surgical Clinics of North America* 51 (1971): 265–88; H. Rudert, "Von der submukosen Septumresektion Killians über Cottles Septumplastik zur modernen plastischen Septumkorrektur und funktionellen Septo-Rhinoplastik," *Hals-Nase-Ohren* 32 (1984): 230–33; D. J. Hauben, "Die Geschichte der Rhinoplastik," *Laryngologie, Rhinologie, Otologie* 62 (1983): 53–55; P. A. Adamson, "Rhinoplasty—Our Past," *Facial Plastic Surgery* 5 (1988): 93–96; C. Walter, "The Evolution of Rhinoplasty," *Journal of Laryngology and Otology* 102 (1988): 1079–85; I. Eisenberg, "A History of Rhinoplasty," *South African Medical Journal* 62 (1982): 286–92; and A. B. Sokol and R. B. Berggren, "Rhinoplasty: Its Development and Present Day Usages," *Ohio State Medical Journal* 68 (1972): 556–62.

29. Joseph, "Operative Reduction," p. 180.

30. Jacques Joseph, *Nasenplastik und sonstige Gesichtsplastik, nebst einem Anhang über Mammaplastik und einige weitere Operationen aus dem Gebiete der äusseren Körperplastik: Ein Atlas und ein Lehrbuch* (Leipzig: C. Kabitzsch, 1931). All quotations are from Jacques Joseph, *Rhinoplasty and Facial Plastic Surgery with a Supplement on Mammaplasty and Other Operations in the Field of Plastic Surgery of the Body,* trans. Stanley Milstein (Phoenix: Columella Press, 1987), here p. 34.

31. Cited by Blair O. Rogers, "John Orlando Roe—not Jacques Joseph—the Father of Aesthetic Rhinoplasty," *Aesthetic Plastic Surgery* 10 (1986): 63–88, quotation on p. 81.

32. Trendelenburg, *Die erste 25 Jahre der Deutschen Gesellschaft für Chirurgie,* pp. 199–200. Trendelenburg's claim of priority has been ignored to date.

33. John O. Roe, "The Correction of Angular Deformities of the Nose by a Subcutaneous Operation," *The Medical Record* (July 18, 1891): 1–7. Cited from McDowell, *Source Book,* pp. 131–35, here p. 131.

34. Robert F. Weir, "On Restoring Sunken Noses without Scarring the Face," *New York Medical Journal* 56 (1892): 449–54, cited in McDowell, *Source Book,* p. 141.

35. Jacques Joseph, "Nasenverkleinerung (mit Krankenvorstellung)," *Deutsche Medi-*

zinische Wochenschrift 30 (1904): 1095. See also Joseph's "Nasenverkleinerungen," *Verhandlungen der deutsche Gesellschaft für Chirugie* 33 (1904): 112–20, and Joseph's *Eine Nasenplastik, ausgeführt in Lokalanesthesie* (Berlin: G. Stilke, 1927).

36. Rogers, "Roe," p. 84.

37. See, for example, the discussion of circumcision as castration in Sándor Ferenczi, "Die psychische Folgen einer 'Kastration' im Kindesalter," *Zeitschrift für Psychoanalyse* 4 (1916–17): 263–66. On the history and culture of circumcision, see S. J. Waszak, "The Historic Significance of Circumcision," *Obstetrics and Gynecology* 51 (1978): 499–501; E. Grossman and N. A. Posner, "Surgical Circumcision of Neonates: A History of Its Development," *Obstetrics and Gynecology* 58 (1981): 241–46; James Boon, *Other Tribes, Other Scribes* (New York: Cambridge University Press, 1982), pp. 162–68, and Boon's *Affinities and Extremes* (Chicago: University of Chicago Press, 1990), pp. 55–60; Elliot A. Grossman, *Circumcision: A Pictorial Atlas of Its History, Instrument Development and Operative Techniques* (Great Neck, N.Y.: Todd & Honeywell, 1982); John J. Collins, "A Symbol of Otherness: Circumcision and Salvation in the First Century," in Jacob Neusner and Ernest S. Frerichs, eds., *"To See Ourselves As Others See Us": Christians, Jews, "Others," in Late Antiquity* (Chico, Calif.: Scholars Press, 1985), pp. 163–85; Desmond Morris, *Bodywatching* (London: Jonathan Cape, 1985), pp. 218–20; Claude Lévi-Strauss, "Exode sur Exode," *Homme* 28 (1988): 106–7; Nigel Allan, "A Polish Rabbi's Circumcision Manual," *Medical History* 33 (1989): 247–54; Moisés Trachtenberg and Philip Slotkin, "Circumcision, Crucifixion, and Anti-Semitism: The Antithetical Character of Ideologies and Their Symbols Which Contain Crossed Lines," *International Review of Psycho-Analysis* 16 (1989): 459–71; Howard Eilberg-Schwartz, *The Savage in Judaism: An Anthropology of Israelite Religion and Ancient Judaism* (Bloomington: Indiana University Press, 1990), pp. 141–76; Moisés Trachtenberg, *Psicanálise da circuncisão* (Porto Alegre: Sagra, 1990); and Malek Chebel, *Histoire de la circoncision: Des origines à nos jours* (Paris: Balland, 1992).

38. Sander L. Gilman, *The Case of Sigmund Freud: Race and Identity at the Turn of the Century* (Baltimore: Johns Hopkins University Press, 1993).

39. Richard Andree, *Zur Volkskunde der Juden* (Leipzig: Velhagen & Klasing, 1881), p. 68.

40. When the Roman general Turnus Rufus confronted Rabbi Akiba over the practice of infant male circumcision ("Why has God not made man just as He wanted him to be?"), Akiba answered: "Everything that God has created was purposely made incomplete, in order that human ingenuity may perfect it. Take, for instance, the acorn and the cake made from it; the cotton plant and the beautiful garments that are made from it. Man is born uncircumcised because it is the duty of man to perfect himself" (*Pesiata Raba and Tanchuma on Tazria*). See Lawrence A. Hoffman, *Covenant of Blood: Circumcision and Gender in Rabbinic Judaism* (Chicago: University of Chicago Press, 1996).

41. Andree, *Zur Volkskunde der Juden*, pp. 152–60.

42. Benedict Spinoza, *The Political Works*, trans. A. G. Wernham (Oxford: Oxford University Press, 1958), p. 63.

43. E. R. Owen and J. L. Kitson, "Plastibell Circumcision," *British Journal of Clinical Practice* 44 (1990): 661.

44. Maxwell Maltz, *Evolution of Plastic Surgery* (New York: Froben, 1946), pp. 278–79.

45. Jody P. Rubin, "Celsus' Decircumcision Operation: Medical and Historical Implications," *Urology* 16 (1980): 121–24.

46. Willard L. Marmelzat, "Celsus (A.D. 25), Plastic Surgeon: On the Repair of Defects of the Ears, Lips, and Nose," *Journal of Dermatologic Surgery and Oncology* 8 (1982): 1012–14.

47. See Francette Pacteau, *The Symptom of Beauty* (London: Reaktion Books, 1994).

48. Edward Wallerstein, "Circumcision: The Uniquely American Medical Enigma," *Urologic Clinics of North America* 12 (1985): 123–32; David L. Gollaher, "From Ritual to Science: The Medical Transformation of Circumcision in America," *Journal of Social History* 28

(1994–95): 5–36; and Daniel Itzkovitz, "Secret Temples," in Jonathan Boyarin and Daniel Boyarin, eds., *Jews and Other Differences: The New Jewish Cultural Studies* (Minneapolis: University of Minnesota Press, 1997), pp. 176–202.

49. Johann Friedrich Dieffenbach, *Die operative Chirugie*, 2 vols. (Leipzig: F. A. Brockhaus, 1845), 1:515–22.

50. A. Müller, "100 Jahre Kieferchirugie in Berlin," *Zahnärzte-Kalender der Deutschen Demokratischen Republik* 22 (1984): 70–77.

51. Eduard Zeis, *Handbuch der plastischen Chirurgie* (Berlin: G. Reimer, 1838). All citations from this will be to the translation by T. J. S. Patterson, *Zeis' Manual of Plastic Surgery* (Oxford: Oxford University Press, 1988), here pp. 182–84.

52. Eduard Streissler, "Posthioplastik bei kongenitaler Verwachsung von Vorhaut und Eichel," *Beiträge zur klinischen Chirurgie* 59 (1908): 206–16, here p. 209.

53. Friedrich August von Ammon and Moritz Baumgarten, "Postthioplastik," in *Die plastische Chirugie nach ihren bisherigen Leistungen* (Berlin: G. Reimer, 1842), pp. 262–67, quotation on p. 262.

54. See my "Indelibility of Circumcision," *Koroth* (Jerusalem) 9 (1991): 806–17.

55. Compare Marc Shell, "The Holy Foreskin; or, Money Relics, and Judeo-Christianity," in Boyarin and Boyarin, *Jews and Other Differences*, pp. 345–59.

56. Gabriel Groddeck, *De Judaeis praeputium attrahentibus ad illustrandum locum I. Cor. VII. 18* (Leipzig: 1690), reprinted in Christianus Schoettgenius, ed., *Horae hebraicae et Talmudicae* (Dresden: Thomam Fritsch, 1733), pp. 1163 (fleshly desires) and 1166 (rareness of decircumcision).

57. Karl Julius Weber, *Demokritos, oder, Hinterlassene Papiere eines lachenden Philosophen* in Weber's *Sämmtliche Werke*, 25 vols. (Stuttgart: Brodhag, 1837–?), 10:235.

58. Douglas Gairdner, "The Fate of the Foreskin: A Study of Circumcision," *British Medical Journal* 2 (1949): 1433–37; and Jacob Oster, "Further Fate of the Foreskin: Incidence of Preputial Adhesions, Phimosis, and Smegma among Danish Schoolboys," *Archives of Disease in Childhood* 48 (1968): 200–202. The debate about the efficacy of circumcision as prophylaxis continues. See Morten Frisch, S{{oslash}}ren Friis, Susanne Kruger Kjaer, and Mads Melbye, "Falling Incidence of Penis Cancer in an Uncircumcised Population: Denmark, 1943–90," *British Medical Journal* 311 (1995): 1471.

59. Susann Heenen-Wolff, *Im Haus des Henkers: Gespräche in Deutschland* (Frankfurt a. M.: Dvorah, 1992), pp. 68–69.

60. Sander L. Gilman, *Jews in Today's German Culture,* the Schwartz Lectures (Bloomington: Indiana University Press, 1995), p. 83. See also Janet Lungstrum's expansion of this discussion in her "Foreskin Fetishism: Jewish Male Difference in *Europa, Europa,*" *Screen* 39 (1998): 53–66.

61. Ernst Brücke, *Schönheit und Fehler der menschlichen Gestalt* (Vienna: Braumüller, 1891), pp. 141–44.

62. See Sander L. Gilman, *The Jew's Body* (New York: Routledge, 1992), pp. 38–59.

63. Jacques Joseph, *Nasenplastik und sonstige Gesichtsplastik, nebst einem Anhang über Mammaplastik und einige weitere Operationen aus dem Gebiete der äusseren Körperplastik: Ein Atlas und ein Lehrbuch* (Leipzig: C. Kabitzsch, 1931). All quotations are from the translation by Stanley Milstein, Jacques Joseph, *Rhinoplasty and Facial Plastic Surgery with a Supplement on Mammaplasty and Other Operations in the Field of Plastic Surgery of the Body* (Phoenix: Columella Press, 1987), here pp. 21–24.

64. Jan Bialostocki, *Dürer and His Critics, 1500–1971: Chapters in the History of Ideas, Including a Collection of Texts* (Baden-Baden: V. Koerner, 1986).

65. Thus Joseph cited and reproduced images (p. 26) from Carl Heinrich Stratz, *Die Darstellung des menschlichen Körpers in der Kunst* (Berlin: J. Springer, 1914).

66. See Stephanie D'Alessandro, "'Über alles die Liebe': The History of Sexual Imagery

in the Art and Culture in the Weimar Republic" (Ph.D. diss., University of Chicago, 1997).

67. Pierre Bourdieu, *Sociology in Question*, trans. Richard Nice (London: Sage, 1993), p. 109.

68. Harold Gillies, *The Development and Scope of Plastic Surgery*, the Charles H. Mayo Lecture for 1934 (Chicago: Northwestern University, 1935), p. 1.

69. L. G. Farkas, J. C. Kolar, and I. R. Munro, "Geography of the Nose: A Morphometric Study," *Aesthetic and Plastic Surgery* 10 (1986): 191–223.

70. Charles Darwin, *The Descent of Man and Selection in Relation to Sex* (New York: D. Appleton, 1897), p. 585. See also John V. Pickstone, "Bureaucracy, Liberalism and the Body in Post-Revolutionary France: Bichat's Physiology and the Paris School of Medicine," *History of Science* 19 (1981): 115–42; as well as C. Heywood, "D. H. Lawrence's 'Blood Consciousness' and the Work of Xavier Bichat and Marshall Hall," *Études Anglaises, Grande-Bretagne–États-Unis* 32 (1979): 397–413.

71. James Hirsch, "Views on Beauty: When Artists Meet Surgeons," *New York Times*, June 20, 1988, p. B2. This view is not yet lost in the training of aesthetic surgeons. See A. D. Morani, "Art in Medical Education: Especially Plastic Surgery," *Aesthetic Plastic Surgery* 16 (1992): 213–18.

72. See my *Seeing the Insane* (Lincoln: University of Nebraska Press, 1996).

73. P. F. Johnson, "Racial Norms: Esthetic and Prosthodontic Implications." *Journal of Prosthetic Dentistry* 67 (1992): 502–8; A. Kiyak, "Psychosocial Predictors and Sequelae of Facial Change," *Journal of the Canadian Dental Association* 58 (1992): 459–62; and N. C. Cons and J. Jenny, "Comparing Perceptions of Dental Aesthetics in the USA with Those in Eleven Ethnic Groups," *International Dental Journal* 44 (1994): 489–94.

74. Charles H. Willi, *Facial Rejuvenation: How to Idealise the Features and the Skin of the Face by the Latest Scientific Methods* (London: Cecil Palmer, 1926), p. 100.

75. Natvig, *Jacques Joseph*, p. 71.

76. See the comments by Eugen Holländer, "Die kosmetische Chirurgie," in Max Joseph, ed., *Handbuch der Kosmetik* (Leipzig: Veit & Comp., 1912), pp. 669–712, here p. 673.

CHAPTER FIVE
NOSES AT WAR

1. Paul Natvig, *Jacques Joseph: Surgical Sculptor* (Philadelphia: W. B. Saunders, 1982), pp. 23–24, 177–80.

2. H. D. Gillies, *Plastic Surgery of the Face* (London: Oxford University Press / Hodder & Stoughton, 1920), p. 49.

3. "Plastic Surgery at the Queen's Hospital, Sidcup," *British Journal of Surgery* 9 (1921–22): 87–90; Reginald Pound, *Gillies, Surgeon Extraordinary* (London: M. Joseph, 1964).

4. Ernst Friedrich, *Krieg dem Kriege!* (1924; rpt. Frankfurt am Main: Zweitausendeins, 1980), pp. 204–27. See the context in Claudia Schmölders, "Welche Visage hat der Feind?" *Freibeuter* 64 (1995): 17–29.

5. Compare the representation of the rebuilt face on the allied side in World War I in Matthew Naythons, ed., *The Face of Mercy: A Photographic History of Medicine at War* (New York: Random House, 1993), pp. 152–58.

6. See the extraordinary images of the Turkish soldier whose face was literally obliterated in Jacques Joseph, "Ungewöhnlich große Gesichtsplastik," *Deutsche medizinische Wochenschrift* 44 (1918): 465–66.

7. Jacques W. Maliniak, *Sculpture in the Living: Rebuilding the Face and Form by Plastic Surgery* (New York: Romaine Pierson, 1934), p. 30.

8. Blair O. Rogers, "The First Pre- and Post-Operative Photographs of Plastic and Reconstructive Surgery: Contributions of Gurdon Buck (1807–1887)," *Aesthetic Plastic Surgery* 15 (1991): 19–33.

9. Kathy Newman, "Wounds and Wounding in the American Civil War: A (Visual) History," *Yale Journal of Criticism* 6 (1993): 63–86.

10. Ernest Hemingway, *A Moveable Feast* (New York: Charles Scribner's Sons, 1964), p. 197. See also D. J. Brain, "Facial Surgery during World War I," *Facial Plastic Surgery* 9 (1993): 157–64.

11. Harold Gillies, *The Development and Scope of Plastic Surgery* the Charles H. Mayo lecture for 1934 (Chicago: Northwestern University, 1935), p. 2.

12. The problem of the damaged body does not vanish in Hemingway's corpus. See John M. McLellan, "The Unrising Sun: The Theme of Castration in Hemingway and Sterne," *Studies in English Literature and Linguistics* 18 (1992): 51–61.

13. The best study of British attitudes on this topic is Joanna Bourke, *Dismembering the Male: Men's Bodies, Britain and the Great War* (London: Reaktion, 1996). On France, see Sophie Delaporte, *Les gueules cassées: Les blessés de la face de la Grande Guerre* (Paris: Noesis, 1996).

14. Carl Ferdinand von Graefe, *Rhinoplastik; oder, Die Kunst den Verlust der Nase organisch zu ersetzen, in ihren früheren Verhältnissen erforscht und durch neue Verfahrensweisen zur höheren Vollkommenheit gefördert* (Berlin: Realschulbuchhandlung, 1818), p. vi.

15. Adalbert G. Bettman, "The Psychology of Appearances," *Northwest Medicine* 28 (1929): 182–85, quotation on p. 184.

16. Hugh McLeave, *McIndoe: Plastic Surgeon* (London: Frederick Muller, 1961); Leonard Mosley, *Faces from the Fire: The Biography of Sir Archibald McIndoe* (London: Quality Book Club, 1962); and Peter Williams and Ted Harrison, *McIndoe's Army: The Injured Airmen Who Faced the World* (Leicester: Charnwood, 1981). See also Richard Battle, "Plastic Surgery in the Two World Wars and in the Years Between," *Journal of the Royal Society of Medicine* 71 (1978): 844–48.

17. Richard Hillary, *The Last Enemy* (1942; rpt. London, Macmillan, 1946). See Sebastian Faulks, *The Fatal Englishman: Three Short Lives* (London: Hutchinson, 1996).

18. Steven Totosy de Zepetnek, "*The English Patient:* 'Truth Is Stranger than Fiction,'" *Essays on Canadian Writing* 53 (1994): 141–53; Geetha Ganapathy-Dore, "The Novel of the Nowhere Man: Michael Ondaatje's *The English Patient*," *Commonwealth Essays and Studies* 16 (1993): 96–100; Geert Lernout, "Michael Ondaatje: The Desert of the Soul," *Kunapipi* 14 (1992): 124–26; and Maureen Garvie, "Listening to Michael Ondaatje," *Queen's Quarterly* 99 (1992): 928–34.

19. Dalton Trumbo, *Johnny Got His Gun* (New York: Monogram, 1939). See Leonard Kriegel, "Dalton Trumbo's *Johnny Got His Gun*," in David Madden, ed., *Proletarian Writers of the Thirties* (Carbondale: Southern Illinois University Press, 1968), pp. 106–13.

20. J. Howard Crum, *The Making of a Beautiful Face or Face Lifting Unveiled* (New York: Walton Book Company, 1928), p. 17.

21. Robert Alan Franklyn (as told to Alyce Canfield), *Beauty Surgeon* (Long Beach, Calif.: Whitehorn Publishing Company, 1960), p. 15. The popular reception of Joseph's very academic study of aesthetic surgery in Germany should not be underestimated. In the mass-circulation magazine *Das Magazin* 6 (April 1930): 4616–19, Werner Friedländer, a physician, published a review essay on noses and legs as the objects of aesthetic surgery under the title "Der liebe Gott wird korrigiert!" In fact, it is a review of Joseph's book.

22. Henry J. Schireson, *As Others See You: The Story of Plastic Surgery* (New York: Macaulay, 1938).

23. Maxwell Maltz, *Doctor Pygmalion: The Autobiography of a Plastic Surgeon* (London: Museum Press Limited, 1954), pp. 16–36, quotation on p. 17.

24. Leslie E. Gardiner, *Faces, Figures and Feelings: A Cosmetic Plastic Surgeon Speaks* (London: Leslie Gardiner, 1959), pp. 46–49.

25. George Sava (a.k.a. George Borodin and George Alexis Bankoff) was the most prolific popularizer of aesthetic surgery during the 1930s and 1940s. He was the author of some 150 volumes, including *Beauty from the Surgeon's Knife* (London: Faber and Faber, 1939); *Surgeon's Symphony* (London: Faber and Faber, [1945]); and *They Come by Appointment* (London: Right Book Club, 1947). His parallel today is the American surgeon Richard Selzer, who has also written on reconstructive surgery. See his "postmodern" version of the origins of rhinoplasty, which relies on the "modern" notion of graft rejection to frame the moral problem presented by Tagliacozzi, in Richard Selzer, "The Sympathetic Nose," in *Rituals of Surgery* (New York: Harper's Magazine Press, 1974), pp. 37–49.

26. Jean Boivin, *Beauty's Scalpel,* trans. Eileen Bigland (London: Jarrolds, 1958), p. 175.

27. Natvig, *Jacques Joseph,* p. 179.

28. Ernest Reinhold, "Martin Gumpert," in John M. Spalek and Joseph Strelka, eds., *Deutschsprachige Exilliteratur seit 1933, II: New York* (Bern: Francke, 1989), pp. 305–20.

29. All quotations are from Martin Gumpert, *Hölle im Paradies: Selbstdarstellung eines Arztes* (Stockholm: Bermann-Fischer, 1939), here on p. 211.

30. A. Noël, *La chirurgie esthétique: Son rôle social* (Paris: Masson, 1926).

31. Blair O. Rogers, "Hippolyte Morestin (1869–1919)," *Aesthetic and Plastic Surgery* 6 (1982): 141–47, quotation on p. 142.

32. Max Thorek, *A Surgeon's World: An Autobiography* (Philadelphia: J. B. Lippincott, 1943), pp. 19–43.

33. The mapping of ethnic identity onto the history of aesthetic surgery in Europe and the United States is part of the project of this study. The work of Sara Bershtel and Allen Graubard, *Saving Remnants: Feeling Jewish in America* (Berkeley and Los Angeles: University of California Press, 1992), presents a short history of ethnic identity in America that has been helpful in structuring my argument.

34. Robert M. Goldwyn, *Beyond Appearance: Reflections of a Plastic Surgeon* (New York: Dodd, Mead & Co., 1986), p. 11.

35. Janine Merlet, *Vénus et Mercure* (Paris: Éditions de la Vie Moderne, 1931), p. 167.

36. All in-text references are to Ludwig Lévy-Lenz, *Erinnerungen eines Sexual-Arztes: Aus den Memorien eines Sexologen* (Baden-Baden: Wadi-Verlagsbuchhandlung, 1954), here p. 455.

37. Rainer Herrn, "'Phantom Rasse: Ein Hirngespinst als Weltgefahr' Anmerkungen zum einem Aufsatz Magnus Hirschfelds," *Mitteilungen der Magnus Hirschfeld-Gesellschaft* 18 (1993): 53–62.

38. Friedrich von Zglinicki, "Die Sprechstunde: Soll ich zum kosmetischen Chirugen gehen?" *Die Ehe* (September 1933): 33.

39. Friedrich von Zglinicki, *Die Wiege der Traumfabrik: von Guckkasten, Zauberscheiben und bewegten Bildern bis zur UFA in Berlin* (Berlin: Transit, 1986).

40. Gertrude Atherton, *Black Oxen* (New York: Boni & Liveright, 1923), p. 215.

41. All quotations are from Ludwig Lévy-Lenz, *Die aufgeklärte Frau: Ein Buch für alle Frauen* (Berlin: Man Verlag, 1928).

42. Jacob Wassermann, *My Life as German and Jew* (London: George Allen & Unwin, 1933), p. 156.

43. Ibid.

44. Ludwig Lévy-Lenz, "Schönheits-Operation," *Die Ehe* (August 1933): 20–21.

45. Jacques Joseph, "Nasenverkleinerungen," *Deutsche medizinische Wochenschrift* 30 (1904): 1095–98, here p. 1095; cited from Frank McDowell, ed., *The Source Book of Plastic Surgery* (Baltimore: Williams & Wilkins, 1977), pp. 174–76, here p. 184.

46. Natvig, *Jacques Joseph,* p. 94.

47. See Fridolf Kudlien and Christian Andree, "Sauerbruch und der Nationalsozialis-mus," *Medizinhistorisches Journal* 15 (1980): 202–22.

48. McLeave, *McIndoe*, pp. 65–66. The original account of this is in Harold Gillies and D. Ralph Millard, *The Principles and Art of Plastic Surgery*, 2 vols. (London: Butterworth, 1957), 1:104–11.

49. See Michael H. Kater, *Doctors under Hitler* (Chapel Hill: University of North Car-olina Press, 1989). See also Fridolf Kudlein, *Ärzte im Nationalsozialismus* (Cologne: Kiepen-heuer & Witsch, 1985); *Medizin im Nationalsozialismus* (Munich: R. Oldenbourg, 1988); Jo-hanna Bleker and Norbert Jachertz, eds., *Medizin im Dritten Reich* (Cologne: Deutscher Ärzte Verlag, 1989); Achim Thom and Genadij Caregorodcev, eds., *Medizin unterm Hak-enkreuz* (Berlin: VEB Volk und Gesundheit, 1989); Gerrit Hohendorf and Achim Magull-Seltenreich, eds., *Von der Heilkunde zur Massentötung: Medizin im Nationalsozialismus* (Hei-delberg: Wunderhorn, 1990); Sabine Fahrenbach and Achim Thom, eds., *Der Arzt als "Gesundheitsführer"* (Frankfurt a. M.: Mabuse, 1991); and Christoph Meinel and Peter Voswinckel, eds., *Medizin, Naturwissenschaft, Technik und Nationalsozialismus: Kontinuitäten und Diskontinuitäten* (Stuttgart: Verlag für Geschichte der Naturwissenschaften und der Technik, 1994).

50. The most recent, detailed account of Hitler's upbringing and his real and imagined experience of Jews in Linz and Vienna is Brigitte Hamann, *Hitlers Wien: Lehrjahre eines Dik-tators* (Munich: Piper, 1996).

51. Gillies, *Development and Scope of Plastic Surgery*, p. 1.

52. The proceedings are printed in *Archiv für klinische Chirugie* 193 (1938); Verschuer et al. on pp. 3–40. See Henry Friedlander, *The Origins of Nazi Genocide: From Euthanasia to the Final Solution* (Chapel Hill: University of North Carolina Press, 1995).

53. Martin Gumpert, *Heil Hunger! Health under Hitler*, trans. Maurice Samuels (New York: Alliance Book, 1940), pp. 105–6.

54. Schireson, *As Others See You*, p. 141.

55. Joseph Goebbels, *The Goebbels Diaries*, trans. Louis P. Lochner (London: H. Hamil-ton, 1948), p. 367. On women in the Third Reich, see Jill Stephenson, *Women in Nazi Soci-ety* (London: Croom Helm, 1975); Martin Broszat, Elke Fröhlich, and Falk Wiesemann, eds., *Bayern in der NS-Zeit: soziale Lage und politisches Verhalten der Bevölkerung im Spiegel vertraulicher Berichte* (Munich: R. Oldenbourg, 1977); Jill Stephenson, *The Nazi Organiza-tion of Women* (London: Croom Helm, 1981); Gerda Szepansky, ed., *Frauen leisten Wider-stand: 1933–1945: Lebensgeschichten nach Interviews und Dokumenten* (1983; rpt. Frankfurt am Main: Fischer Taschenbuch, 1994); Renate Bridenthal, Atina Grossmann, and Marion Kaplan, *When Biology Became Destiny: Women in Weimar and Nazi Germany* (New York: Monthly Review Press, 1984); Claudia Koonz, *Mothers in the Fatherland: Women, the Fam-ily and Nazi Politics* (New York: St. Martin's Press, 1987); Atina Grossmann, *Reforming Sex: The German Movement for Birth Control and Abortion Reform, 1920–1950* (New York: Oxford University Press, 1995); and Alison Owings, ed., *Frauen: German Women Recall the Third Reich* (New Brunswick, N.J.: Rutgers University Press, 1995).

56. "Promoting Pulchritude under Nazism," *Journal of the American Medical Association* 114 (1940): 70.

57. All quotations are from Natvig, *Jacques Joseph*, here p. 95.

58. Wilhelm Stekel, *Compulsion and Doubt*, trans. Emil A. Gutheil (New York: Liveright, 1949), 2:587–88.

59. Alfred Berndorfer, "Aesthetic Surgery as Organopsychic Therapy," *Aesthetic Plastic Surgery* 3 (1979): 143–46, quotation on pp. 144–45.

60. Georg Mannheimer, *Lieder eines Juden* (Prague: Neumann & Co., 1937), p. 31.

61. Hans Franck in a memorandum quoted in G. M. Gilbert, *The Psychology of Dictator-ship: Based on an Examination of the Leaders of Germany* (New York: Ronald Press Co., 1950), p. 48.

62. Edgar Hilsenrath, *The Nazi and the Barber,* trans. Andrew White (Garden City, N.Y.: Doubleday, 1971); and Hilsenrath, *Der Nazi und der Friseur* (Cologne: Literarischer Verlag Braun, 1977). See my "Hilsenrath und Grass Redivivus," in Thomas Kraft, ed., *Edgar Hilsenrath: Das Unerzählbare erzählen* (Munich: Piper, 1995), pp. 119–27.

63. Dick Sheridan, "Finally, Justice on the Gallows," *Daily News* (New York), May 14, 1995, p. 26.

64. Press Association Newsfile, April 20, 1993.

65. M. G. Lord, "A Hitler in Their Own Backyard?" *Newsday,* March 3, 1991, p. 38.

66. Richard Cohen, "GOP Played Race Card and Won David Duke," *St. Louis Post-Dispatch,* October 24, 1991, p. 3C.

67. "Didn't Kill Doctor, Nazi Sympathizer Says," *Times-Picayune,* September 23, 1993, p. A7.

Chapter Six
Assimilation in the Promised Lands

1. Rudolf Virchow, "Gesamtbericht über die Farbe der Haut, der Haare und der Augen der Schulkinder in Deutschland," *Archiv für Anthropologie* 16 (1886): 275–475.

2. George L. Mosse, *Toward the Final Solution: A History of European Racism* (New York: Howard Fertig, 1975), pp. 90–91.

3. This report was submitted to Congress on December 3, 1910, and issued on March 17, 1911. Columbia University Press published a full text in 1912. Franz Boas summarized his findings (and chronicled the objections to this report) in his *Race, Language and Culture* (New York: Macmillan, 1940), pp. 60–75.

4. Boas, *Race, Language and Culture,* p. 83.

5. Karl Shapiro, "Jew," in *V Letter and Other Poems* (New York: Harcourt, Brace & Co., 1944), p. 27.

6. Carl Rakosi, *The Collected Poems of Carl Rakosi* (Orono, Maine: National Poetry Foundation, University of Maine, 1986), p. 116.

7. Paul Celan, "Eine Gauner- und Ganovenweise," from *Die Niemandsrose* (1963), reprinted in Paul Celan, *Gesammelte Werke,* 5 vols. (Frankfurt: Suhrkamp, 1986), 1:229.

8. Hugh McLeave, *McIndoe: Plastic Surgeon* (London: Frederick Muller, 1961), p. 62.

9. "Retouching Nature's Way: Is Cosmetic Surgery Worth It?" *Toronto Star,* February 1, 1990.

10. Robert M. Goldwyn, *Beyond Appearance: Reflections of a Plastic Surgeon* (New York: Dodd, Mead & Co., 1986), p. 92.

11. Philip Roth, *American Pastoral* (Boston: Houghton Mifflin, 1997).

12. Ernest Hemingway, *The Sun Also Rises* (New York: Charles Scribner's Sons, 1954), p. 4. See Michael S. Reynolds, *The Sun Also Rises: A Novel of the Twenties* (Boston, Mass.: Twayne Publishers, 1995).

13. Maurice Fishberg, *The Jews: A Study of Race and Environment* (London: Walter Scott Publishing Co., 1911).

14. Joseph Jacobs, *Studies in Jewish Statistics, Social, Vital and Anthropometric* (London: D. Nutt, 1891), p. xxxii.

15. John R. Baker, *Race* (New York: Oxford University Press, 1974), p. 241.

16. Gordon Allport and Bernard M. Kramer, "Some Roots of Prejudice," *Journal of Psychology* 22 (1946): 9–39. See also Frederick H. Lund and Wilner C. Berg, "Identifiability of Nationality Characteristics," *Journal of Social Psychology* 24 (1946): 77–83; Launor F. Carter, "The Identification of 'Racial' Membership," *Journal of Abnormal and Social Psychology* 43 (1948): 279–86; Gardner Lindzey and Saul Rogolsky, "Prejudice and Identification of Minority Group Membership," *Journal of Abnormal and Social Psychology* 45 (1950): 37–53; and

Donald N. Elliott and Bernard H. Wittenberg, "Accuracy of Identification of Jewish and Non-Jewish Photographs," *Journal of Abnormal and Social Psychology* 51 (1955): 339–41.

17. Leonard D. Savitz and Richard F. Tomasson, "The Identifiability of Jews," *American Journal of Sociology* 64 (1958): 468–75.

18. Alvin Scodel and Harvey Austrin, "The Perception of Jewish Photographs by Non-Jews and Jews," *Journal of Abnormal and Social Psychology* 54 (1957): 278–80.

19. Frances Cooke Macgregor, "Social, Psychological and Cultural Dimensions of Cosmetic and Reconstructive Plastic Surgery," *Aesthetic Plastic Surgery* 13 (1989): 1–8, here p. 1.

20. See the discussion in Joseph G. McCarthy, ed., *Plastic Surgery,* 4 vols. (Philadelphia: W. B. Saunders, 1990), 1:122–24.

21. Eugene Meyer, Wayne E. Jacobson, Milton T. Edgerton, and Arthur Canter, "Motivational Patterns in Patients Seeking Elective Plastic Surgery," *Psychosomatic Medicine* 22 (1960): 193–203, quotation on p. 197.

22. Herbert Lindenberger, "Between Texts: From Assimilationist Novel to Resistance Novel," *Jewish Social Studies* 1 (1995): 48–68, quotation on p. 51.

23. See my *Smart Jews: The Construction of the Idea of Jewish Superior Intelligence at the Other End of the Bell Curve,* the inaugural Abraham Lincoln Lectures (Lincoln: University of Nebraska Press, 1996).

24. Immanuel Jakobovits, "Jewish Views on Cosmetic Surgery," *Eye, Ear, Nose and Throat Monthly* 41 (1962): 133–34, 142, and 220–21; quotation on pp. 133–34.

25. J. David Bleich, *Judaism and Healing: Halakhic Perspectives* (New York: KTAV, 1981), pp. 126–28, here p. 127.

26. Ibid., p. 126.

27. Douglas Danoff, "Jews Lose Tattoos Taboos," *Jerusalem Post,* February 7, 1996, p. 7.

28. P. Morrisroe, "Forever Young: Plastic Surgery on the Fast Track," *N.Y. Magazine,* June 9, 1989, pp. 43–50, quotation on p. 47. See also the discussion in David A. Hyman, "Aesthetics and Ethics: The Implications of Cosmetic Surgery," *Perspectives in Biology and Medicine* 33 (1990): 190–202.

29. Frances Cooke Macgregor, *Transformation and Identity: The Face and Plastic Surgery* (New York: Quadrangle Press / New York Times Book Company, 1974), pp. 89–90.

30. Helen Fielding, "If the Face Doesn't Fit Is Plastic Too Drastic?" *Sunday Times,* February 3, 1991, p. E7.

31. Matt Moffett, "In Mexico, the Rich Hasten to Turn Up Noses—Surgically," *Wall Street Journal,* October 27, 1988, section 1, p. 1.

32. "Riding the New Mexican Wave, Latin-Style Thatcherism Helps Forge an Economic Miracle," *Sunday Telegraph,* February 14, 1993, p. 18.

33. Mark Gorney, "Patient Selection and Medicolegal Responsibility for the Rhinoplasty Patient," in Thomas D. Ress, ed., *Rhinoplasty: Problems and Controversies* (St. Louis: C. V. Mosby, 1988), p. 2.

34. Jean-Paul Sartre, *Anti-Semite and Jew,* trans. George J. Becker (New York: Schocken Books, 1965), p. 119.

35. Marissa Piesman, *Heading Uptown* (New York: Dell, 1993), p. 13.

36. Sue Fishkoff, "Body Beautiful," *Jerusalem Post,* October 11, 1996, p. 8.

37. Orthodox Jews are for the most part freed from military obligation. They also recognize the ban on aesthetic surgery. Thus the discussion about altering the body prior to military service does not include them. Secularized Jews are generally unconcerned by such religious prohibitions against aesthetic surgery.

38. Rafael Moses, "Projection, Identification, Projective Identification: Their Relation to the Political Process," in Joseph Sandler, ed., *Projection, Identification, Projective Identification* (London: Karnac, 1989), pp. 133–51.

39. Judy Siegel Itzkovich, "Do Our Patients Heal More Slowly?" *Jerusalem Post,* April 12, 1990, p. 1.

40. Agence France Presse, February 18, 1997, 18:13 GMT.

41. For example, see the discussion of "special considerations" in Eugene H. Courtiss, ed., *Male Aesthetic Surgery* (St. Louis: Mosby, 1991), pp. 159–88; as well as Elisabeth Rosenthal, "Ethnic Ideals: Rethinking Plastic Surgery," *New York Times,* September 25, 1991, p. C1.

42. Leslie A. Fiedler, "The Tyranny of the Normal" (1978), reprinted in Carol Donley and Sheryl Buckley, eds., *The Tyranny of the Normal: An Anthology* (Kent, Ohio: Kent State University Press, 1996), p. 9.

43. *Too Jewish? Challenging Traditional Identities,* ed. Norman L. Kleeblatt (New York: Jewish Museum, 1996).

44. Rae Burczyk, "Ugliness Is in the Eyes of the Beholder," *Charleston Gazette,* January 22, 1997, p. 7.

45. Quoted in the *Washington Times,* January 3, 1997, p. A2

46. Dave Eggers, "Jews R Us," *SF Weekly,* December 4, 1996.

47. Victoria Dalkey, "Too Jewish?' Raises Provocative Questions," *Sacramento Bee,* November 10, 1996, p. C7.

48. During the Philadelphia tryout of "I Can Get It for You Wholesale," the featured performer playing "Miss Marmelstein" asked her agent: "Should I get a nose job?" "No," he claims to have said to Streisand. Richard L. Coe, "Press Agentry Made Easy," *Washington Post,* August 14, 1977, p. E1.

49. Henry J. Schireson, *As Others See You: The Story of Plastic Surgery* (New York: Macaulay, 1938), p. 87.

50. Norman Katkov, *The Fabulous Fanny* (New York: Alfred A. Knopf, 1953), p. 141; *New York Times,* August 15, 1923, section 10, p. 3.

Chapter Seven
After the Nose

1. Eduard Zeis, *Handbuch der plastischen Chirurgie* (Berlin: G. Reimer, 1838). All citations from this will be to the translation by T. J. S. Patterson, *Zeis' Manual of Plastic Surgery* (Oxford: Oxford University Press, 1988), p. 55.

2. See my *Sexuality: An Illustrated History* (New York: John Wiley, 1989).

3. "The construction of stable bodily contours relies upon fixed sites of corporeal permeability and impermeability. . . . The deregulation of such (heterosexual) exchanges accordingly disrupts the very boundaries that determine what it is to be a body at all." (pp. 132–33) "If gender is not tied to sex, either casually or expressively, then gender is a kind of action that can potentially proliferate beyond the binary limits imposed by the apparent binary of sex" (p. 112). Judith Butler, *Gender Trouble: Feminism and the Subversion of Identity* (New York: Routledge, 1990).

4. Daniel Boyarin, *A Radical Jew: Paul and the Politics of Identity* (Berkeley and Los Angeles: University of California Press, 1994).

5. Christina von Braun, "Die Erotik des Kunstkörpers," in Irmgard Roebling, ed., *Lulu, Lilith, Mona Lisa . . . Frauenbilder der Jahrhundertwende* (Pfaffenweiler: Centaurus-Verlagsgesellschaft, 1988), pp. 1–17.

6. Harold Gillies, *The Development and Scope of Plastic Surgery,* the Charles H. Mayo lecture for 1934 (Chicago: Northwestern University, 1935), pp. 26, 31.

7. H. W. Losken, "Psychological Aspects of Breast Surgery," *Aesthetic Plastic Surgery* 14 (1990): 107–9, quotation on p. 109.

8. "Dance: Ten; Looks: Three," from Marvin Hamlisch and Edward Kleban, *A Chorus Line* (New York: E. H. Morris; C. Hansen, distributor, 1975).

9. Charles Darwin, *The Descent of Man and Selection in Relation to Sex* (New York: D. Appleton, 1897), p. 579.

10. The debates about the meaning of the mammae and their defining force in determining the very nature of the "mammal" has been well documented by Londa Schiebinger in her *Nature's Body: Gender in the Making of Modern Science* (Boston: Beacon Press, 1993).

11. See the anonymous "Sahrah, die Hottentottenvenus," *Die Ehe* 7 (April 1, 1933): 102–4. According to the note, this is most probably by Hirschfeld, who edited this journal.

12. Bernadette Bucher, *Icon and Conquest: A Structural Analysis of the Illustrations of de Bry's Great Voyages,* trans. Basia Miller Gulati (Chicago: University of Chicago Press, 1981).

13. Havelock Ellis, *Studies in the Psychology of Sex,* volume 7, *Eonism and Other Supplementary Studies* (Philadelphia: F. A. Davis, 1928), pp. 126–99.

14. See my *Difference and Pathology: Stereotypes of Sexuality, Race, and Madness* (Ithaca, N.Y.: Cornell University Press, 1985); as well as Jean Luc Hennig, *The Rear View: A Brief and Elegant History of Bottoms through the Ages,* trans. Margaret Crosland and Elfreda Powell (London: Souvenir Press, 1995).

15. J. Agris, "Use of Dermal Fat Suspension Flaps for Thigh and Buttock Lift," *Plastic and Reconstructive Surgery* 59 (1977): 817.

16. Ivo Pitanguy, *Aesthetic Plastic Surgery of Head and Body* (Berlin—Heidelberg—New York: Springer, 1981).

17. Martha Gil-Montero, "Ivo Pitanguy: Master of Artful Surgery," *Americas* 43 (1991): 24.

18. Ricardo Baroudi, "Why Aesthetic Plastic Surgery Became Popular in Brazil?" *Plastic Surgery* 27 (1991): 396–97.

19. Raul Loeb, *História da cirugia plástica brasileira* (Sao Paulo: Medsi, 1993).

20. C. M. Lewis, "Early History of Lipoplasty in the United States," *Aesthetic Plastic Surgery* 14 (1990): 123–26; and B. E. Burnham, "Notes on the History of the Adoption of Liposuction," *Plastic and Reconstructive Surgery* 97 (1996): 258–59.

21. Francis M. Otteni and Pierre F. Fournier, "A History and Comparison of Suction Techniques until Their Debut in North America," in Gregory P. Hetter, *Lipoplasty: The Theory and Practice of Blunt Section Lipectomy* (Boston: Little, Brown, 1984) , pp. 19–23.

22. A detailed history of "Thighplasty" with comments is to be found in Frederick M. Grazer and Jerome R. Klingbeil, *Body Image: A Surgical Perspective* (St. Louis: C. V. Mosby, 1980), pp. 238–44, here p. 238.

23. Lewis, "Early History of Lipoplasty in the United States," p. 123.

24. Yves-Gerard Illouz, "The Origins of Lipolysis," in Hetter, *Lipoplasty,* pp. 25–33, quotation on p. 25. See also Illouz's *La sculpture chirurgicale de la silhouette* (Edinburgh: Churchill Livingstone, 1988).

25. All quotations are from Ricardo Baroudi and Mario Moraes, "Philosophy, Technical Principles, Selection, and Indication in Body Contouring Surgery," *Aesthetic Plastic Surgery* 15 (1991): 1–18, here p. 1.

26. Raymond Vilain and Jean-Claude Dardour, "Aesthetic Surgery of the Medial Thigh," *Annals of Plastic Surgery* 17 (1986): 176–83; and Stephen C. Drukker, "Transverse Flank-Thigh-Buttock Lift with Superficial Fascial Suspension," *Plastic and Reconstructive Surgery* 87 (1991): 1019–27.

27. Marilyn Yalom, *A History of the Breast* (New York: Knopf, 1997), pp. 205–40.

28. Hans May, "Scope and Problems of Plastic Surgery," *Pennsylvania Medical Journal* 42 (1939): 1457–58.

29. Maxwell Maltz, *New Faces, New Futures: Rebuilding Character with Plastic Surgery* (New York: Richard R. Smith, 1936), p. 34.

30. *People,* December 4, 1994, p. 12.

31. *Sunday Mirror* (London), July 28, 1996, p. 12.

32. Ernst Brücke, *Schönheit und Fehler der menschlichen Gestalt* (Vienna: Wilhelm Braumüller, 1893), p. 71.

33. Friedrich S. Krauss, *Die Anmut des Frauenleibes* (Leipzig: A. Schumann, 1904).

34. All quotations are from Heinrich Ploss and Max Barthel, *Das Weib in der Natur- und Völkerkunde,* 2 vols., 9th ed. (Leipzig: Th. Grieben, 1908). See also Paula Weideger, *History's Mistress: A New Interpretation of a Nineteenth-Century Ethnographic Classic* (Harmondsworth: Penguin Books; New York: Viking Penguin, 1985).

35. Hans Friedenthal, "Muttersprache and Mutterbrust," *Die Ehe* 2 (1927): 135–39. See also Friedenthal's *Menschheitskunde* (Leipzig: Quelle & Meyer, 1927).

36. Jacques Joseph, *Rhinoplasty and Facial Plastic Surgery with a Supplement on Mammaplasty and Other Operations in the Field of Plastic Surgery of the Body,* trans. Stanley Milstein (Phoenix: Columella Press, 1987), p. 743.

37. Hans F. K. Günther, *Rassenkunde des jüdischen Volkes* (Munich: J. F. Lehmann, 1930), pp. 164–65.

38. Simona de Logu, "Plastic Surgery Gets Boost in Brazil," *Reuters,* December 6, 1996.

39. Michael George Hanchard, *Orpheus and Power: The Movimento Negro of Rio de Janeiro and Sao Paulo, Brazil, 1945–1988* (Princeton, N.J.: Princeton University Press, 1994); and Gregor Burkhart, *Die Kinder Omulus: der Einfluss afrobrasilianischer Kultur auf die Wahrnehmung von Körper und Krankheit* (Frankfurt am Main; New York: P. Lang, 1994).

40. Aesthetic surgery in the United States continues to be a sort of holiday present, if just to oneself. The American Academy of Facial Plastic and Reconstructive Surgery found its members performed 7,140 nose jobs nationwide in the last two weeks of 1993, compared with 3,920 in the average two-week period. The increase has been attributed to the seasonal vacation time, but it has also to be seen in terms of the idea of aesthetic surgery as a gift. "Outliers: Asides and Insides on Healthcare," *Modern Healthcare* (January 6, 1997): 60.

41. Quoted by William R. Long, "Rio Cultists: Good Looks at the Beach," *Los Angeles Times,* August 15, 1987, section 1, p. 1. See also Roberto Da Matta, *Carnivals, Rogues, and Heroes: An Interpretation of the Brazilian Dilemma,* trans. John Drury (Notre Dame, Ind.: University of Notre Dame Press, 1991).

42. Robert M. Goldwyn, *Beyond Appearance: Reflections of a Plastic Surgeon* (New York: Dodd, Mead & Co., 1986), p. 175.

43. *Le Monde,* September 2, 1988, cited by Yalom, *A History of the Breast,* p. 236.

44. Amaranta Wright, "In Argentina, Cosmetic Surgery Tops Popular Conversation Topics," *Dallas Morning News,* May 26, 1996.

45. Luis Majul, *Las mascaras de la Argentina: Cambios esteticos, patrimoniales, psicologicos e ideologicos de los argentinos que estan en la vidriera* (Buenos Aires: Atlantida, 1995).

46. See the general discussion in J. P. Lalardrie and R. Mouly, "History of Mammaplasty," in Mario González-Ulloa, ed., *The Creation of Aesthetic Plastic Surgery* (New York: Springer, 1976), pp. 135–44.

47. *The Seven Books of Paulus Agineta. With a commentary embracing a complete view of the knowledge possessed by the Greeks, Romans, and Arabians on all subjects connected with medicine and surgery,* trans. Frances Adams, 3 vols. (London: Printed for the Sydenham Society, 1844–47), here 2:329.

48. Theodor Billroth, *Chirurgische Klinik, Wien, 1868 [1869–1876] Erfahrungen aus dem Gebiete der praktischen Chirurgie,* 3 vols. (Berlin: Hirschwald, 1870–79).

49. [Alfred] Pousson, "De la mastopexie," *Bulletins et mémoires de la société de chirurgie de Paris* 23 (1897): 507–8.

50. Hippolyte Morestin, "De l'ablation esthétique des tumeurs bénignes du sein," *Presse médicale* 10 (1902): 975–77.

51. The history of breast reduction is given in Joseph, *Rhinoplasty and Facial Plastic Surgery*, pp. 748–52; and in Antony F. Wallace, *The Progress of Plastic Surgery: An Introductory History* (Oxford: Willem A. Meeuws, 1982), pp. 155–59. On the history of nipple transplantation, see Antonio Duarte Cardoso, Mario Cezar Pessanha, and Julio Montalvan Peralta, "Three Dermal Pedicles for Nipple-Areola Complex Movement in Reduction of Gigantomastia," *Annals of Plastic Surgery* 12 (1984): 419–27. On the history of surgical procedures, see T. D. Rees, "Plastic Surgery of the Breast," in John Marquis Converse, ed., *Reconstructive Plastic Surgery*, 7 vols. (Philadelphia: W. B. Saunders, 1977), 7:3661–3710.

52. Jacques Joseph, "Für Operation der Hipertrophichen Hängebrust," *Deutsche Medizinische Wochenschrift* 51 (1925):1103–5.

53. Goldwyn, *Beyond Appearance*, p. 194.

54. Ludwig Lévy-Lenz, "Schönheits-Operation," *Die Ehe* (August 1933): 20–21.

55. Richard Klein, *Eat Fat* (New York: Pantheon, 1996). See also Susan Bordo, *Unbearable Weight: Feminism, Western Culture, and the Body* (Berkeley and Los Angeles: University of California Press, 1993); Kim Chernin, *The Obsession: Reflections on the Tyranny of Slenderness* (New York: Harper Perennial, 1994); and Sharlene Hesse-Biber, *Am I Thin Enough Yet: The Cult of Thinness and the Commercialization of Identity* (New York: Oxford University Press, 1996).

56. See my *Franz Kafka: The Jewish Patient* (New York: Routledge, 1995).

57. Paule Regnault, "The History of Abdominal Dermolipectomy," in González-Ulloa, *Creation of Aesthetic Plastic Surgery*, pp. 145–55.

58. H. A. Kelly, "Excessive Growth of Fat," *Bulletin of the Johns Hopkins Hospital* 10 (1899): 197. A detailed follow-up on Kelly's patient is to be found in Lindsay Peters, "Resection of the Pendulous, Fat Abdominal Wall in Cases of Extreme Obesity," *Annals of Surgery* 33 (1901): 299–304. All subsequent quotations are from the Peters follow-up article.

59. Hans F. K. Günther, *Rassenkunde des jüdischen Volkes* (Munich: J. F. Lehmann, 1930), p. 247.

60. Fritz Felgenhauer, *Willendorf in der Wachau: Monographie der Paläolith-Fundstellen I-VII*, 3 vols. (Vienna: R. M. Rohrer, 1956–59), 1:11.

61. Albert Edward Wiggam, *The Fruit of the Family Tree* (Garden City, N.Y.: Garden City Publishing, 1924), pp. 262, 272.

62. Peters, "Resection of the Pendulous, Fat Abdominal Wall," p. 303.

63. A detailed history of "Abdominoplasty" with comments is to be found in Grazer and Klingbeil, *Body Image*, pp. 63–80, quotation on p. 63.

64. Max Thorek, "Possibilities of the Reconstruction of the Human Form," *New York Medical Journal* 116 (1922): 572–75.

65. Max Thorek, *A Surgeon's World: An Autobiography* (Philadelphia: J. B. Lippincott, 1943), p. 167.

66. S. Vernon, "Umbilical Transplantation Upward and Abdominal Contouring in Lipectomy," *American Journal of Surgery* 94 (1957): 490–92.

67. I. Pitanguy, "Abdominal Lipectomy: An Approach to It through an Analysis of 300 Consecutive Cases," *Plastic Reconstructive Surgery* 40 (1967): 383–91.

68. John F. Pick, *Surgery of Repair: Principles, Problems, Procedures*, 2 vols. (Philadelphia: J. B. Lippincott, 1949), 2:445.

69. Suzanne Moore, "Rip the `Real' Roseanne," *The Guardian*, May 28, 1993, p. 14.

70. Illouz, "Origins of Lipolysis," p. 25.

71. Many of the claims for the "happiness" of the augmentation mammaplasty patient prior to the discussions about the implants are to be found in Judith Collins Knight, "Body,

Image, Self-Concept and the Effects of Augmentation Mammaplasty" (Ph.D. diss., University of South Florida, 1982); Laurie A. Stevens, "The Psychological Aspects of Breast Surgery," in Richard S. Blacher, ed., *The Psychological Experience of Surgery* (New York: John Wiley & Sons, 1987), pp. 87–97; Losken, "Psychological Aspects of Breast Surgery"; and Sandra Birtchnell, Patrick Whitfield, and J. Hubert Lacey, "Motivational Factors in Women Requesting Augmentation and Reduction Mammaplasty," *Journal of Psychosomatic Research* 34 (1990): 509–14.

72. *U.S. News & World Report* 117 (October 17, 1994): 15.

73. Henry Junius Schireson, *As Others See You: The Story of Plastic Surgery* (New York: Macaulay, 1938), pp. 218–26.

74. Marguerite Clark, "Breast Surgery," *McCalls* 75 (1948): 2.

75. H. O. Bames, "Breast Malformations and a New Approach to the Problem of the Small Breast," *Plastic and Reconstructive Surgery* 5 (1950): 499.

76. A. S. Braley, "The Use of Silicone in Plastic Surgery: A Retrospective View," *Plastic Reconstructive Surgery* 51 (1973): 280–88.

77. E. S. Truppman and B. M. Schwarz, "Aesthetic Breast Surgery," *Journal of the Florida Medical Association* 76 (1989): 609–12.

78. These are the American Society for Plastic and Reconstructive Surgery's statistics, which only cover procedures undertaken by the members of that society. From the society's website: www.plasticsurgery.org.

79. "1996 ASPRS National Plastic Surgery Procedural," *PR Newswire,* April 28, 1997.

80. Diana Sugg, "Breast Implants, Illness Linked, UCD Study Hints," *Sacramento Bee,* March 15, 1993, p. A1.

81. "FDA Bowed to Media Hype in Banning Implants," *San Diego Union-Tribune,* January 11, 1992, p. B13.

82. Jane Gross, "Recipients of Breast Implants Split on Need for U.S. Controls," *New York Times,* November 5, 1991, p. A1.

83. See Gordon Letterman and Maxine Schurter, "A History of Augmentation Mammaplasty," in Nicolas G. Georgiade, Gregory S. Georgiade, and Ronald Riefkohl, eds., *Aesthetic Surgery of the Breast* (Philadelphia: W. B. Saunders, 1990), pp. 41–48, here p. 44. See also Joan Austoker, "The 'Treatment of Choice': Breast Cancer Surgery, 1860–1985," *Society for the Social History of Medicine Bulletin* 37 (1985): 100–107; Pamela Sanders-Goebel, "Crisis and Controversy: Historical Patterns in Breast Cancer Surgery," *Canadian Bulletin of Medical History* 8 (1991): 77–90; as well as Jean Coates Cleary, "Myth, Misogyny and the Mastectomy: The Bad Breast in Women's Fiction and Culture, 1761–1814," *Transactions of the International Congress on the Enlightenment* 8 (1992): 818–21.

84. Tom Steadman, "Man Reveals His Story of Breast Cancer," *News & Record* (Greensboro, N.C.), October 31, 1996, p. A1.

85. S. Rosenfeld, "Penile Implant Maker Sued: Health Problems, Defects Concealed, Three Men Allege," *San Francisco Examiner,* May 21, 1994, p. A1.

86. "Explosive Market Growth Forecast in Soft Tissue Implant Industry," *Hospitals* 59 (1985): 74.

87. See Marcia Angell, *Science on Trial: The Clash of Medical Evidence and the Law in the Breast Implant Case* (New York: W. W. Norton, 1996).

88. Quotations are from D. A. Kessler, R. B. Merkatz, and R. Shapiro, "A Call for Higher Standards for Breast Implants," *Journal of the American Medical Association* 270 (1993): 2607–8. The alternative view was stated in a collective piece by the American Medical Association's Council on Scientific Affairs, "Silicone Breast Implants," *Journal of the American Medical Association* 270 (1993): 2602–6.

89. Lennart Meyer, "On Acceptance of Appearance and Shape after Plastic Surgery. The Use of Psychiatric and Psychosocial Evaluation in Plastic Surgery: Methodological As-

pects and Clinical Applications (Mastectomy, Adaptation)" (Diss., University of Malmo, 1987).

90. Audre Lorde, *The Cancer Journals* (Argyle, N.Y.: Spinsters, Ink, 1980). See also Theresa Laurel Brown, "Storytelling and Trauma: Gender, Identity, and Testimony in a Contemporary Context" (Ph.D. diss., University of Chicago, 1995); Elizabeth Alexander, "`Coming Out Blackened and Whole': Fragmentation and Reintegration in Audre Lorde's *Zami* and *The Cancer Journals*," *American Literary History* 6 (1994): 695–715; G. Thomas Couser, "Autopathography: Women, Illness, and Lifewriting," *A/B: Auto/Biography Studies* 6 (1991): 65–75; and Jeanne Perreault, "`That the pain not be wasted': Audre Lorde and the Written Self," *A/B: Auto/Biography Studies* 4 (1988): 1–16.

91. Jean Dykstra, "Putting Herself in the Picture: Autobiographical Images of Illness and the Body," *Afterimage* 23 (1995): 16–20.

92. Don Hopey, "Saying Thanks to the Activists: Breast Cancer Victims Gain Another Voice," *Pittsburgh Post-Gazette*, April 11, 1994, p. A7.

93. Elizabeth Predeger, "Womanspirit: A Journey into Healing through Art in Breast Cancer," *Advances in Nursing Science* 18 (1996): 48.

94. Gina Kolata, "Judge Dismisses Implant Evidence," *New York Times*, December 19, 1996, p. 1.

95. S. E. Gabriel et al., "Risk of Connective-Tissue Diseases and Other Disorders after Breast Implantation," *New England Journal of Medicine* 330 (1994): 1697–1702.

96. Marsha L. Vanderford and David H. Smith, *The Silicone Breast Implant Story* (Mahwah, N.J.: Lawrence Erlbaum, 1996), p. 25.

97. Ibid., p. 16.

98. Robert Gersuny, "Über eine subcutane Prothese," *Zeitschrift für Heilkunde* 21 (1900): 199–204.

99. Robert Gersuny, "Über einige kosmetische Operationen," *Wiener Medizinische Wochenschrift* 53 (1903): col. 2253–57, here col. 2256. See G. Matton, A. Anseeuw, and F. De Keyser, "The History of Injectable Biomaterials and the Biology of Collagen," *Aesthetic Plastic Surgery* 9 (1985): 133–40.

100. Martin Bartels, "Zur Fetttransplantation in die Orbita," *Archiv für Augenheilkunde* 67 (1910): 1–24 (with a survey of the earlier literature); and Charles H. Willi, *Facial Rejuvenation: How to Idealise the Features and the Skin of the Face by the Latest Scientific Methods* (London: Cecil Palmer, 1926), pp. 86–93. See L. J. Ludovici, *Cosmetic Scalpel: The Life of Charles Willi, Beauty-Surgeon* (London: Moonraker Press, 1981).

101. Vincenz Czerny, "Plastischer Ersatz der Brustdrüse durch ein Lipom," *Beilage zum Centralblatt für Chirurgie*, no. 27 in *Centralblatt für Chirurgie* 22 (1895): 72; and Czerny, "Drei Plastische Operationen," *Verhandlungen der deutschen Gesellschaft für Chirugie* 24 (1895): 216–17. See the discussion about the priority of this operation in Robert M. Goldwyn, "Vincenz Czerny and the Beginnings of Breast Reconstruction," *Plastic and Reconstructive Surgery* 61 (1978): 673–81.

102. Gustav Neuber, "Fetttransplantation," *Verhandlungen der deutschen Gesellschaft für Chirugie* 1 (1893): 66.

103. Ludovici, *Cosmetic Scalpel*, pp. 36–38.

104. See the detailed discussion in Letterman and Schurter, "History of Augmentation Mammaplasty."

105. Leopold Schönbauer, *Das medizinische Wien* (Berlin/Wien: Urban & Schwarzenberg, 1944), p. 294.

106. Robert Gersuny, "Subkutane Paraffineinspritzungen," *Wiener klinische Wochenschrift* 36 (1923): 726–27.

107. Hugo Eckstein, "Über subkutane und submukose Hartparaffinprothesen," *Deutsche Medizinische Wochenschrift* 28 (1902): 573; Eckstein, "Therapeutische Erfolge durch Hartparaffininjektionenen aus dem Gesammtgebiet der Chirurgie," *Berliner kli-*

nische Wochenschrift 40 (103): 266–68, 302–4; and Eckstein, "Vaselin- oder Hartparaffin-prothesen?" *Deutsche medizinische Wochenschrift* 29 (1903): 993–95.

108. Gersuny, "Subkutane Paraffineinspritzungen," citing his earlier paper from 1900, "Über eine subcutane Prothese."

109. See the bibliography on paraffin in Thomas J. S. Patterson, *The Patterson Index of Plastic Surgery 1864 A.D. to 1920 A.D.*, vol. 3 of Frank McDowell, ed., *The McDowell Indexes of Plastic Surgical Literature*, 5 vols. (Baltimore: Williams & Wilkins, 1977–81, here 1978), pp. 415–24.

110. Martin Gumpert, *Hölle im Paradies: Selbstdarstellung eines Arztes* (Stockholm: Bermann-Fischer, 1939).

111. Stephen Paget, "The Use of Paraffin Injections in Surgery," *West London Medical Journal* 9 (1904): 89–96; quotation on p. 90.

112. Roland Barthes, *Camera Lucida*, trans. Richard Howard (New York: Hill and Wang, 1981), p. 105.

113. Adalbert G. Bettman, "The Psychology of Appearances," *Northwest Medicine* 28 (1929): 182–85, quotation on pp. 183–85.

114. Frederick Strange Kolle, *Plastic and Cosmetic Surgery* (New York: D. Appleton, 1911), p. 213.

115. James Brough, *Consuelo: Portrait of an American Heiress* (New York: Coward, McCann & Geoghegan, 1979). See here the insightful analysis by Robert M. Goldwyn, "The Paraffin Story," *Plastic and Reconstructive Surgery* 65 (1980): 517–24.

116. T. T. Alagaratnam and W. F. Ng, "Paraffinomas of the Breast: An Oriental Curiosity," *Australian and New Zealand Journal of Surgery* 66 (1996): 138–40.

117. P. Basse and B. Alsbjorn, "Paraffinoma of the Male Breast," *Acta chirurgiae plasticae* 33 (1991): 163–65; and I. E. Doney and D. L. Ranson, "Unusual Breast Findings in a Transsexual," *American Journal of Forensic Medical Pathology* 8 (1987): 342–45.

118. T. Lee, H. R. Choi, Y. T. Lee, and Y. H. Lee, "Paraffinoma of the Penis," *Yonsei Medical Journal* 35 (1994): 344–48.

119. Sue Fishkoff, "Body Beautiful," *Jerusalem Post*, October 11, 1996, p. 8.

120. Kolle, *Plastic and Cosmetic Surgery*, pp. 213–14.

121. Charles Conrad Miller, *Rubber and Gutta Percha Injections* (Chicago: n.p., 1923).

122. Vilray Papin Blair and James Barrett Brown, "Nasal Abnormalities, Fancied and Real. The Reaction of the Patient: Their Attempted Correction," *Surgery, Gynecology, Obstetrics* 53 (1931): 797–819, here p. 818.

123. Elaine Showalter, *Hystories: Hysterical Epidemics and Modern Culture* (New York: Columbia University Press, 1997).

CHAPTER EIGHT
THE WRONG BODY

1. Londa L. Schiebinger, *Nature's Body: Gender in the Making of Modern Science* (Boston: Beacon Press, 1993); and (from a popular culture perspective) Katherine Dunn, *Why Do Men Have Nipples? And Other Low-Life Answers to Real-Life Questions* (New York, N.Y.: Warner Books, 1992).

2. Jacques Joseph, *Nasenplastik und sonstige Gesichtsplastik, nebst einem Anhang über Mammaplastik und einige weitere Operationen aus dem Gebiete der äusseren Körperplastik: Ein Atlas und ein Lehrbuch* (Leipzig: C. Kabitzsch, 1931). All quotations are from Jacques Joseph, *Rhinoplasty and Facial Plastic Surgery with a Supplement on Mammaplasty and Other Operations in the Field of Plastic Surgery of the Body*, trans. Stanley Milstein (Phoenix: Columella Press, 1987), p. 747.

3. Robert H. Springer, S. J., "Transsexual Surgery: Some Reflections on the Moral Issues

Involved," in Earl E. Shelp, ed., *Sexuality and Medicine*, 2 vols. (Dordrecht: Reidel, 1987), 2:233–47.

4. *Toronto Sun*, August 3, 1995, p. 61.

5. T. J. Rissanen, H. P. Makarainen, M. J. Kallioinen et al., "Radiography of the Male Breast in Gynecomastia," *Acta Radiologica* 33 (1992): 110–14.

6. See the discussion in Arthur J. Barsky, Sidney Kahn, and Bernard E. Simon, "The Development of a Technique for the Surgical Correction of Gynecomastia," in A. B. Wallace, ed., *Transactions of the International Society of Plastic Surgeons, Second Congress* (Edinburgh: E. & S. Livingstone, 1960), pp. 527–30, quotation on p. 527.

7. Naoyuki Ohtake and Nobuyuki Shioya, "Aesthetic Breast Surgery in Orientals," in Nicolas G. Georgiade, Gregory S. Georgiade, and Ronald Riefkohl, eds., *Aesthetic Surgery of the Breast* (Philadelphia: W. B. Saunders, 1990), pp. 639–53, quotation on p. 651.

8. See Samuel Wilson Fussell, *Muscle: Confessions of an Unlikely Bodybuilder* (London: Poseidon, 1995).

9. K. F. Burnett and M. E. Kleiman, "Psychological Characteristics of Adolescent Steroid Users," *Adolescence* 29 (1994): 81–89.

10. See the discussion in Ronald Riefkohl and Eugene H. Courtiss, "Gynecomastia," in Georgiade, Georgiade, and Riefkohl, *Aesthetic Surgery of the Breast*, pp. 657–67.

11. Christopher Derek Kenway, "Kraft und Schönheit: Regeneration and Racial Theory in the German Physical Culture Movement, 1895–1920" (Ph.D. diss., University of California, Los Angeles, 1996).

12. Sue Fishkoff, "Body Beautiful," *Jerusalem Post*, October 11, 1996, p. 8.

13. T. W. Adorno et al., *The Authoritarian Personality* (New York: Harper [1950]), p. 261.

14. All quotations are from Alan M. Klein, *Little Big Men: Bodybuilding Subculture and Gender Construction* (Albany: State University of New York Press, 1993), here p. 164.

15. *The Seven Books of Paulus Agineta. With a commentary embracing a complete view of the knowledge possessed by the Greeks, Romans, and Arabians on all subjects connected with medicine and surgery*, 3 vols., trans. Frances Adams (London: Printed for the Sydenham Society, 1844–47), 2:334.

16. Peter Francis Hall, *Gynaecomastia* (Glebe, Australia: Australasian Medical Publishing Co., 1959), p. 147. See also Martin Kirschner and Otto Nordmann, *Die Chirurgie: Eine zusammenfassende Darstellung der allgemeinen und der speziellen Chirurgie*, 6 vols. (Berlin: Urban & Schwarzenberg, 1926–30), 3:83–89; Russell Ross Williams, "Gynecomastia" (M.S. thesis, University of Minnesota, 1949); Karl Gunnar Tillinger, *Testicular Morphology: A Histo-Pathological Study, with Special Reference to Biopsy Findings in Hypogonadism with Mainly Endocrine Disorders and in Gynecomastia. Acta endocrinologica.* Supplementum 30 (Copenhagen: Periodica, 1957); Bernadine Z. Paulshock, "Tutankhamun and His Brothers: Familial Gynecomastia in the Eighteenth Dynasty," *Journal of the American Medical Association* 244 (1980): 160–64; and Ole Scheike, *Male Breast Cancer* (Copenhagen: Munksgaard, 1975).

17. Hall, *Gynaecomastia*, p. 147.

18. Louis Dartigues, "Mammectomie totale et autogreffe libre aréolomamelonaire: Mammectomie bilatérale esthétique," *Bulletins et mémoires de la société nationale de chirugie* 20 (1928): 739–44. See also Dartigues's *Les directions actuelles et les destinées de la chirurgie* (Paris: O. Doin, 1925).

19. See the discussion in Barsky, Kahn, and Simon, "Development of a Technique for the Surgical Correction of Gynecomastia."

20. F. Samdal, G. Kleppe, P. F. Amland, and F. Abyholm, "Surgical Treatment of Gynaecomastia: Five Years' Experience with Liposuction," *Scandinavian Journal of Plastic and Reconstructive Surgery and Hand Surgery* 28 (1994): 123–30.

21. All quotations are from Alfred Adler, *The Neurotic Constitution: Outlines of a Com-*

parative Individualistic Psychology and Psychotherapy, trans. Bernard Glueck and John E. Lind (New York: Moffat, Yard, and Co., 1917), pp. 198–202. See Edward Hoffman, *The Drive for Self: Alfred Adler and the Founding of Individual Psychology* (Reading, Mass.: Addison-Wesley, 1994); Hannes Bohringer, *Kompensation und common sense: Zur Lebensphilosophie Alfred Adlers* (Königstein: Hain Verlag bei Athenaum, 1985); Paul E. Stepansky, *Adler in Context* (Hillside, N.J.: Analytic Press, 1983); Henry Jacoby, *Alfred Adlers Individualpsychologie und dialektische Charakterkunde* (Frankfurt am Main: Fischer-Taschenbuch, 1974); and Almuth Bruder-Bezzel, *Alfred Adler: Die Entstehungsgeschichte einer Theorie im historischen Milieu Wiens* (Göttingen: Vandenhoeck & Ruprecht, 1983).

22. Elizabeth Gail Haiken, "Body and Soul: Plastic Surgery in the United States, 1914–1990" (Ph.D. diss., University of California, Berkeley, 1994), pp. 191–245.

23. Alfred Adler, *Study of Organ Inferiority and Its Psychical Compensation: A Contribution to Clinical Medicine,* trans. Smith Ely Jelliffe (New York: Nervous and Mental Disease Publishing Company, 1917). Translation of Alfred Adler, *Studie über Minderwertigkeit von Organen* (Berlin: Urban & Schwarzenberg, 1907).

24. All quotations are from Maxwell Maltz, *New Faces, New Futures: Rebuilding Character with Plastic Surgery* (New York: Richard R. Smith, 1936), here p. ix.

25. All quotations are from Philip Roth, *The Breast* (New York: Vintage, 1972). See Norbert Greiner, "Parodie der Verwandlung oder: Der Komparatist als Romanheld: Philip Roth's *The Breast,*" *Arcadia* 21 (1986): 190–202; Alice R. Kaminsky, "Philip Roth's Professor Kepesh and the 'Reality Principle,'" *Denver Quarterly* 13 (1978): 41–54; Julian C. Rice, "Philip Roth's *The Breast:* Cutting the Freudian Cord," *Studies in Contemporary Satire* 3 (1976): 9–16; Daniel A. Dervin, "Breast Fantasy in Barthelme, Swift, and Philip Roth: Creativity and Psychoanalytic Structure," *American Imago* 33 (1976): 102–22; Pierre Michel, "Philip Roth's *The Breast:* Reality Adulterated and the Plight of the Writer," *Dutch Quarterly Review of Anglo-American Letters* 5 (1975): 245–52; Arnold E. Davidson, "Kafka, Rilke, and Philip Roth's *The Breast,*" *Notes on Contemporary Literature* 5 (1975): 9–11; and Elizabeth J. Sabiston, "A New Fable for Critics: Philip Roth's *The Breast,*" *International Fiction Review* 2 (1975): 27–34.

26. This discussion is indebted to M. Vanini and G. Weiss, "Contributo clinico allo studio dei disturbi della corporeità psicotica," *Revista sperimentale di freniatria e medicine legale della alienzioni mentali* 96 (1972): 32–55; Katharine A. Phillips, "Body Dysmorphic Disorder: The Distress of Imagined Ugliness," *American Journal of Psychiatry* 148 (1991): 1138–49; and German E. Berrios, *The History of Mental Symptoms: Descriptive Psychopathology since the Nineteenth Century* (Cambridge, Eng.: Cambridge University Press, 1996), pp. 276–81.

27. Enrico Morselli, "Sulla dismorfofobia e sulla tefefobia: Due forme non per anco descritte di Pazzia con idee fisse," *Bolletinno dell R. accademia di Genova* 6 (1891): 110–19.

28. The *Diagnostic and Statistical Manual of Mental Disorders* of the American Psychiatric Association sets forth the standard American (and, in general, now European) diagnostic criteria for mental illness. The DSM has appeared in five editions: *Diagnostic and Statistical Manual of Mental Disorders* (Washington, D.C.: American Psychiatric Association, 1st ed., 1952; 2d. ed., 1968; 3d ed., 1980; 3d ed.–R[evised], 1987; 4th ed., 1994).

29. Katharine A. Phillips, "An Open Study of Buspirone Augmentation of Serotonin-Reuptake Inhibitors in Body Dysmorphic Disorder," *Psychopharmacology Bulletin* 32 (1996): 175–80. See also Eric Hollander, David Neville, Maxim Frankel, and Stephen Josephson, "Body Dysmorphic Disorder: Diagnostic Issues and Related Disorders," *Psychosomatics* 33 (1992): 156–65.

30. Michael Haederle, "Specializing in Sexual Healing," *Chicago Tribune,* February 3, 1995, p. C1.

31. Marjorie B. Garber, *Vested Interests: Cross-Dressing and Cultural Anxiety* (New York:

Routledge, 1992), pp. 101, 110. See also Bernice Louise Hausman, *Changing Sex: Transsexualism, Technology, and the Idea of Gender* (Durham, N.C.: Duke University Press, 1995), and Leslie Feinberg, *Transgender Warriors: Making History from Joan of Arc to Dennis Rodman* (Boston: Beacon Press, 1997).

32. Vamik D. Volkan and Stanley Berent, "Psychiatric Aspects of Surgical Treatment for Problems of Sexual Identification (Transsexualism)," in John G. Howells, ed., *Modern Perspectives in the Psychiatric Aspects of Surgery* (New York: Brunner / Mazel, 1976), pp. 447–67, quotation on p. 449.

33. All references are to Gary T. Marx, "Fraudulent Identity and Biography," in David Altheide, ed., *New Directions in the Study of Justice, Law, and Social Control* (New York: Plenum, 1990), pp. 143–65.

34. John Money and Patricia Tucker, *Sexual Signatures: On Being a Man or a Woman* (Boston: Little, Brown, 1975), p. 3.

35. John Money and Anke A. Ehrhardt, *Man and Woman, Boy and Girl* (Baltimore: Johns Hopkins University Press, 1972), pp. 1–23.

36. See the discussion throughout John Money and Herman Musaph, eds., *The Handbook of Sexology* (Amsterdam: Excerpta medica, 1977), for example on pp. 171, 487, 1295, and 1309.

37. This argument concerning autonomy is made in outlining the legal and ethical question concerning the relationship between aesthetic surgery and transgender surgery by E. Quadri, "Profili contrattuali e reponsabilità nell'attività di chirugo plastico," *Rivista italiana di chirugia plastica* 22 (1980): 385–408, and D. Rouge et al., "Évolution de la jurisprudence en matière de contrat médical en chirurgie esthétique," *Annales de chirurgie plastique et esthétique* 35 (1990): 297–302.

38. Thus, there is a rubric for transgender surgery in *The McDowell Indexes of Plastic Surgical Literature* vol. 5, *The Honolulu Index of Plastic Surgery, 1971 A.D. to 1976 A.D.* (Baltimore: Williams & Wilkins, 1977), pp. 796–97.

39. C. G. Jung, "Zur Frage der ärztlichen Intervention," C. G. Jung, *Das symbolische Leben: Verschiedene Schriften,* ed. Lilly Jung-Merker and Elisabeth Ruf (Olten: Walter, 1995), pp. 375–76.

40. Ronald R. Garet, "Symposium on Biomedical Technology and Health Care: Social and Conceptual Transformations: Article: Self-Transformability," *Southern California Law Review* 65 (1991–92): 121–203, quotation on p. 121.

41. Felix Abraham, "Genitalumwandlung an zwei männlichen Transvestiten," *Zeitschrift für Sexualwissenschaft und Sexualpolitik* 28 (1931): 223–26. See also Ludwig Lévy-Lenz, *Praxis der kosmetischen Chirurgie, Fortschritte und Gefahren* (Stuttgart: Hippokrates, 1954).

42. Richard Mühsam, "Chirurgische Eingriffe bei Anomalien des Sexuallebens," *Therapie der Gegenwart* 28 (1926): 451–55. The patient accounts in this paper are more extensive, and include the follow-up to the earlier case reported in Mühsam's earlier paper on the treatment of "homosexuality" through castration, "Der Einfluß der Kastration der Sexualneurotiker," *Deutsche Medizinische Wochenschrift* 6 (1921): 155–56. All quotations are from these two articles, identified in the text by year and page number. See also Eduard Sonnenburg and Richard Mühsam, *Compendium der Operations- und Verbandstechnik* (Berlin: Hirschwald, 1903). See Vern L. Bullough, "A Nineteenth-Century Transsexual," *Archives of Sexual Behavior* 16 (1987): 81–84.

43. Karl A. Menninger, "Polysurgery and Polysurgical Addiction," *Psychoanalytic Quarterly* 3 (1934): 173–99.

44. There is a very good survey of the literature that includes many such cases in Franz von Neugebauer, "58 Beobachtungen von periodischen genitalen Blutungen menstruellen

Anschein, pseudomenstruellen Blutungen, Menstruatio vicaia, Molimina menstrualia usw. bei Scheinzwitter," *Jahrbuch für sexuallen Zwischenstufen* 6 (1904): 277–326.

45. See, for example, Magnus Hirschfeld, *Geschlechts-Übergänge: Mischungen männlicher und weiblicher Geschlechtscharaktere* (Leipzig: Max Spohr, 1913), and Franz Ludwig von Neugebauer, *Hemaphroditismus beim Menschen* (Leipzig: Werner Klinhardt, 1908).

46. Abraham, "Genitalumwandlung," p. 225.

47. Niels Hoyer, ed., *Man into Woman: An Authentic Record of a Change of Sex. The True Story of the Miraculous Transformation of the Danish Painter Einar Wegener,* trans. H. J. Stenning (London: Jarrolds, 1933). The original is Niels Hoyer, ed., *Lili Elbe: Ein Mensch wechselt sein Geschlecht* (Dresden: Carl Reissner, 1932). See Vern L. Bullough, "Transsexualism in History," *Archives of Sexual Behavior* 4 (1975): 561–71, on the tradition of seeing the transsexual, including the Lili Elbe case.

48. Carlson Wade, *She-male: The Amazing True-Life Story of Coccinelle* (New York: Epic, 1963); Marcelo Lopes, *Meu nome e Marcelo* (Sao Paulo: L. Oren, 1969); Christine Jorgensen, *A Personal Autobiography* (New York: Eriksson, 1967); Dawn Langley Simmons, *Man into Woman: A Transsexual Autobiography* (London: Icon Books, 1970); Barbara Buick, *L'Étiquette* (Paris: La Jeune Parque, 1971); Patricia Morgan (as told to Paul Hoffman), *The Man-maid Doll* (Secaucus, N.J.: Lyle Stuart, 1973); Jan Morris, *Conundrum* (London: Faber and Faber, 1974); Canary Conn, *Canary: The Story of a Transsexual* (Los Angeles: Nash, 1974); Mario Martino, *Emergence: A Transsexual Autobiography* (New York: Crown Publishers, 1977); Duncan Fallowell, *April Ashley's Odyssey* (London: Cape, 1982); Liz Hodgkinson, *Michael Née Laura* (N.p.: Columbus Books, 1989) (about Michael Dillon, 1915–62); Peter Stirling, *So Different: An Extraordinary Autobiography* (Sydney: Simon & Schuster Australia, 1989); Louis Sullivan, *From Female to Male: The Life of Jack Bee Garland* (Boston: Alyson Publications, 1990); Caroline Cossey, *My Story* (London: Faber and Faber, 1991); Erica Rutherford, *Nine Lives: The Autobiography of Erica Rutherford* (Charlottetown, P.E.I.: Ragweed, 1993); and Jennifer Spry, *Orlando's Sleep: An Autobiography of Gender* (Norwich, Vt.: New Victoria Publishers, 1997).

49. Jean Boivin, *Beauty's Scalpel,* trans. Eileen Bigland (London: Jarrolds, 1958), p. 58.

50. Ibid., p. 54.

51. N. O. Body, *Aus eines Mannes Mädchenjahren,* reprint with an afterward by Hermann Simon (1907; rpt. Berlin: Hentrich, 1993). See Andreas Hartmann, "Im falschen Geschlecht: Männliche Scheinzwitter um 1900," in Michael Hagner, ed., *Der "falsche" Körper: Beiträge zu einer Geschichte der Monstrositäten* (Göttingen: Wallstein 1995), pp. 187–220.

52. Caryle Murphy, "Can an Infant's Sex Be Changed? Researchers Report That Boy Raised as a Girl Was Miserable until Learning His True Identity," *Washington Post,* March 18, 1997, p. Z7.

53. All quotations are from Mark Rees, *Dear Sir or Madam: The Autobiography of a Female-to-Male Transsexual* (London: Cassell, 1996).

54. On the alteration of the voice, see P. J. Donald, "Voice Change Surgery in the Transsexual," *Head and Neck Surgery* 4 (1982): 433–37; D. Gunzburger, "An Acoustic Analysis and Some Perceptual Data Concerning Voice Change in Male-Female Trans-Sexuals," *European Journal of Disorders of Communication* 28 (1933): 13–21; and V. I. Wolfe, D. L. Ratusknik, F. H. Smith, and G. Northrop, "Intonation and Fundamental Frequency in Male-to-Female Transsexuals," *Journal of Speech and Hearing Disorders* 55 (1990): 43–50.

55. Berhard Blechmann, *Ein Beitrag zur Anthropologie der Juden* (Dorpat: Wilhelm Just, 1882), p. 8.

56. All quotations are from Paul Hewitt with Jane Warren, *A Self-Made Man: The Diary of a Man Born in a Woman's Body* (London: Headline, 1995), here p. 3.

57. A. Kaczynski, P. K. McKissock, T. Dubrow, and M. A. Lesavoy, "Breast Reduction in the Male-to-Female Transsexual," *Annals of Plastic Surgery* 23 (1989): 323–36.

58. All quotations are from R. Blanchard, B. W. Steiner, L. H. Clemmensen, and R. Dickey, "Prediction of Regrets in Postoperative Transsexuals," *Canadian Journal of Psychiatry* 34 (1989): 43–45.

59. Michael Z. Fleming, B. R. MacGowan, L. Robinson, J. Spitz, and P. Salt, "The Body Image of Postoperative Female-to-Male Transsexuals," *Journal of Consulting and Clinical Psychology* 50 (1982): 461–62.

60. Molly Walsh, "To Circumcise or Not: A Complicated Decision," *Burlington Free Press/Gannett News Service*, April 25, 1995.

61. Edward O. Laumann, Christopher M. Masi, and Ezra W. Zuckerman, "Circumcision in the United States: Prevalence, Prophylactic Effects, and Sexual Practice," *Journal of the American Medical Association* 277 (1997): 1052–57. Compare the earlier discussions in E. N. Preston, "Wither the Foreskin? A Consideration of Routine Neonatal Circumcision," *Journal of the American Medical Association* 216 (1970): 1853–58, and E. A. Grossman and N. A. Posner, "The Circumcision Controversy: An Update," *Obstetrics and Gynecological Annual* 13 (1984): 181–95.

62. Leonard Tushnet, "Uncircumcision," *Medical Times* 93, no. 6 (June 1965): 588–93. See also D. Griffiths and J. D. Frank, "Inappropriate Circumcision Referrals by GPs," *Journal of the Royal Society of Medicine* 85 (1992): 324–25.

63. Alice Miller, *Banished Knowledge: Facing Childhood Injuries,* trans. Leila Vennewitz (New York: Doubleday, 1990), pp. 135–39. See Lawrence Birken, "From Seduction Theory to Oedipus Complex: A Historical Analysis," *New German Critique* 43 (1988): 83–96.

64. Laumann, Masi, and Zuckerman, "Circumcision in the United States."

65. J. R. Taylor, A. P. Lockwood, and A. J. Taylor, "The Prepuce: Specialized Mucosa of the Penis and Its Loss to Circumcision," *British Journal of Urology,* 77 (1996): 291–95.

66. He cites W. Goodwin, "Uncircumcision: A Technique for Plastic Reconstruction of a Prepuce after Circumcision," *Journal of Urology* 144 (1990): 1203–5.

67. *New Republic,* June 26, 1995, p. 6.

68. Cherrill Hicks, "They Took My Foreskin, and I Want It Back," *The Independent,* August 3, 1993, p. 11.

69. Samuel Holdheim, *Über die Beschneidung zunächst in religiös-dogmatischer Beziehung* (Schwerin: C. Kürschner, 1844).

70. Ronald Goldman, *Questioning Circumcision: A Jewish Perspective* (Boston: Vanguard, 1998).

71. Jack Penn, "Penile Reform," *British Journal of Plastic Surgery* 16 (1963): 287–88. See Asher Dubb, "Jack Penn: 1909–1996, A Tribute," *Adler Museum Bulletin* 23 (1997): 1–3.

72. T. Schneider, "Circumcision and 'Uncircumcision,'" *South African Medical Journal* 50 (1976): 556–58. See also S. Levin, "Brith Milah: Ritual Circumcision," *South African Medical Journal* 39 (1956): 1125–27.

73. Alec Russell, "Ancient Practice of Tribal Circumcision Divides South Africa," *Daily Telegraph,* January 23, 1997, p. 17.

74. Jim Bigelow, *The Joy of Uncircumcising!* (Aptos, Calif.: Hourglass Book Publishing, 1992), pp. 193–204, and *Awakenings: A Preliminary Poll of Circumcised Men, Revealing the Long-Term Harm and Healing the Wounds of Infant Circumcision* (San Francisco: NOHARMM, National Organization to Halt the Abuse and Routine Mutilation of Males, [1994]).

75. A good overview of the movement is the long essay by Jeffrey Felshman, "The Foreskin Flap," *The Reader* (Chicago), March 10, 1995, section 1, pp. 12–34.

76. Terence Monmaney with George Raine, "Doubts about Circumcision," *Newsweek,* March 30, 1987, p. 74.

77. G. Walter and J. Streimer, "Genital Self-Mutilation: Attempted Foreskin Reconstruction," *British Journal of Psychiatry* 156 (1990): 125–27.

Chapter Nine
Dreams of Youth and Beauty

1. Becca Ruth Levy, "Shifting Stereotypes by Culture and Priming: The Dynamic between Stereotypes of Old Age and Memory" (Ph.D. diss., Harvard University, 1996), and Lois W. Banner, *Full Flower: Aging Women, Power, and Sexuality: A History* (New York: Knopf, 1992).

2. Fritz Koch, *Hässliche Gesichts-und Körperformen und ihre Verbesserung: Neue Methoden und Erfolge der Umformung von Gesicht und Körper, sowie der Erscheinungen des Alterns im Lichte der Naturgeschichte, Kunst und Medizin* (Berlin: Leese, 1914).

3. Mirko D. Grmek, *On Aging and Old Age: Basic Problems and Historic Aspects of Gerontology and Geriatrics* (The Hague: W. Junk, 1958); Eric J. Trimmer, *Rejuvenation: The History of an Idea* (London: Robert Hale, 1967); Sharon Romm, "Rejuvenation Revisited," *Aesthetic Plastic Surgery* 7 (1983): 241–48; Chandak Sengoopta, "Rejuvenation and the Prolongation of Life: Science or Quackery?" *Perspectives in Biology and Medicine* 37 (1993): 55–66; and Jessica Jahiel, "Rejuvenation Research and the American Medical Association in the Early Twentieth Century: Paradigms in Conflict" (Ph.D. diss., Boston University, 1992).

4. P. A. Adamson and M. L. Moran, "Historical Trends in Surgery for the Aging Face," *Facial Plastic Surgery* 9 (1993): 133–42.

5. Alex Kuczynski, "Pursuing Potions: Fountain of Youth or Poisonous Fad?" *New York Times*, April 14, 1998, p. B9.

6. C. E. Brown-Séquard, "The Effects Produced on Man by Subcutaneous Injections of a Liquid Obtained from the Testicles of Animals," *Lancet* 137 (1889): 105, as well as Brown-Séquard's "Des effets produits chez l'homme par les injections sous-cuntanées d'un liquide retiré des testicules frais de cobaye et de chien," *Comptes rendus des séances et mémoires de la société de biologie* 41 (1889): 415–19. See Merriley Borell, "Brown-Séquard's Organotherapy and Its Appearance in America at the End of the Nineteenth Century," *Bulletin of the History of Medicine* 50 (1976): 309–20, as well as Borell's "Organotherapy and the Emergence of Reproductive Endocrinology," *Journal of the History of Biology* 18 (1985): 1–30.

7. Norman Haire, *Rejuvenation: The Work of Steinach, Voronoff and Others* (New York: Macmillan, 1925).

8. David Hamilton, *The Monkey Gland Affair* (London: Chatto and Windus, 1986), pp. 67–68; and Robert Youngson and Ian Schott, *Medical Blunders* (London: Robinson, 1996), pp. 164–70. See also Voronoff's standard handbook on bone grafts: Serge Voronoff, *Traité des greffes humaine* (Paris: Octave Doin, 1916).

9. Eugen Steinach, *Sex and Life* (New York: Viking Press, 1940).

10. The most detailed account of the disease is Sharon Romm, *The Unwelcome Intruder: Freud's Struggle with Cancer* (New York: Praeger, 1983). See also Jose Schavelzon, *Freud, un paciente con cancer* (Buenos Aires: Editorial Paidos, 1983); and Sharon Golub, "Coping with Cancer: Freud's Experiences," *Psychoanalytic Review* 68 (1981): 191–200. I have used also the excerpt from Romm's book included in her *Symposium on Historical Perspectives of Plastic Surgery* (Philadelphia: Saunders, 1983), pp. 709–14, and the commentary on it in that same volume by Edward A. Luce, "The Ordeal of Sigmund Freud," pp. 715–16, as well as C. T. Brown, "Freud and Cancer," *Texas Medicine* 70 (1974): 62–64. In addition I have used the following biographical studies: Max Schur, *Freud: Living and Dying* (New York: International Universities Press, 1972); and Jacob Meitlis, "The Last Days of Sigmund Freud," *Jewish Frontier* 18 (1951): 20–22. Of special interest, as it provides one of the first readings of Freud's cancer, is the parallel drawn between the oral bleeding resulting from Freud's cancer and the oral bleeding in the case of Emma Eckstein by Madelon Sprengnether, *The Spectral Mother: Freud, Feminism, and Psychoanalysis* (Ithaca, N.Y.: Cornell University Press, 1990), pp. 169–71.

11. Ernest Jones, *The Life and Works of Sigmund Freud,* 3 vols. (New York: Basic Books, 1957), 3:99.

12. Sigmund Freud, *Standard Edition of the Complete Psychological Works of Sigmund Freud,* ed. and trans. J. Strachey, A. Freud, A. Strachey, and A. Tyson, 24 vols. (London: Hogarth, 1955–74), here 18:171.

13. Wilhelm Fliess, "Steinach," in *Zur Periodenlehre: Gesammelte Aufsätze* (Jena: Eugen Dietrichs, 1925), pp. 98–117, quotation on p. 98.

14. Serge Voronoff, *Life: A Study of the Means of Restoring Vital Energy and Prolonging Life* (New York: E. P. Dutton, 1920), pp. 116–17.

15. All quotations are from Max Thorek, *A Surgeon's World* (Philadelphia: J. B. Lippincott, 1943), here p. 180. See Robert L. Ruberg and Rajerdra R. Shah, "Max Thorek: A Surgeon for All Seasons," *Clinics in Plastic Surgery* 10 (1983): 611–17.

16. Max Thorek, *The Human Testis* (Philadelphia: J. B. Lippincott, 1924), p. 444.

17. All quotations are from Gertrude Atherton, *Black Oxen* (New York: Boni and Liveright, 1923). See Laura Hapke, "The Problem of Sensual Womanhood: Three Late Nineteenth-Century Fictional Solutions," *The Nassau Review: The Journal of Nassau Community College* 4 (1981): 86–95, and Carolyn Forrey, "Gertrude Atherton and the New Woman," *California Historical Society Quarterly* 55 (1976): 194–209.

18. All quotations are from Bruce Sterling, *Holy Fire* (New York: Bantam, 1996). See Veronica Hollinger, "Cybernetic Deconstructions: Cyberpunk and Postmodernism," *Mosaic: A Journal for the Interdisciplinary Study of Literature* 23 (1990): 29–44.

19. Susan E. Mackinnon, "What's New in Plastic Surgery," *Journal of the American College of Surgeons* 182 (1996): 150–61.

20. On the relationship between aesthetic surgery and cloning, see Hillel Schwartz, *The Culture of the Copy: Striking Likenesses, Unreasonable Facsimiles* (New York: Zone Books, 1996), pp. 345–51.

21. Aldous Huxley, *Brave New World* (Mattituck, N.Y.: Amereon House, 1979).

22. Ben Bova, *The Multiple Man: A Novel of Suspense* (Indianapolis: Bobbs-Merrill, 1976).

23. Nancy Freedman, *Joshua, Son of None* (New York: Delacorte Press, 1973).

24. Ira Levin, *The Boys from Brazil* (New York: Random House, 1976).

25. George B. Johnson, "One Small Step for Man; A Giant Leap with a Sheep," *St. Louis Post-Dispatch,* March 20, 1997, section G, p. 1.

26. Otto Mangold, *Hans Spemann, ein Meister der Entwicklungsphysiologie, sein Leben und sein Werk* (Stuttgart: Wissenschaftlich Verlagsgesellschaft, 1953).

27. Ian Dow, "Is Dolly the First Step to Creating Master Race? Fears of Nazi-Style Master Race Experiments over New Cloned Sheep," *Daily Record,* February 24, 1997, p. 8.

28. Gustav Niebuhr, "Suddenly, Religious Ethicists Face a Quandary on Cloning," *New York Times,* March 1, 1997, p. A1.

29. All quotations are from Nathaniel Hawthorne, *Tales and Sketches* (New York: The Library of America, 1982): "Dr. Heidegger's Experiment," pp. 470–79; "The Birth-Mark," pp. 764–80.

30. Marie Mulvey Roberts, "'A Physic against Death': Eternal Life and the Enlightenment—Gender and Gerontology," in Marie Mulvey Roberts and Roy Porter, eds., *Literature and Medicine during the Eighteenth Century* (London: Routledge, 1993), pp. 151–67.

31. Max Thorek, *The Face in Health and Disease* (Philadelphia: J. B. Lippincott, 1946), and Thorek's *Camera Art as a Means of Self-Expression* (Philadelphia: J. B. Lippincott, 1947).

32. Thorek, *Surgeon's World,* p. 166.

33. See his accounts in Eugen Holländer, "Die kosmetische Chirugie," in Max Joseph, ed., *Handbuch der Kosmetik* (Leipzig: Veit, 1912), p. 688, and in Holländer, "Plastische (Kosmetische) Operation: Kritische Darstellung ihres gegenwärtigen Standes," in Georg

Klemperer und Felix Klemperer, eds., *Neue deutsche Klinik: Handwörterbuch der praktischen Medizin mit besonderer Berücksichtigung der inneren Medizin, der Kinderheilkunde und ihrer Grenzgebiete,* 11 vols. (Berlin: Urban und Schwarzenberg, 1928–32), 9:1–17.

34. Erich Lexer, *Die gesamte Wiederherrstellungschirugie,* 2 vols. (Leipzig: J. A. Barth, 1931), 2:548.

35. Antony F. Wallace, *The Progress of Plastic Surgery: An Introductory History* (Oxford: Willem A. Meeuws, 1982), pp. 104–5.

36. David M. Reifler, ed., *The American Society of Ophthalmic Plastic and Reconstructive Surgeons (ASOPRS): The First Twenty-Five Years: 1969–1994; History of Ophthalmic Plastic Surgery: 2500 B.C.–A.D. 1994* (Winter Park, Fla.: American Society of Ophthalmic Plastic and Reconstructive Surgery, 1994), pp. 1–105; Blair O. Rogers, "History of Oculoplastic Surgery: The Contributions of Plastic Surgery," *Aesthetic Plastic Surgery* 12 (1988): 129–52; L. B. Katzen, "The History of Cosmetic Blepharoplasty," *Advances in Ophthalmic, Plastic and Reconstructive Surgery* 5 (1986): 89–97; and Blair O. Rogers, "History of Cosmetic Blepharoplasty," *Third International Symposium of Plastic and Reconstructive Surgery of the Eye and Adnexa,* ed. S. J. Aston et al. (Baltimore: Williams & Wilkins, 1982), pp. 276–81.

37. Cited by Sharon Romm, *The Changing Face of Beauty* (St. Louis: Mosby Year Book, 1992), p. 181

38. A. Noël, *La chirurgie esthétique* (Paris: Masson, 1926), pp. 6–7.

39. Jacques Joseph, "Verbesserung meiner Hängewangenplastik (Melomioplastik)," *Deutsche medizinische Wochenschrift* 54 (1928): 567–68.

40. See the detailed discussion by Mario González-Ulloa, "The History of Rhytidectomy," in his *The Creation of Aesthetic Plastic Surgery* (New York: Springer, 1985), pp. 41–87.

41. Charles H. Willi, *Facial Rejuvenation: How to Idealise the Features and the Skin of the Face by the Latest Scientific Methods* (London: Cecil Palmer, 1926), p. 91. See also K. M. Cameron and A. F. Wallace, "'Dr. Willi' (1882?–1972?), Disciple of Jacques Joseph," *Plastic and Reconstructive Surgery* 88 (1991): 363–64.

42. Charles Conrad Miller, *Cosmetic Surgery: The Correction of Featural Imperfections* (Philadelphia: F. A. Davis, 1924), p. 256.

43. All quotations are from J. Howard Crum, *The Making of a Beautiful Face or Face Lifting Unveiled* (New York: Walton Book Company, 1928).

44. Philip Roth, *American Pastoral* (Boston: Houghton Mifflin Company, 1997).

45. Crum, *Making of a Beautiful Face,* p. 10.

46. T. E. Cook, "Rhytidectomy," *Dallas Medical Journal* 30 (1944): 60–62, quotation on p. 61.

47. Crum, *Making of a Beautiful Face,* p. 82.

48. See the detailed discussion by Mario González-Ulloa, "The History of Rhytidectomy," p. 81.

49. "Technological Advances Lead Many to Undergo Smaller Procedures in Facial Plastic Surgery, New Survey Shows," *PR Newswire,* October 8, 1996, Tuesday.

50. "'Mad Cow' Fever Infects Cosmetic Industry," *Agence France Presse,* April 1, 1996, 02:00 GMT.

51. All quotations are from Fay Weldon, *The Life and Loves of a She-Devil* (London: Hodder and Stoughton, 1983). See Patricia Juliana Smith, "Weldon's *The Life and Loves of a She-Devil,*" *Explicator* 51 (1993): 255–57.

52. All references are to Mary Higgins Clark, *Let Me Call You Sweetheart* (New York: Pocket Books, 1995).

53. Wolfgang Mühlbauer, "Plastic Surgery on Identical Twins," *Annals of Plastic Surgery* 26 (1991): 30–39.

54. Duncan McCorquodale, ed., *Orlan: This Is My Body . . . This Is My Software . . .* (London: Black Dog, 1996); Rosie Millard, "Pain in the Art: This Is My Body . . . This Is My Software: Zone Gallery, Newcastle, England; Exhibit," *Art Review* (London, England) 48 (1996): 52–53; David Moos, "Memories of Being: Orlan's Theater of the Self," *Art & Text* 54 (1996): 66–73; Orlan, "I Do Not Want to Look Like . . . : Orlan on Becoming-Orlan," *Women's Art Magazine* 64 (1995): 5–10; and Barbara Rose, "Is It Art? Orlan and the Transgressive Act," *Art in America* 81 (1993): 82–87.

55. Quoted from the "Orlan Project," in McCorquodale, ed., *Orlan,* p. 91.

56. These references are from Candice Breitz's paper "Orlan: The Pain of Beauty," delivered at the College Art Association in 1997. I am grateful to Ms. Breitz for sharing her insightful paper with me.

57. Quoted from Orlan's statement in McCorquodale, ed. *Orlan,* pp. 81–93, here p. 93.

58. Pontus Hulten, comp., *The Arcimboldo Effect: Transformations of the Face from the 16th to the 20th Century* (New York: Abbeville, 1987). Dali's portrait is reproduced on p. 313.

59. Pierre Bourdieu, *Sociology in Question,* trans. Richard Nice (London: Sage, 1993), p. 148.

60. "Explorations: Suffering for Art," *The Economist,* July 6, 1996, U.S. edition, p. 76.

61. Adrian Searle, "Changing Face of Modern Art; Orlan: Portfolio Gallery, Edinburgh," *The Guardian,* June 6, 1996, p. 2.

62. Richard Schechner, "From Perform-1: The Future in Retrospect; E-Mail Messages about the First Annual Performance Studies Conference Held in March 1995 at New York University," *TDR* 39 (December 22, 1995): 142.

63. Simon Holden, "Orlan Turns Cosmetic Surgery into an Art Form," *Press Association Newsfile,* March 18, 1996.

64. Elizabeth Lenhard, "The Changing Face of Orlan," *Atlanta Journal and Constitution,* April 19, 1994, p. 5.

65. *New York Times,* September 13, 1996.

66. Quoted from Orlan's statement in McCorquodale, ed., *Orlan,* p. 92.

67. Sarah Wilson, "L'histoire d'O, Sacred and Profane," in McCorquodale, ed., *Orlan,* pp. 7–29, here p. 14.

68. Reuters, Monday, 8 May 1995 11:42:47 -0700 (PDT).

69. Quoted from the "Orlan Project," in McCorquodale, ed., *Orlan,* p. 91.

70. Searle, "Changing Face of Modern Art," p. 2.

71. Dalya Alberge, "How Plastic Surgery Adds to the High Temple of Art," *The Times* (London), March 15, 1996, p. A3.

72. Sarah Wilson, "L'histoire d'O, Sacred and Profane," in McCorquodale, ed., *Orlan,* pp. 7–29, here p. 8.

73. Kathy Davis, "'My Body Is My Art': Cosmetic Surgery as Feminist Utopia," *European Journal of Women's Studies* 4 (1997): 23–37, here p. 31.

74. All quotations are from Sage Sohier, *Artist's Statement* accompanying the exhibit "About Face," Friends of Photography Exhibition, San Francisco, 1996.

75. David Bonetti, "Photo Exhibit Peeks into Private Lives," *San Francisco Examiner,* July 5, 1996, p. D7.

CONCLUSION
"PASSING" AS HUMAN

1. Rainer Maria Rilke, *Selected Poems,* trans. C. F. MacIntyre (Berkeley and Los Angeles: University of California Press, 1962), p. 93.

2. Ashley Bickerton, "On Passing," *Documents* 3 (1993): 62–64, quotation on p. 62.

3. Robert Frost, "Mending Wall," in Oscar Williams, ed., *A Little Treasury of Modern Poetry* (New York: Scribner's, 1952), p. 135.

4. Mark C. Taylor, *Nots* (Chicago: University of Chicago Press, 1992), p. 215.

5. William Butler Yeats, "A Woman Young and Old," in *The Collected Poems of William Butler Yeats,* ed. Richard J. Finneran (New York: Scribner's, 1996), p. 270.

INDEX